SCIENCE
in Nursing

SCIENCE
in Nursing
Third Edition Revised

Laurie Cree Teach. Cert., B.Sc., M.Sc.
Sandra Rischmiller R.N., B.Sc.N.

University of Technology, Sydney (Kuring-gai)

W.B. Saunders
Baillière Tindall

Harcourt Brace & Company
Sydney Philadelphia London Toronto

For
Heloise, Vanessa, Andrew and Stephen;
and
Keith, Simon and David

W. B. Saunders/Baillière Tindall

An imprint of
Harcourt Brace & Company, Australia
30–52 Smidmore Street,
Marrickville, NSW 2204

Harcourt Brace & Company
24–28 Oval Road, London NW1 7DX

Harcourt Brace & Company
Orlando, Florida 32887

National Library of Australia Cataloguing-in-Publication Data

Cree, L. A. (Laurie A.).
  Science in nursing.

  3rd ed.
  Bibliography.
  Includes index.
  ISBN 0 7295 1257 6.

  1. Science. 2. Human biology. 3. Nursing. I.
  Rischmiller, Sandra. II. Title.

502.4613

Cover design: Sheren Farag
Printed in Australia by Star Printery

Contents

Preface

TO THIRD EDITION

This edition has been updated and amended where necessary or where we believe improvements could be made. This includes a section on the hormones which are involved in metabolism. We have done this because the treatment of this topic in most texts tends to concentrate on the overall effects of each hormone. Our treatment brings together those effects which are related specifically to metabolism, which we trust the reader will find useful.

The diagrams have also been upgraded in a uniform style.

It is particularly satisfying to us that readers find this book so helpful.

TO SECOND EDITION

This text has been substantially revised for this edition. Chapters 4 and 9 have been completely rewritten and the old Chapter 9 has been divided into two separate chapters, with the inclusion of additional material.

We are particularly grateful to all those colleagues and readers who supplied helpful comments and constructive criticism. Naturally, it has not been possible to meet everyone's wishes.

We will continue to welcome comments and suggestions. However, readers are reminded of our basic philosophy as indicated in the original preface, i.e. we are firmly committed to the concept of integration and consideration of the needs of students in their chosen field of study.

We trust that our readers will find this text informative and stimulating.

TO FIRST EDITION

The emphasis in this book is on nursing. The basis of the text is the identification of those aspects of nursing whose foundations lie in scientific principles and concepts and the examination of those principles and concepts.

Thus our objective is to further the understanding of nursing care in order to meet the needs of the modern nurse who is using a planned and holistic approach to patient care.

The style is one of integration. Our intention was not to have separate areas of 'science' and 'nursing' but to integrate the two areas to demonstrate more clearly their close interrelationships. We hold the view that the separation of these is artificial in the nursing process. You can no more separate the foundations of a building from the rest of the structure and expect it to stand than you can separate the foundations of nursing theory from its practice. One cannot survive and progress without the other. Therefore, the reader will not find a body of science theory followed by a list of nursing applications.

We have endeavoured to present ideas in an interesting and relevant manner. At times the student nurse may find more detail than is required at a given stage in his/her programme of study. However the information is built up gradually and the reader may stop at a chosen point. The text may then continue to be used for reference and be utilised again at another level.

The writing and preparation of this text has been a challenging and interesting task. We hope it will increase and extend the student's knowledge of nursing practice and thus contribute to a high quality of nursing care.

Any suggestions for improvement that readers care to make so that the text will better serve their needs will be warmly received.

We wish our readers well in their chosen careers.

Acknowledgments

The authors and publisher would like to express thanks to a number of people who have helped in various ways in the preparation of this manuscript.

W.B. Saunders Company, Philadelphia, kindly gave permission to use illustrations adapted from: F. Brescia, S. Mehlman, F.C. Pellegrini and S. Stambler, *Chemistry. A Modern Introduction*, 2nd ed., copyright © 1978 W.B. Saunders; A.C. Guyton, *Physiology of the Human Body*, 5th ed., copyright © 1984 W.B. Saunders; A.C. Guyton, *Textbook of Medical Physiology*, 6th ed., copyright © 1981 W.B. Saunders; C.R. Nave and B.C. Nave, Physics for the Health Sciences, 3rd ed., copyright © 1985 W.B. Saunders; E.P. Solomon and P.W. Davis, Human Anatomy and Physiology, copyright © 1983 W.B. Saunders.

Holt Rinehart and Winston, Inc., kindly gave permission to use illustrations adapted from: A.C. Giese, *Cell Physiology*, copyright © 1979 Holt Rinehart and Winston. Inc.

Pergamon Press kindly gave permission to use illustrations adapted from: L. Cree and J.B. Webb, *Biology Outlines*, copyright © 1984 Pergamon Press.

Alice McKay helped in manuscript preparation in a number of ways; the late Stuart Tyler, biomedical engineer at the Royal North Shore Hospital, gave valuable assistance; and Struan K. Sutherland of Commonwealth Serum Laboratories provided very

useful information on venoms. Many others gave help and
encouragement.

We are also most grateful to the following reviewers for their
many helpful comments and suggestions which have been
incorporated in the manuscript.

First edition: Stephen Beveridge of Newcastle College of
Advanced Education; Jean Deck, Aileen McCauliffe, John
Bullivant and Peter Carroll of Sydney College of Advanced
Education; Jim Keith of Kuring-gai College of Advanced Educa-
tion; and Jill O'Connor of Prince Henry Hospital.

Second edition: Tony DiMichiel and John Rayner of Can-
berra College of Advanced Education; Fazlul Huq and Jennifer
Lingard of Cumberland College of Health Sciences; Susan Rhind
and A.D. Needham of Western Australian College of Advanced
Education; Tat Beng Cheah of Hunter Institute of Higher
Education; R. Fleming and Robyn Nash of Queensland Institute
of Technology; John A. Harris and Phill Higgins of Gippsland
Institute of Advanced Education; R. Newby and (Darby) Dor-
othy B. Paull of Capricornia Institute of Advanced Education;
John Bullivant of Sydney College of Advanced Education; Penny
Little and Vikki Hardy of Macarthur Institute of Higher
Education; Elizabeth Deane of Nepean College of Advanced
Education; Stephen Collins of Footscray Institute of Technology;
Rod Sutherland of Hawkesbury College of Advanced Education;
J. Thyer of Ballarat College of Advanced Education; and J. B.
Bapat of Chisholm Institute of Technology.

Third edition: Patricia Fitzgerald of School of Nursing
Studies, Australian Catholic University; Lyn Stockhausen of
Queensland University of Technology; J. Banks-Hughes of
Department of Nursing, Royal Melbourne Hospital; David
Kershaw of Department of Applied Science, Australian Catholic
University — Mercy Campus, Melbourne; Robyn Carroll of
Department of Nursing, Mercy Hospital; Andrew Yung of Edith
Cowan University; Pam Storer of Flinders University, Sturt
campus, SA; A. J. Sperring of University of Sydney; Martin Caon
of Flinders University, Sturt campus; Charu Mishra of La Trobe
University, Wodonga; John Beard of Charles Sturt University —
Mitchell; Lea Budden of James Cook University; Dr Beng Cheah
of University of Newcastle; Beverley Green of University of
Western Sydney — Milperra; Mr. R. W. Vinen of Victoria
University of Technology — Footscray; Dr G. McKenzie of
Charles Sturt University — Riverina; H. Cleland of Manuwatu
Polytechnic, N.Z.; J. Gardiner of Hawkes Bay Polytechnic, N.Z.;
K. Ahern of Edith Cowan University; Patricia Gentile of
Queensland University of Technology; L. Kelleher of Auckland
Technical Institute; Dr Jan Wilson of Australian Catholic

University, McAuley campus — Brisbane; Mr Allan Ballard of Ballarat University College; Carol Sheldrake of University of Western Sydney — Macarthur; Dr H. M. Miller of Southland Polytechnic, N.Z.; Dr Bashir Sumar of University of Western Sydney — Hawkesbury; Dr Tofts of University of South Australia; Rhonda Albini of North Syndey College of TAFE; Mal Herron of James Cook University; Ian Blue of University of South Australia; Bob Lyall of Monash University College, Gippsland.

The authors would like to pay particular tribute and express sincere gratitude to the editor of the third edition, Denise O'Hagan, whose meticulous checking, attention to detail, thorough professionalism and pleasant personality have all contributed most significantly to the final product.

Finally, the authors and publisher acknowledge Craig Sahlin, whose photograph we use on the cover.

Note on non-sexist language

The lack of a non-sexist singular personal pronoun in the English language has posed problems for the authors.

We have consequently called the nurse 'she' and the patient 'he' on a number of occasions. No sexist implications are intended, the authors being just as aware of the existence of male nurses as the existence of female patients.

1

Introduction – homeostasis

OBJECTIVES

After studying this chapter the student should be able to

1. Explain the concept of homeostasis.
2. Describe homeostatic mechanisms and explain how these cope with stress.
3. Distinguish between negative and positive feedback and explain the operation of each.

INTRODUCTION

Nursing has changed so much in recent times that nurses of previous generations might fail to recognise it. Probably the greatest change has been the shift in the focus of care. The move from an approach which focuses on the obvious physical needs of sick people to one encompassing the total needs of an individual in health and in sickness, has meant that radical changes have occurred in all aspects of nursing. For example, the role of the nurse in promoting the attainment and maintenance of health has been widely expanded, particularly in the community.

Together with this progress in nursing has been the explosion of scientific knowledge and technological advancement, dramatic increases in the cost and complexity of health services and a greater awareness in the community of health care.

What are the implications of all these changes for the nurse? We will point out only a few which are relevant to this text. Nursing has had to assume more responsibility for patient care and has had to search independently for ways not only to meet patient's needs but also the needs of nursing itself. Nursing has begun to develop into an independent discipline, while increasing its role in the teamwork of modern health care.

Like other disciplines or professions, nursing has come to recognise the need for a solid foundation, a scientific basis upon which to build the whole subject of nursing care. As a result, the nursing profession has instituted its own research programmes and has recognised other fields of study, from which it borrows many scientific concepts, laws and principles. It is no longer a sufficiently good reason to do things because 'we have always done it this way', with no solid, reasoned justification for the practice.

The recognition of the patient as a unique individual and the emphasis on preventive care means that the nurse can no longer learn things by rote. Instead, the nurse needs to be educated in such a way that the main emphasis is on the understanding of both health and illness and the nature of professional intervention in both. Thus one key to modern nursing care is adaptability in a changing situation.

In this text we are going to examine those aspects of biology, chemistry and physics which provide a basis for many of the practices and approaches used in nursing care. We hope to expand the reader's knowledge and understanding, so that he or she will be able to gain as much as possible from the study of diverse fields such as physiology, disease processes, etc, and to develop those vital skills necessary for the professional nurse.

HOMEOSTASIS

This is a concept that has been developed to describe the internal workings of living things. It is now used to describe the relationship between the internal and external environments of the living organism as well. Some people are even using the concept to describe the relationship between mind and body in humans. Homeostasis is a concept applicable in many fields, but in the body it refers to the existence of a relatively constant environment. A small quantity of fluid surrounds every cell of the body and the normal function of the cell depends upon the maintenance of its fluid environment within a narrow range of conditions. These conditions include temperature, volume and chemical composition. Any variation outside these narrow limits may cause the cell to die.

All of the organ systems in the body make a contribution towards the maintenance of a constant cellular environment and the control of these organ systems often is effected by the nervous and endocrine systems. However, it must be remembered that organ systems and, indeed, individual cells in the body are very dependent upon one another. It follows then, that a problem with one cell, as above, may rapidly develop into a problem for many cells, for tissues and organs and ultimately for the individual as a whole.

Homeostasis is sometimes referred to as 'dynamic equilibrium' or 'a state of dynamic balance'. For our purposes in this text we will limit the definition of homeostasis to the following one, which reflects the original meaning of the term.

Homeostasis is the tendency of the body to maintain the stability of the internal environment. A number of points need to be made about homeostasis before we proceed.

1. Homeostasis is dynamic and active. We will use the term 'dynamic' when we discuss chemical systems (p. 257), and the term has similar implications here. The point is that things are happening – the body's systems are not static. Everything that is happening in the body is constantly being monitored by the nervous system, and small adjustments are constantly being made. Furthermore, metabolism is constantly occurring in cells, thus requiring oxygen; carbon dioxide is constantly being produced and must be removed; energy is being produced, which is being used or stored, and so it goes on.

The whole body is an incredibly complex machine and many of its components must be kept within certain operating constraints to keep on functioning satisfactorily. Even when we are asleep, a great deal is happening within the body and homeostatic adjustments are constantly occurring. The system which is monitoring body temperature, for example, is constantly busy, and may operate in conjunction with the system which is monitoring metabolism or may operate independently.

It is also an *active* process rather than a passive one, since the body constantly and actively pursues the maintenance of the internal environment. The concept of homeostasis applies particularly to self-regulating systems, such as the temperature-regulating system in the body.

2. The 'balance' which is maintained by the body is open-ended rather than closed. By this we mean that because various substances are entering and leaving the system, that is the body, we do not have a self-contained or closed system, but an open-ended one. Open at both ends, in fact!

3. This dynamic balance is critical to the body. It is now believed that when the body is not able to maintain that state of affairs and restore the body to that dynamic balance, then the

health of the individual is threatened and sickness or disease may develop.

4. If imbalance does occur the medical and nursing professions can intervene. Obviously it is even better if this intervention can occur in time to prevent an imbalance from arising – hence the modern emphasis on preventive medicine.

Many of the topics discussed in this text relate to the state of homeostasis in the body. Some examples of this include:

- heat and cold   : body temperature regulation
- electrolytes   : electrolyte and fluid balance
- acids and bases : acid/base balance in body fluids
- food   : energy production in the cell

These are a few of the thousands of intricate, delicate and sensitive homeostatic situations which exist in the body. Since this concept will be referred to in many parts of this text, it is appropriate to briefly explain some of the characteristics and workings of the mechanisms which help to maintain homeostasis, so that the student will better understand how various factors contribute to this state of affairs.

The **extracellular fluid** or the fluid outside the cells of the body, is in a constant state of motion and is supplied and serviced by the lungs, the gastrointestinal tract, the skin and the kidneys. It enables all body cells to function properly. The cells of the body live in this same extracellular fluid environment – one which has been called the 'internal environment' of the body.

As long as constant conditions of temperature and the necessary ions and nutrients are provided in this internal environment and wastes are removed, cells are able to fulfil their special functions and grow and live. The key to this lies in the maintenance of optimum concentrations and conditions in this internal environment.

As we have already seen, most organs and tissues in the body contribute to the maintenance of homeostasis. They make this contribution because of the constant necessity for that organ to play its part in the renewal of much-needed supplies. The lungs, for example, have to continually provide oxygen to the extracellular fluid, to replace that which is constantly being used by the cells. In a similar manner, the gut has to provide nutrients to replenish the supply that the cells use up.

The various waste products produced by the cells of the body must be removed from the extracellular fluid. For example, the kidneys play a part in removing unwanted materials and those in excess of requirements, while the lungs remove carbon dioxide, a waste product of cell function.

Thus we have an overall pattern of a vast number of variables which are kept in a state of active or dynamic balance by control systems of the body. The individual cells are thus able to function without having the worry of raw material supply or waste removal problems!

What are these 'control systems' to which we refer? They are the multitude of mechanisms by which the body is able to control the state of the internal environment. These are known as **homeostatic mechanisms**, a number of which will be discussed in this book, while others will be treated in physiology and other texts.

One example is the regulation of the carbon dioxide concentration in the blood which affects breathing rates. High carbon dioxide levels, within certain limits, cause an increase in the rate of breathing, which serves to lower the carbon dioxide concentration, to return carbon dioxide concentration to the correct level and thus restore homeostasis.

Homeostatic mechanisms are those processes and means by which the human body is able to adapt to stresses and yet maintain its inner balance. Note also that 'stress' in this context 'refers to anything which threatens or upsets homeostasis'.

Homeostatic mechanisms, while very large in number, tend to have many characteristics in common. These include:

- self-regulation or automaticity;
- negative feedback – in most cases;
- positive feedback – in just a few cases since this usually leads to illness or disaster.

Homeostatic mechanisms help to counterbalance or minimise any variation from those conditions which are most normal and/or optimal for the individual concerned at the time. Thus the body needs a means by which a control system can sense to what degree, if any, it is deviating from the set norm or pattern, and make the needed adjustments to correct the variation or deviation. Feedback provides that means.

As indicated above, two types of feedback exist:

negative feedback, which brings the body's internal environment back to its normal or optimum state, and *compensates* for the stress situation which prevails; and

positive feedback, which directs the body's internal environment away from its normal or optimum state.

Negative Feedback

Most control systems act by this process. One example of this is blood-sugar levels. The glucose in the blood is a necessary nutrient, but its concentration in the blood has to be kept at the correct levels, within a specified range of values (see Appendix III).

When blood sugar levels rise above normal levels, typically after meals, a series of reactions occur which are sensed by control systems – for example, the pancreas. Action is then instituted by several systems to restore the blood-sugar concentration to the normal or optimal level. Since this *restoration acts in a direction opposite* to the abnormality, that is, *back* towards the normal value, it is called *negative* feedback. Thus, if the blood-sugar level is high, then the negative feedback acts to lower this level. If the level is low, then the negative feedback acts so that the level is raised.

In the blood sugar example and that previously mentioned involving carbon dioxide, the response by the body has been in a *negative* or opposite direction, to *compensate* for the abnormality, not to compound the problem.

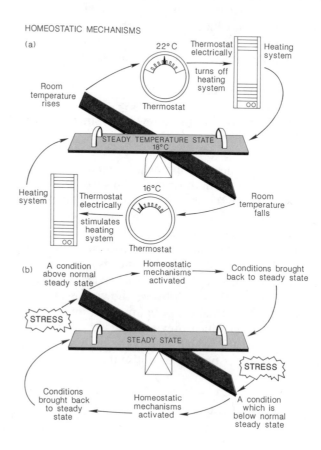

HOMEOSTATIC MECHANISMS

Figure 1.1. Homeostasis: the process of maintaining steady states. (a) The heating system and thermostat illustrate the concept of negative feedback in maintaining a steady state. When the temperature rises, the thermostat is triggered to turn off the heating system. When the temperature falls below the set level, the thermostat is triggered to turn the heating system on. (b) Stressful stimuli disrupt homeostasis. In the body, any deviation from the steady state is regarded as stress. Stress activates an appropriate homeostatic mechanism that brings conditions back towards the steady state. (Adapted from Solomon & Davis: *Human Anatomy & Physiology*. New York. Saunders College Publishing, 1983.)

A number of organs, tissues or systems may be involved in the effort to correct the deviation or abnormality. In fact, it normally requires a coordinated response, so that a factor which affects one part of the body can, in the long run, influence the functioning of other parts of the body.

These mechanisms are *self regulating* or *automatic*, as opposed to voluntary responses, which are those responses over which we normally have direct control. It would be impossible to voluntarily manage all these control systems since many operate simultaneously, and all would require a state of continual alertness.

Fig. 1.1 illustrates the general concept of homeostasis – note the definition of stress, which is discussed in more detail later – and Fig. 1.2 illustrates the principle of regulation of body temperature by negative feedback mechanisms.

Figure 1.2. How body temperature is regulated by negative feedback mechanisms. An increase in body temperature above the normal range is a signal that activates homeostatic mechanisms that bring body temperature back to normal. Increased circulation of blood in the skin and increased sweating are mechanisms that help the body get rid of excess heat. When body temperature falls below the normal range, blood vessels in the skin constrict so that less body heat is carried to the skin. Shivering, in which muscle contractions generate heat, may also occur. (From Solomon & Davis: *Human Anatomy & Physiology*. New York. Saunders College Publishing, 1983.)

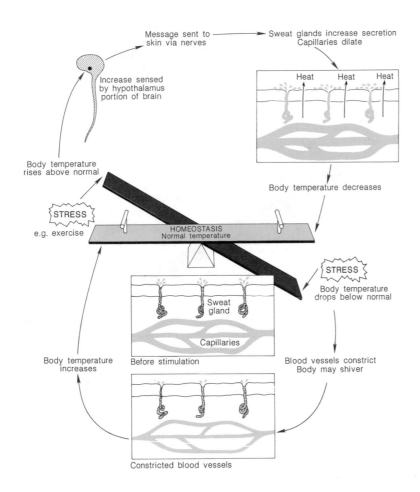

Message sent to skin via nerves → Sweat glands increase secretion Capillaries dilate

Increase sensed by hypothalamus portion of brain

Heat   Heat   Heat

Body temperature rises above normal

Body temperature decreases

STRESS
e.g. exercise

HOMEOSTASIS
Normal temperature

STRESS
Body temperature drops below normal

Sweat gland

Capillaries

Body temperature increases

Before stimulation

Blood vessels constrict
Body may shiver

Constricted blood vessels

Positive Feedback

Positive feedback systems *act in the direction of the change or abnormality* – compounding the situation. Some positive feedback mechanisms are useful. These include uterine contractions during birth, whereby one contraction induces further contractions which keep on building up until the baby is expelled from the uterus. Another example is the clotting of blood following an injury – the first stages of clotting induce further clotting, etc.

Most positive feedback situations are undesirable. They are often induced by irregular functioning of a mechanism, or instability, and can be very serious or even fatal. In this case the stimulus produces a condition similar to that which already exists. The mechanism thus enters a very nasty and sometimes deadly cycle. If the positive feedback is mild, this can normally be offset by the normal negative feedback mechanisms of the body. However, if these systems cannot cope or fail, severe distress will occur and perhaps death will follow.

As an example we will look at the question of circulatory shock, which is a general inadequacy of blood flow throughout

Figure 1.3. Homeostatic mechanisms that increase cardiac output in non-progressive circulatory shock. (From Solomon & Davis: *Human Anatomy & Physiology*. New York. Saunders College Publishing, 1983.)

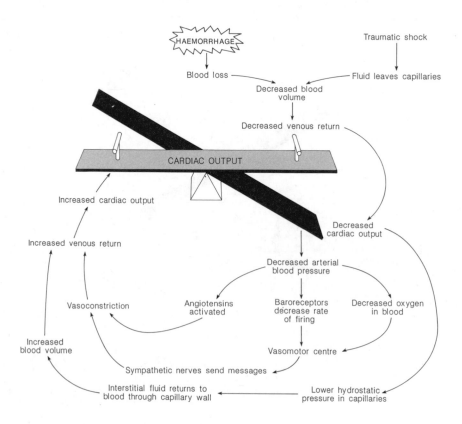

the body, leading to tissue damage through oxygen starvation. The causes may include haemorrhage and any factors which reduce cardiac output – the output of blood from the heart – such as heart attacks.

Fig. 1.3 illustrates *non-progressive shock* – shock which is not severe enough to either cause its own progression or to make the shock worse and from which the patient normally recovers. At this stage the reader may not be familiar with many of the terms which are used in the diagram, but the important thing here is the overall pattern, which we will now discuss.

The significant fact in this case is that negative feedback mechanisms compensate for the decreased blood volume and thus the decreased venous return – the return of blood through the veins – and the decreased cardiac output. As a result of these mechanisms the blood volume increases, venous return increases and cardiac output increases so that homeostasis is restored, as shown.

In *progressive shock*, the structures of the circulation system itself, the blood vessels and the heart, begin to deteriorate and the negative feedback mechanisms can no longer compensate. For example, the coronary blood flow, that which supplies the

Figure 1.4. In progressive circulatory shock, positive feedback mechanisms develop and act to deepen the shock. (From Solomon & Davis: *Human Anatomy & Physiology*. New York. Saunders College Publishing, 1983.)

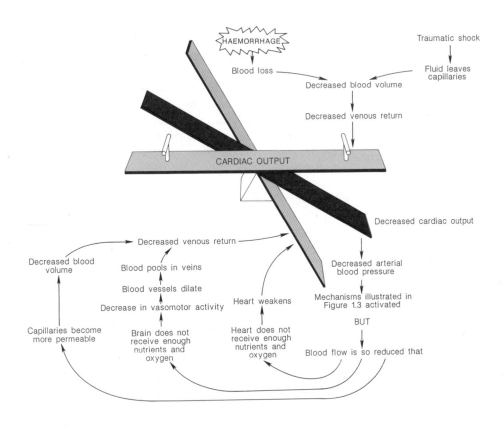

heart itself, decreases to such an extent that the heart does not receive adequate nutrition, which further weakens the heart, which in turn decreases the cardiac output still more and a vicious cycle of positive feedback occurs and shock intensifies. Thus we see that the problem is increasing because it is reinforcing or compounding itself: we then have a reduced flow, which weakens the heart, which further reduces the flow, which weakens the heart further, which results in even less flow, etc.

While this explanation and even Fig. 1.4 is an oversimplification, the reader should be able to grasp the general principles involved and the fact that progressive shock, where the negative feedback mechanisms can no longer cope, is fatal without intervention.

In some cases, positive feedback and overshoots or over-correction, can result in the overproduction of a normal body chemical and bring about such conditions as allergies, epilepsy, cirrhosis of the liver and nephritis.

In a malignant condition, homeostatic mechanisms have gone away and therefore the normal inhibitions of cell division do not function. This means that the cells will continue to divide and produce new, unwanted growth.

Speed of Homeostatic Mechanisms

Because homeostatic feedback mechanisms tend to be slower than voluntary responses and automatic reflexes, there is always a lag time between *the stimulus* – the factor causing the change or response – and *the response*. The nerve fibres involved in homeostatic mechanisms often have a considerably lower rate of transmission than voluntary nerve fibres. Also many of the information transmission mechanisms involve such chemical messengers as hormones and carbon dioxide in the blood. Since these rely on the circulatory system for their effectiveness, some time delay is involved. However, the time delay is not normally significant, since it is not normally necessary that these mechanisms should be as rapid as, for example, the blink reflex.

As a result of this time lag, the adjustments made through homeostatic mechanisms are not always perfect. If the lag is too great, the compensating mechanisms:

- may be too great;
- may occur at the wrong time and be out of phase with the mechanism being regulated;
- may thus produce an overkill or overshoot.

Thus the system overcompensates because of the time lag involved and may keep doing this, resulting in responses of increasing magnitude each time the stimulus enters the homeostatic mechanism and goes around the stimulus-response-effect cycle.

Any overshoot is itself an error, which may then require a new correction, with a new time lag, which in turn may result in another overshoot in the opposite direction. This can lead to fluctuations backwards and forwards around the normal value. While this is normal in human beings, since some degree of fluctuation always happens in homeostatic systems, it usually occurs within very narrow limits.

However, if fluctuations or overshoots increase in size, then the situation becomes unstable and a problem results. The whole system will collapse if the body cannot correct it, and it is at this time that some intervention in the form of medical and nursing care may halt or modify a potential or real disaster.

Stress

Stress may be defined as *any condition that tends to disturb the homeostasis of the body.* A more comprehensive definition of stress could be: the sum of the biological reactions, physiological as well as psychological, to any adverse stimulus, physical, mental, or emotional, internal or external, which tends to disturb the homeostasis of an organism.

Such reactions may lead to disease states, if they are inappropriate.

The body and the mind are normally able to cope with the stresses of life, new situations, etc., by homeostatic mechanisms, which can operate in such a way as to assist the individual to cope with a particular problem. Sometimes, the normal value for a particular variable, for example the blood-sugar level or temperature, may vary, either temporarily or permanently, to allow the individual to keep functioning, even in a limited way. However, there are very real limits. Continued stress may lead to a breakdown, which may be either physiological or psychological or both. The limit to which an individual can cope with a given stress situation will obviously vary from one person to another.

In addition, one type of stress can often lead to another. A physical stress may cause a psychological stress, as is the case where a person loses a limb. Similarly, psychological stress may cause physical stress. Many students are familiar with the physical stress which becomes apparent when students are sitting for exams, in the form of increased perspiration, shaking hands, nausea – even vomiting, frequent need to urinate, dry mouth and so on.

As a further example, the point could be made that most anaesthetists will refuse to administer an anaesthetic to patients who are in a very depressed state or who are convinced that they are not going to survive surgery, because people in such states have died during or after surgery for no apparent reason.

The many kinds of stress can be divided into two principal types. The body reacts to these two types of stress in different ways.

The first type is *acute* stress, which arises as a result of a situation which poses an immediate threat, such as an accident or near accident in a car, or an injury or wound of some type. In a similar way, acute psychological stress can arise from such situations as the sudden, unexpected death of a loved one, or witnessing a murder, for example. In such acute situations, the adrenal glands release hormones such as adrenalin (epinephrine) to stimulate a 'fight or flight' response.

The second type of stress is *continuing* stress, both physical and psychological, which may be caused by such factors as the onset of puberty, pregnancy, menopause, chronic disease or continuing exposure to such things as excessive noise, vibration, fumes or chemicals.

When a problem occurs, the adrenal glands can act in a continuous fashion to increase the body's tendency to fight the problem. This supplements specific defences which fight disease and infection by producing antibodies. If the stress is very severe, such as an uncontrollable disease, the adrenal glands become exhausted, other homeostatic mechanisms break down, and death may follow.

Stress and Homeostasis

Thus we have established a relationship between stress and homeostasis. Any stress situation which arises activates homeo-static mechanisms which endeavour to compensate for that stress. In Fig. 1.5 we have the example of blood-sugar levels, figuratively represented by a level seesaw. Stress may then be regarded as any factor which causes the seesaw to be other than level. At the left hand side of the diagram, the stress of a high blood-sugar level is represented by an elevated end of the seesaw and a low blood-sugar level by the lowering of the other end.

The nurse is continually involved in stress situations and, in general terms, her chief function can be described as the task of restoring homeostasis. This book is designed to help to provide some of the knowledge, understanding and insight necessary to help him or her to do just that as efficiently and effectively as possible.

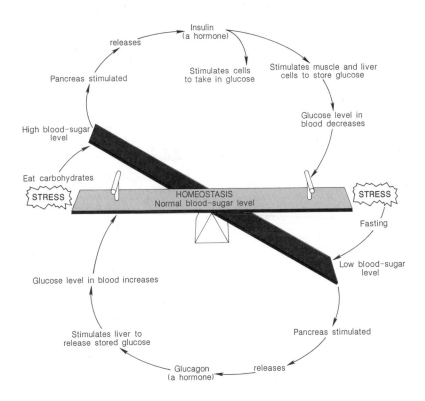

REVIEW

1. Describe the meaning of the term 'homeostasis', using the body's response to a rise in blood-sugar level as an example.
2. Define 'stress' as the term is used in its correct physiological sense.
3. Identify one mechanism (other than the example used in Question 1) which meets the criteria of a homeostatic mechanism.
4. Using an appropriate example, discuss the advantage of negative feedback mechanisms.
5. Using progressive and non-progressive shock as example, distinguish between negative and positive feedback.

Figure 1.5 Homeostatic mechanisms regulate blood-sugar level. When the blood-sugar level rises above the steady state, the pancreas releases the hormone insulin, which stimulates glucose uptake by cells, causing the blood-sugar level to fall. When the level decreases below the steady state, the pancreas releases another hormone, glucagon, which causes the glucose level to rise. (From Solomon & Davis: *Human Anatomy & Physiology*. New York. Saunders College Publishing. 1983.)

2

Humans and heat

OBJECTIVES

After studying this chapter the student should be able to:

1. State the difference between the temperature of an object and the amount of heat contained by the object.
2. List the factors which affect body temperature.
3. Describe the mechanisms which increase and decrease normal body temperature as part of the body's system of temperature regulation.
4. List the major causes of abnormal body temperature.
5. Define metabolic rate.
6. Distinguish between hypothermia and hyperthermia.
7. Describe the three methods of heat transfer, giving examples of relevance to nursing.
8. Outline the factors which affect rate of evaporation.
9. Define latent heat and use a knowledge of this concept to explain the devastating effect of steam on human tissue.

INTRODUCTION

One of the earliest procedures which the student nurse learns is how to take a patient's temperature, Methods by which that temperature may be altered, when necessary, are among some of the first nursing skills developed. However, these skills form only part of the care of the patient with respect to body temperature. Nursing involves not only performing tasks, but assessing and planning a programme of care to achieve the best possible results. In order to fulfil this comprehensive approach to the care of a patient, it is essential to understand the mechanics of heat loss and gain by the body and its need to maintain homeostasis with respect to temperature. It is from this understanding that we can proceed to assess, anticipate, make decisions, and choose the appropriate tools to assist in the care of the patient.

Heat is a form of energy. What does this mean? In scientific terms it means that heat is able to do work. For example, it can be used to raise the temperature of water to produce steam, which can then drive a steam engine.

In the body, heat which is produced by metabolism of food is used to maintain the temperature of the body in the normal range of 36.1 to 37.1 °C.

Before proceeding further, we need to distinguish between heat and temperature. Consider a situation where we have two containers – say a 250 mL beaker and a 200 L drum – each filled with water at 80°C.

The temperature is the same in both cases, but the amount of heat stored in the drum is much larger than the amount of heat in the beaker. This arises because the amount of heat required to raise the temperature of the large mass of water in the drum to 80°C is much greater than that required to raise the temperature of the small mass of water in the beaker to 80°C. Another way of saying this is that the amount of heat depends upon both the temperature and the mass of the water. The heat increase is thus defined as the *quantity of energy required to raise the temperature of the mass of that substance (in kg) through a given number of Celsius degrees*. This is stated in *joules*. *Temperature* may be regarded as the degree of 'hotness' or 'coldness' of a body.

THE CELSIUS SCALE

In nursing and most scientific work, the Celsius scale of temperature is used. Note that the kelvin scale of temperature is the scale used in the SI system, and the kelvin (K) is the SI unit of temperature. *The Celsius degree is equivalent to the kelvin* (but a given temperature does not have the same numerical value on the two scales – temperature in K equals temperature in °C plus 273).

To convert a kelvin reading to Celsius, we simply *subtract* 273.

To convert a Celsius reading to kelvin, we simply *add* 273.

The fixed points on the Celsius scale relate to simple properties of pure water, thus:

1. The lower fixed point of a thermometer on the Celsius scale is the *freezing point* of pure water and is called 0 degrees Celsius (0°C).

2. The upper fixed point of a thermometer on the Celsius scale is the *boiling point* of pure water and is called 100 degrees Celsius (100°C).

3. The interval between these is divided into one hundred equal parts, each being equal to one Celsius degree.

MEASUREMENT OF BODY TEMPERATURE

The sites used most frequently for this purpose are the mouth, axilla (armpit) and rectum. Other areas which are sometimes used, particularly during anaesthesia, include the nasopharynx, the oesophagus and the aural canal. It should be noted that temperature changes in the rectum have the greatest time lag of all areas used for temperature measurement.

The most useful instruments for measurement of body temperature are the mercury or clinical thermometer and the thermistor.

The Clinical Thermometer

The clinical thermometer is the most common and most simple tool used to measure body temperature in the human being (Fig. 2.1).

The clinical thermometer is special for two reasons:

1. It is able to measure temperature only over a narrow range (usually about 35°C to 45°C).

2. The fine tube which is filled with mercury has a constriction, so that a temperature reading, once obtained, is maintained. With ordinary thermometers, the temperature would start dropping as soon as the thermometer was removed from the patient.

After a temperature has been taken, read and recorded, the mercury has to be shaken down past the constriction, to prepare the thermometer for the next reading. If this is not done, inaccuracy in the next measurement may occur. Note that the thermometer will also have to be disinfected prior to another reading being taken to reduce the risk of germs (bacteria) being carried to the patient.

Why Use Mercury?
Mercury is used for a number of reasons:

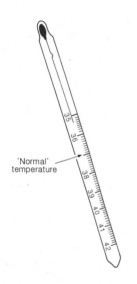

'Normal' temperature

Figure 2.1. The clinical thermometer covers the range of observed body temperatures. It has a constriction in the fine glass column which serves to maintain the mercury at the level attained while it is being read. After the reading is taken, the mercury is shaken down, ready for the next reading.

1. It is *opaque* and thus can be easily seen. Most clinical thermometers are constructed in such a way that the fine column of mercury is magnified by the stem, making reading easier.

2. It is a good conductor of heat – it readily permits the transfer of heat from one point to another.

3. It expands in a regular manner – in a thermometer this means that the length of the mercury column increases uniformly as the temperature increases.

4. It does not stick to the glass.

Mercury is poisonous if the vapour is inhaled over a long period and all compounds of mercury should also be regarded as poisonous.

The mercury used must be pure, since compounds of mercury are poisonous and produce symptoms of insanity because of their long-term effect on the central nervous system. Indeed, mercury (11) nitrate used to be used to soften the felt from which hats were made and the consequent effects on people involved in this work led to the expression 'mad as a hatter'.

Mercury is a liquid over a wide range of temperature, from $-39°C$ to $357°C$.

The only satisfactory way to measure a patient's temperature is with a clinical thermometer or one of the devices described below. It is very easy to gain an incorrect impression of a patient's temperature by using one's hand. As an example lukewarm water can feel quite warm when your hands are cold. However, the same water can feel coolish if your hands have been previously immersed in hot water.

Mercury thermometers with a wider temperature range than clinical thermometers are used as solution thermometers, for example, for enema solutions.

Mercury thermometers capable of registering temperatures below 35°C are available for such situations as profound hypothermia – very low body temperature. However, it is preferable in this case to use the *thermistor*, also called the thermistor probe or temperature probe.

A variety of disposable thermometers is also available on the market. Some of these are dependent upon chemical changes in specially prepared paper and indicate temperature changes by means of colour changes.

Note: If a mercury thermometer is broken, every effort must be made to clean up the mercury as well as the broken glass.

The Thermistor or Temperature Probe

This device consists of a blunt-ended, heat-sensitive, flexible, covered wire connected to a recording device which gives a

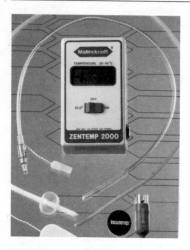

Figure 2.2 A range of temperature probes used in medical applications, together with a digital thermometer. (*Courtesy of Mallinckrodt Australia Pty. Ltd.*)

digital readout of temperature, or an indication by means of a rod. It is extremely accurate in reflecting the core temperature of the body – so important in some situations. It is used in hypothermia therapy, with unconscious patients and in situations requiring frequent and highly accurate measurement, such as post-cardiac or neural surgery and anaesthesia.

The particular value of this device is that it can be inserted into regions where a clinical thermometer cannot go or cannot reach and which are able to give a truer indication of core temperature. These probes can be left in place for extended periods of time, thus providing constant monitoring of body temperature without disturbing the patient or requiring active patient participation. This procedure can then facilitate nursing, as well as medical and surgical care.

The probes are usually inserted into the rectum or nasopharynx, but can be inserted into the oesophagus or even placed on the end of a urinary catheter and inserted into the bladder.

They do however require care, since they are in fact foreign bodies situated inside the human body, often for a considerable period of time. One problem that arises is irritation, since the probe generates friction by rubbing against highly sensitive tissues, although the probe feels very smooth and is flexible to a degree. Irritation can also result from stress on the probe caused by pulling.

Another problem that can arise is damage during insertion. Probes should be lubricated and properly anchored in position and the entry points checked frequently for signs of irritation.

Body Temperature
There is no single temperature level which can be considered to be normal, since a range of values is observed in and between healthy people. In addition, temperature varies between different regions of the body in response to various factors in those regions. These include the level of chemical activity, contact with the external environment and a regulatory system which is not always completely effective. However, *the average temperature of the interior of the body (the core), is kept almost exactly constant, within plus or minus 0.6°C*, except when a person has developed a febrile illness. For example, a nude person can be exposed to temperatures as low as 13°C or as high as 60°C in dry air and still maintain an almost constant body temperature.

It is the *surface temperature* – that of the skin – which rises and falls with the temperature of the surroundings. This is why it is most important, before taking body temperature, to choose an instrument and a body site which will reflect the actual temperature of the internal core as accurately as possible.

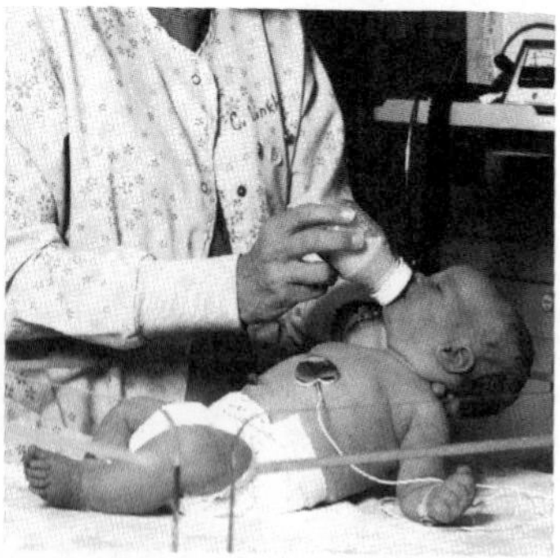

In the healthy person at rest:

Figure 2.3. A surface probe being used to measure skin temperature. (*Courtesy of Mallinckrodt Australia Pty. Ltd.*)

- oral body temperature averages between 36.6 and 37.0°C;
- axillary temperature is usually 0.6°C lower than oral temperature;
- rectal temperature is usually about 0.6°C higher than oral temperature. This reading is considered to be the most accurate of the three, since it is closer to the body core and is less susceptible to influence by external factors.

It is interesting to note that the temperature of the liver averages about 40.6°C as a result of the high level of chemical activity in that organ.

A number of factors affect body temperature, some in a regular, normal pattern in the healthy individual. These include:

1. *Time of day* – the normal body temperature of mature individuals varies in a regular pattern each day by as much as plus or minus 0.5°C, all other things being equal. One's temperature is usually lowest during sleep, particularly towards early morning. This should be borne in mind in hospital work where workloads often result in temperature readings being taken at this time, for example between 4 a.m. and 5 a.m.

2. In females, normal body temperature varies with the *menstrual cycle* over a range of about one Celsius degree. A sharp drop in temperature, usually of the order of 0.6°C, is observed a few days before ovulation and a further 0.2°C just before ovulation.

3. *Age* – children generally have higher oral and rectal temperatures (37.5 to 38.0°C) than adults, whereas elderly people often have temperatures around 36.3 to 36.4°C.

4. Factors such as *prolonged exposure* to high or low air temperatures, *fever, emotional stress, some non-febrile diseases* and *exercise* are all important in causing temperature variations.

Finally, it is most important to remember the reason why body temperature is maintained within a narrow range. It is simply that chemical reactions in cells and the enzymes (proteins) which assist these reactions function best at normal body temperatures. Thus the maintenance of normal body temperature is vital to preserve homeostasis.

PRODUCTION OF HEAT IN THE BODY

All heat in the body is produced by the processes which occur in cells, that is by *cellular metabolism*. This process is called *thermogenesis*. This means the changing of chemical energy ingested as food into other forms of energy. Some 75 to 85 per cent is released as heat or thermal energy. Furthermore, the rate at which heat is *produced by the body* is a measure of the rate *at which energy is released from foods.* This is called the *metabolic rate.*

This may be as low as 250 to 300 kJ per hour (note that the kilojoule has replaced the old unit which was the kilocalorie). However, this was often simply called the Calorie, or the Diet Calorie in diet therapy. The Calorie, which has been replaced by the kilojoule, is unfortunately still quoted as such in much of the literature – particularly American texts (see also Appendix I, Joule).

An individual walking steadily may have a metabolic rate of 900 kJ per hour and if untrained, could have a metabolic rate of 6000 kJ per hour or more during a few minutes of strenuous activity.

Production of heat is a function of *all* tissues but those in which rapid chemical reactions occur produce most of the heat. The heart, brain and liver, and most of the endocrine glands generate large quantities of heat in the resting state. As a result of this, the temperature of these organs is approximately one degree higher than most of the rest of the body.

The production of heat by resting muscles is low, but accounts for about 30 per cent of the total heat output of the body, since half of the body's mass is composed of muscles. Thus the state of muscle tone and the level of exercise at any time will affect the amount of heat produced. During extreme exercise, heat output in the muscles can rise to about 50 times that produced in all other tissues combined. This fact is utilised by the body in the regulation of body temperature, as in shivering.

Let us digress for a moment to look at the heat energy which is available from the food we eat.

Food Values

The amount of heat energy released by oxidation (that is, conversion to heat energy) of one gram of each of the following food types is as follows:

	kilojoules
carbohydrates	16
fats	17
proteins	17
alcohol	29

These are the Atwater values adopted by the Royal Society and recommended in *Metric Tables of Composition of Australian Foods,* (Thomas, S. and Corden, M. Canberra, AGPS, 1977).

Note the high energy value of fats compared to carbohydrates and proteins. However, because fats produce too many waste products and because the amount of oxygen required for fat metabolism is high they are not preferred as body fuels. The means by which food is stored and releases energy is discussed later.

Body Temperature Regulation

Normal regulation of the body's temperature is effected by centres in the **hypothalamus,** a small structure in the centre portion of the brain near the midbrain. Blood flowing through these centres has its temperature constantly monitored and information is also constantly supplied by receptors in the skin. Temperature is then adjusted in response to this information.

Thus the hypothalamus may be regarded as a *thermostat*, i.e. an instrument which keeps temperature constant – the thermostat of an oven is an example. The hypothalamus is a remarkably efficient thermostat, since an unclothed individual is able to survive for several hours in dry air temperatures as low as 10°C and as high as 65°C.

As part of the temperature control mechanism of the hypothalamus, a 'set-point' exists. All temperature control mechanisms then act in such a way as to bring the body's temperature back to this set-point, whenever variations occur above or below this temperature.

Chills

Chills are an attack of shivering accompanied by the sensation of coldness, and pallor of the skin.

A number of factors, such as dehydration, can give rise to a sudden elevation of the set-point, or body thermostat setting. The body may take several hours to elevate the core temperature to this setting, although mechanisms start operating to increase the core temperature immediately. The individual feels cold although the core temperature is already being elevated, since a temperature difference still exists between that core temperature and the body thermostat setting. The sensation of feeling cold will continue for that individual until the core temperature and the hypothalamic thermostat temperature are equal. Furthermore, the skin will also feel cold because of vasoconstriction (which decreases the supply of warm blood to the skin) and the person will shake vigorously because of shivering. Shivering is a homeostatic mechanism which causes muscles to produce heat and thereby assist the process of increasing body temperature.

Chills continue until the body temperature reaches the set point. Chills then cease and a new homeostatic situation prevails, during which the person feels neither cold nor hot. This new situation continues until the body's response to the original cause of the problem (for example, dehydration) causes the set point suddenly to fall back to the initial correct level. The patient then feels very hot and sweats profusely. This is the 'crisis' or 'flush' of febrile diseases.

Heat Balance In The Body

The concept of homeostasis dictates that the following relationship holds true:

heat loss = heat gain.

This is an idealised relationship which is oversimplified but it is the basis of the overall regulation of heat in the body. It is not necessary for the body to retain all the heat which it produces. In fact it could be disastrous if that were always the case. Therefore it is essential that the body has various mechanisms by which it can lose heat. At times very large quantities of heat are lost from the body, but under normal circumstances heat loss occurs at a fairly steady rate. Since, in some circumstances, large quantities of heat can be lost by exposure to extreme cold, or insufficient heat may be produced, it is also necessary to have mechanisms which promote heat gain.

Body temperature is *increased* by such mechanisms as:

1. *Vasoconstriction within the skin.* This refers to the constriction of the very fine blood vessels which penetrate the skin. Blood flow to the skin is thus reduced and loss of heat from the blood, through the skin, is reduced. The consequence of this is that blood temperature is kept high and this assists in increasing body temperature.

2. *Sympathetic stimulation of metabolism.* Body cells can increase their rate of heat production as a result of signals from the nervous system, or as a result of higher adrenalin and noradrenalin levels in the blood. This can account for an increase in heat production of 10 to 15 per cent in adults and up to 100 per cent in infants.

3. *Shivering.* This mechanism arises as a result of an increase in muscle tone of the skeletal muscles of the body. Contractions of skeletal muscles occur at a rapid rate, but the energy which is then available changes into heat rather than mechanical work. At a maximum level, it can increase heat production by as much as four or five times the normal rate.

4. *Hairs standing on end (piloerection).* This mechanism is obviously not as significant in humans as it is in furry animals but it has the effect of enclosing a layer of air which acts as an insulator (see below) and cuts down heat losses.

5. *Increased thyroid hormone production.* Hormone activity

can lead to an increase in production of thyroxine, which in turn increases the rate of cellular metabolism throughout the body. This process normally requires several weeks, as an acclimatisation process.

Some readers may be interested in the effect of extreme cold on human beings. For example, the Australian Aborigines in their native state are able to sleep out at night in near-freezing conditions with no body covering. No increase in metabolic rate is observed, but body heat is increased by running activity in the early morning. Eskimos, however, have high metabolic rates and the same effect appears to occur with members of Antarctic expeditions if they spend a period of time under such conditions. This appears to be associated with increased thyroid activity.

Similarly, body temperature is *decreased* by such mechanisms as:

1. *Vasodilation.* This is a process which increases the size of blood vessels in the skin. It is controlled by the hypothalamus and affects almost all areas of the body. It can increase the rate of heat transfer to the skin as much as eight times. This then provides the body with a very effective cooling process.

2. *Sweating.* This process is initiated by the sympathetic nervous system or by the action of hormones, adrenalin or noradrenalin, or by sweat glands in the skin all over the body. These glands secrete a watery fluid which contains sodium and chloride ions (refer to Chapter 4 for a discussion of these), as well as potassium ions, urea and lactic acid. The concentration of sodium and chloride ions in sweat lost in some extreme conditions can be as high as 60 millimoles per litre.

The maximum volume of sweat secreted by an individual in normal circumstances is about 700 mL per hour, but under some conditions this can rise to as much as 1500 mL per hour.

It is interesting to observe that sweat, which is water containing dissolved salts, is very effective as a cooling agent because a small amount of water requires a large quantity of heat to cause it to evaporate.

The cooling effect of sweat is achieved by the body supplying heat for evaporation. As the body supplies heat, so it becomes cool. Evaporation of 1500 mL of sweat per hour can remove body heat at *more than ten times* the normal basal rate of heat production. In fact, a rise of 1°C above normal core temperature for an individual will generate a heat loss of ten times the basal rate.

In contrast, animals such as dogs do not possess sweat glands and rely on panting as a cooling mechanism. This process relies

on evaporation of saliva to achieve cooling. However, it is not as
effective as sweating.

3. The production of heat by shivering and chemical mechanisms is inhibited.

Behavioural Control
*This is the most potent weapon which human beings possess to
regulate body temperature.* When we feel cold we seek shelter, put
on more clothes (thus building up an insulating layer around our
bodies), use heaters or perform exercise. When we feel hot, we
seek shade, open windows to take advantage of a breeze,
minimise clothing, turn on a fan or air-conditioner, and ingest
cool drinks. Drinks not only have a cooling effect, but serve to
replace fluid which is lost by sweating.

IMBALANCES IN BODY TEMPERATURE HOMEOSTASIS

In spite of the body's ability to regulate its temperature to a
relatively high degree, circumstances arise in which temperature
regulation mechanisms are overcome. These result in either
hyperthermia or hypothermia (Fig. 2.4).

Hyperthermia is a condition in which body temperature is
raised above the normal range. This is also referred to as *fever or
pyrexia.*

Hypothermia is a condition in which body temperature is
lowered below the normal range. To remember which is which of
these terms, bear in mind that 'hypo' rhymes with 'below'.
Hypothermia includes such terms as 'profound hypothermia',
which usually refers to very low temperatures from 26.0 to 24°C
or below, which are induced in cardiovascular and neurological
surgical procedures, for example.

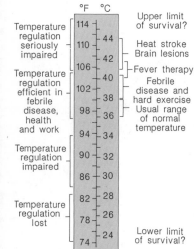

Figure 2.4 Body temperatures under
different conditions. (From DuBois: *Fever.* St
Louis. Charles C Thomas.)

Major Causes of Abnormal Body Temperature

These include:

1. *Malfunction of the thermoregulatory centres in the hypothalamus.* This can occur:

- as a result of cerebral oedema, i.e. leakage of accumulated
  excess fluid into brain tissues, causing pressure to be exerted
  on these centres, as a result of head injuries;
- following intracranial surgery (surgery on brain tissue);
- following cerebrovascular accidents – disturbance of blood
  flow to brain tissues.

2. As a result of *toxic substances* – such as those released during bacterial or viral infections; pollens; dust; vaccines and certain chemicals, including drugs to which some people are sensitive. In some individuals donated human plasma is chemically changed to become toxic.

3. *Dehydration.* This is a state in which the body has insufficient water to maintain correct fluid balance. As a result of this, water is not available for sweating and thus cooling. Furthermore, the thermoregulatory centres in the hypothalamus are directly affected by dehydration.

4. *Prolonged exposure* of the individual to extreme temperatures.

Excessive or prolonged hyperthermia or hypothermia can have quite devastating effects on the human body, even to the point of death.

Hyperthermia
As the body's temperature rises, a point may be reached at which heat cannot be dissipated as fast as it is being produced or received from the environment. Heat gain will consequently then far exceed heat loss. There is a limit to the rate at which heat can be lost from the body and body temperature will therefore continue to rise. In addition, when the hypothalamus becomes excessively heated, its ability to regulate heat is depressed.

As a consequence of this:

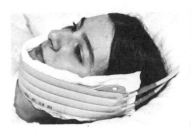

- cooling mechanisms such as sweating decrease;
- cellular metabolism may become too rapid: for example, at 42°C, cell metabolism is increased to a rate 50 per cent higher than in tissues at normal temperature;
- oxygen demand can be excessive: for example, for each 1°C rise in temperature, oxygen requirements rise by approximately 17 per cent.

Figure 2.5. This patient is being treated with hyperthermia/hypothermia equipment, which includes a temperature controller. (*Courtesy of Baxter Health Care P/L.*)

These factors can give rise to a constantly increasing temperature as a result of positive feedback, leading to tissue damage, particularly to brain tissues through protein losses, as well as lack of sufficient oxygen and nutrients to maintain body cells. Without intervention or assistance, death can result.

One example of this type of effect is *heat stroke* which occurs when body temperature rises into the range 41–44°C. This results in changes to the central nervous system, causing headache, dizziness, visual disturbances, nausea and vomiting, and sometimes delirium, loss of consciousness, circulatory effects such as a rapid, bounding pulse, changes in blood pressure and increased heart rate together with increases in respiration rate.

Immediate treatment is required as this is a life-threatening situation. Note that heat exhaustion or heat cramps are not the same, as a marked rise in body temperature does not occur.

It should be noted that heat effects are not always negative or undesirable. In fact, recent research is strongly challenging the need to reduce all fevers. A number of physicians, including paediatricians, are now suggesting that moderate fevers, that is below 40°C, be allowed to run their course. Research suggests that fever may be a very important part of the body's defence mechanism against bacterial or viral invasion. New studies are showing that moderate fever mobilises the body's immunological defences against infectious organisms and, in some cases, directly inhibits their growth. Therefore, fever may shorten the illness, improve the action of antibiotics and reduce the chances of spreading the infection to others.

However, for some patients fever would not be safe. Groups such as the elderly, people with heart disease or newborn infants may suffer unnecessary stress, especially if the fever is prolonged. *High* fevers are not well tolerated by any group because of the levels of stress put on most systems of the body and the likelihood of causing more harm than benefit. There appears to be an optimum range of function (see Fig. 2.4).

Hypothermia
This can also be a stressful problem, as it reduces cellular activity, depresses central nervous system performance and impairs the functioning of the hypothalamus. This causes drowsiness or sleepiness and in extreme circumstances, coma may result. As body temperature drops, circulation slows, thus slowing down metabolism, and nervous activity slows – leading to a similar vicious circle (a positive feedback mechanism) as that described for hyperthermia.

A decrease in temperature of *local* areas of the body, such as results from prolonged exposure of fingers, feet and face to very cold temperatures, can have such harmful effects as frostbite. This is an actual freezing of the surface areas involved which, if prolonged, causes permanent damage of local tissues and circulation. Gangrene often occurs in frostbitten areas after thawing because of this impaired circulation.

A decrease in *general* body temperature to low levels, 30–24°C or lower, which can occur for example, if a person falls into very cold water, usually results in heart standstill (cardiac arrest) or heart fibrillation (abnormal rhythm) and death, after 20–30 minutes exposure. However, rapid re-warming can often save the person's life.

Cold, which is really the relative absence of heat, is *not* always detrimental, especially when used with care on local areas. This will be discussed under heat transference mechanisms.

THE MOVEMENT OF HEAT

An understanding of the physical processes by which heat is actually lost from or gained by the body at its surfaces is probably much more essential to nursing care, in terms of treatments and observations, than we usually realise. A good example is that of a nurse following a written order to sponge a patient when the body temperature reaches a certain value. The nurse can easily go ahead and follow the order blindly, accepting little or no responsibility if the patient starts shivering and complaining of cold, because the temperature may still be above the specified value. What of that quality 'care', however? Does the written order excuse the nurse from the responsibility of making accurate observations, re-assessing the situation, understanding the processes which are operating and acting accordingly? This chapter will help provide the necessary knowledge to enable the nurse to act appropriately in this situation.

Heat is *transferred* (lost or gained) to or from the body in four ways:

1. conduction
2. convection
3. radiation
4. evaporation

In the case of a patient suffering from a moderately elevated temperature, for example 38.4°C, surface cooling methods are utilised starting with the simplest methods, such as removing blankets and excess clothing, perhaps to the extent of using only a light sheet or a breast and loin cloth. Keeping room temperature below that of the body's, if possible, and increasing the circulation of air surrounding the body are necessary adjuncts. Should the patient's temperature continue to rise or fail to drop, more active or rigorous treatments may be required, such as bathing, sponging, cold cloths or special cooling apparatus such as hypothermic blankets.

It should also be noted here that drugs such as aspirin, antipyrine and aminopyrine are called *antipyretics* and reduce elevated body temperature, although only by a degree or so.

All of the various methods described above, other than the use of antipyretics, are dependent for their effectiveness on one or more of these four processes of heat transfer.

Conduction

This is a process by which *heat is transmitted through a solid* or from one solid to another when the solids are in contact. A *conductor* of heat is thus *any substance which allows heat to pass through it.*

It should be noted that much of the heat transfer which occurs in the body takes place by conduction through cells and cell fluids, assisted by the circulation of these fluids and the blood.

In this process, the particles which make up the solid, called *molecules*, pass heat energy from one to another. (Molecules will be more fully discussed in Chapters 4 and 5.) For the moment, let us just regard molecules as small particles in a solid which have a mean or average position in that solid. However, molecules vibrate about that mean position, comparatively little at low temperatures and with greater energy at high temperatures. Thus the heat energy gained by conduction, is stored as more energetic vibrations of the molecules of the solid.

What causes a solid to act as a conductor anyway? If we bear in mind that water tends to run downhill, that mountains are worn away to provide material to fill valleys etc., we can come to the conclusion that nature is a great leveller. In the situation where conduction is taking place, one locality has a higher temperature than the other and heat tends to flow 'downhill' as it were, to correct this imbalance, from the hotter locality to the colder one.

When a part of the body, say the hand, comes into contact with a metal, heat passes from the hand to the metal, which is a good conductor. Heat is then rapidly conducted away from the hand, making the hand feel cold. This tends to be interpreted as the coldness of the metal, but the *metal is at room temperature.* The tendency of metals to feel cold is simply due to the fact that they *are very good conductors of heat.* The nurse who is aware of this and warms metal objects before placing them on a patient's body is much more popular than the one who doesn't!

Wood, which is a poor conductor, does not feel as cold. Such poor conductors of heat as wood, glass, water and asbestos are often described as *heat insulators.* Note that this term is also used in electrical work, as we shall see later, to refer to substances which do not conduct electricity. A number of good heat insulators, such as those above, are also good electrical insulators, but this is not always the case.

The insulation of ceilings of homes, of ovens and refrigerators depends upon an insulating material which limits the transfer of heat. The body does the same thing using layers of fat (e.g. Eskimos).

Maintaining Body Heat

To assist the body, we use clothes and blankets to help keep us warm in cold weather. Once again, clothes and blankets act as insulators, not keeping the cold out but keeping the warmth of our bodies in. This is achieved partly by the nature of the material itself and partly by virtue of the fact that a layer of air, which is a poor conductor and thus a good insulator, is trapped within the fibres, such as in a woollen blanket. People camping out in cold weather sometimes claim that they could feel the 'cold' coming up out of the ground. What is really happening, of course, is that they are losing body warmth down through the ground. Sheepskin rugs in a bed help to prevent patients losing body heat down through the mattress of the bed, by setting-up an insulating layer which acts as a heat barrier, thus keeping the patient's body heat where it should be – in the patient's body!

Losing Body Heat

In contrast to this, if we wish to assist the patient to *lose* heat, in order to be cooled, it is necessary to remove any insulating layers. Apart from the obvious ones, such as clothing and blankets, the air layer around the body can be 'removed' by placing the patient in tepid or cool water. We are then replacing a poor conductor – air, with a 25-times better conductor – water. Heat loss from the body is then increased, the heat escaping out to water molecules rather than air molecules. This method is often more effective than sponging and is easier with children, who are frequently too irritable or upset to lie still for sponging.

In situations where the patient must remain in bed, the use of towels or cloths saturated with water that is cold to tepid, applied to the groin and trunk areas, will assist the cooling by the heat conduction process. In an extreme emergency, such as heat stroke, some authorities recommend very cold to ice water baths. However, ice or very cold water frequently induces uncontrolled shivering, with the result that heat production increases, as discussed previously. Therefore, the *gradual* cooling of skin surfaces in such a case is supported by other authorities, for moderate temperature elevations.

Conduction Devices

Types of devices which facilitate heat loss by conduction include hypothermic mattresses and blankets made from special heat-absorbing materials or else by circulating a solution of alcohol and water. This solution absorbs heat and then is moved away to be replaced by a fresh solution which can absorb more heat. The solution is maintained at the required temperature by a machine, thus ensuring a continual cooling of the body. A hypothermic mattress or blanket is the favoured device for treating hyperthermia related to hypothalamic damage.

Internal surface cooling takes advantage of the same conduction concepts, but they are applied to the internal surfaces of the body-tissues. The reason for cooling internal surfaces of the body directly can be the same as that for cooling external surfaces – to reduce body temperature. Examples of such procedures are ice water enemas, cold saline solutions introduced into abdominal or thoracic cavities, and ventricular cooling – introducing a hypothermic physiologic solution into a cavity in the brain called a cerebral ventricle. These procedures are rarely done, they require strict supervision by a physician and can cause many complications.

However, extracorporeal cooling, which involves the use of a heart-lung machine to cool blood passed to it from a large vessel in the body, is utilised more frequently, in heart surgery for example. The blood is returned to the body, thus maintaining a continuous circulation of cooled blood, which lowers body temperature as the internal tissues are exposed to it. The result of this cooling is to reduce cellular metabolism and its associated needs such as the supply of oxygen and nutrients and the removal of blood and waste products; and also to lessen the quantity of anaesthetic required. Surgery can take place with greater ease and patient safety, and over an extended time. The patient is rewarmed after surgery in the same way.

A second reason for internal cooling may be to decrease or stop bleeding as in intragastric cooling. This involves circulating ice-cold water in a balloon inflated in the stomach to treat gastrointestinal bleeding such as that arising from ulcers. Careful and accurate observation and reporting is required.

Induced hypothermia – removing heat from the body to bring a normal temperature to well below the normal range – of the order of 32–34°C, is used in order to carry out some forms of treatment, for example surgery. This takes advantage of heat loss by conduction into ice packed around the body, or to one of the types of apparatus, or procedures, already discussed.

Accidental hypothermia can often arise from conduction of body heat into water beds or into solutions such as those used in dialysis for the treatment of renal failure. This has been known to occur especially in older patients, who have been put on water beds to prevent or ease the development of pressure areas and sores. Low room temperatures at night and during winter months can cause the water temperature in the mattress to drop. The patient can lose too much body heat and develop hypothermia. The temperature of water beds under susceptible patients should always be checked at intervals to avoid this problem.

Local Use of Conduction Principles
Making use of conduction principles, 'cold' and heat can be applied to body surface areas to achieve effects other than that of body temperature. 'Cold' can facilitate blood clotting, slow down fluid movement and inhibit inflammation, suppuration and microbial activity in the early stages of an infection. It is therefore useful in a variety of local situations such as controlling bleeding, e.g. nose bleeds, preventing or controlling swelling after sprains, contusions and muscle strains, and reducing local discomfort.

Heat applied locally can increase the tendency of the blood to flow, increase circulation, vasodilation and the flow of lymph fluid. All these effects can improve the removal of waste or toxic products, the delivery of nutrients and the relief of congestion in some circumstances. Heat can also be used to increase comfort, decrease some muscle tension and treat hypothermia following surgery or frostbite, for example.

Both heat and 'cold' can be applied locally through dressings. Wet or moist ones are most effective, or else through heating pads or blankets, in baths, or with hot wax. These methods all effectively transmit heat through conduction.

Cautionary Factors
It should be pointed out that cooling procedures, particularly baths, sponges and cloths, where more room for temperature error exists, *need to be carried out carefully and properly*. If not properly administered, (with liquid which is too cold or not changed as required, or treatment which is too short or too long), shivering may be induced and the nurse may have achieved nothing but unnecessary discomfort for the patient. The goals of treatment during surface cooling should be not only to lower the temperature but to keep the patient as comfortable as possible, to protect the patient from any injury and to prevent shivering.

Shivering can present a very difficult problem during cooling procedures because it increases the metabolic rate, increases heat production, raises oxygen requirements, increases circulation and may produce low blood sugar levels (hypoglycaemia) by using up muscle and liver glycogen. It may also produce hyperventilation and respiratory alkalosis – a rapid respiratory rate can reduce carbon dioxide levels in the body causing an imbalance in the acid and base concentrations in the blood.

Extreme caution should always be used in applying heat or 'cold' to patients who are elderly, young, unconscious, have impaired circulation, or those not able to respond properly, e.g. the disoriented patient. There have certainly been a number of patients in the past who have suffered burns from hot water bottles and hot wet dressings because sufficient care and correct application procedures were not followed, or allowance was not made for the state of the particular individual.

There are *contraindications to the use of heat* in some situations:

- acute inflammation where it may increase spread;
- trauma where it may promote bleeding; or
- in the presence of some malignancies where it may facilitate growth or spread.

Neither heat nor 'cold' should be applied for long periods. Short intervals of this type of treatment are more effective since prolonged applications can reverse the effects or have negative effects. 'Cold' can reduce circulation to such an extent that tissue injury results.

Convection

On very hot and humid days people are to be found searching for relief from the heat, to cool down and become more comfortable. Thus they are found at the beach, in a pool, in front of fans or perhaps in front of open windows searching for that elusive breeze. Do any of these activities really work? Or is it just a case of mind over matter? Could we possibly take advantage of some of these techniques to facilitate the reduction of an elevated temperature in a patient?

Heat is being transferred from the surface of the body into the environment during all these activities but some promote this transference better than others. Any of these procedures which involve *the movement of air*, particularly the movement of air over water, are frequently utilised as simple and effective ways of aiding temperature reduction. The process involved is called **convection**.

This method of heat transfer applies only to fluids (gases and liquids) not to solids. In this case, *the movement of molecules* causes *the transfer of heat*.

As an example, if a room heater is operating, the air above the heater becomes hot. This causes it to expand and thus become less dense, more spread-out than the cooler air in the room, causing it to rise. As it does so, cooler air replaces the heated air, setting up a cycle as shown in Fig. 2.6. This cycle is called a *convection current*.

The same effect is observed in a container of water which is being heated. The formation of sea breezes in summer is another example. Hot air rises over the land causing cooler air from the sea to take its place and another convection current is set up as in Fig. 2.7., causing a sea breeze.

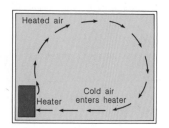

Figure 2.6. Convection air currents in a room, formed by a heating appliance.

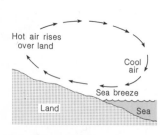

Figure 2.7. Formation of a sea breeze on a hot day, a convection current.

Heat loss from the body follows a similar pattern to these examples. Heat is conducted away from the surface into the adjacent air molecules which rise as they are warmed. Although this process of convection is constantly occurring, it is not really fast enough and does not involve a large enough quantity of air to be of great benefit to a patient with an elevated temperature. However, if we could speed up the convection process and move the heated molecules away from the body faster, allowing cooler molecules to continually replace them, then we would have a method which could be effective in the treatment of hyperthermia. This is the reason why windows are often opened and fans are utilised, sometimes with bowls of iced water in front of them to cool the air flow.

Furthermore, a patient having a tepid or cool bath loses some heat by convection within the water, once the heat has been transferred to the adjacent water molecules by conduction. Shivering can be a complication of these measures. Direct cold draughts should be avoided for this reason and careful observation maintained.

Radiation

Approximately 60 per cent of the total heat loss of an unclothed person in a room at normal temperature is by radiation. The net amount of heat radiated depends on the difference in temperature between the body and its surroundings. It then follows that the rate of heat loss will increase as the surroundings become cooler.

This is a method of heat transfer which does not depend on any substance, i.e. on the movement of molecules. Infra-red radiant energy is a form of heat and is transmitted through space in the form of waves called electromagnetic waves (which are discussed in Chapter 12). Heat is able to pass through a vacuum in this way. Heat coming from the sun through space is passing through a vacuum.

Heat loss from the skin can occur by radiation and varies according to the state of dilation of blood vessels in the skin – the greater the dilation, the greater the heat loss.

Effects of Radiation

It is appropriate at this stage to say a few words about the effects on the body of two particular forms of radiation – infra-red and ultra-violet.

Infra-red radiation is given off by all bodies which possess any heat, including our own. However, we are more concerned with infra-red radiation which *falls* on our bodies. It is often called heat radiation or thermal radiation because it generates heat in any object on which it falls. If our bodies are exposed to too much of this radiation, either from the sun or another heat source such as infra-red lamps, heat stroke and/or severe burning may result. In this case, *heat and burning are closely associated.* This is *not always* the case, as may be seen in the next paragraph.

Ultra-violet radiation has a shorter wavelength (simply the length of one wave) than visible light, which is shorter in turn than infra-red light. It is emitted by very hot bodies. An ordinary electric light bulb at 2300°C emits very litle ultra-violet radiation, but the sun (at approximately 6000°C on the surface), *emits sufficient ultra-violet radiation to sunburn exposed skin* on Earth some 150 million kilometres away!

Sunburn produces exactly the same effects as any other agents which cause tissue damage, such as excessive heat or cold. These effects include blisters, loss of the upper layers of the skin and build-up of fluid. However, one should not confuse the effects with the cause, because sunburn, despite its name, has nothing to do with heat. In fact, it is more liable to occur in cool surroundings, such as a cloudy day at the beach or on the snowfields, because the heat of the sun is not noticed and the person concerned is not aware of the effect of ultra-violet rays on the skin. These rays, unlike heat rays, are able to penetrate cloud and cause the skin damage with which we are all probably familiar.

In summary, then, *infra-red radiation* causes us to feel warm on the beach on a clear day, but this radiation is decreased by clouds. Furthermore, it does not lead to sunburn. *Ultra-violet radiation*, on the other hand, does not make us feel warm, is unaffected by clouds and *causes sunburn* – whether it is clear or cloudy.

The inflammation, or erythema, caused by sunburn, is followed in people with some skin types by an increase in the concentration of one pigment, melanin. This in turn gives rise to a colour change or tan, and an increase in the thickness of the corneum, the horny layer of the skin, which in turn gives very limited protection against further exposure. It is considered by some experts that these effects decrease the capacity of the individual to manufacture vitamin D, which is of particular significance during the winter months. Of even greater significance is the apparently well-establishcd link between over-exposure to the sun and *skin cancer*.

Members of the nursing profession should be aware of the dangers of skin cancer, particularly in a country such as Australia. We are now fortunate that we have very effective sunscreens which are able to provide 99 per cent protection by screening out harmful ultra-violet rays.

Applications of Radiation

Objects which are dull and/or black make the best radiators of heat, i.e. they give off a greater quantity of heat as radiation than objects which are shiny and/or white. Note that elements in stoves or electric heaters are usually a dark, dull material. The shiny or white objects do not radiate heat as effectively, but make much better heat reflectors than dull objects. The aluminium foil blanket which is used by ambulance officers makes use of the fact that shiny surfaces reflect radiant heat, and this helps to retain body heat and maintain the temperature of the patient. Portable infant and new-born baby carriers make use of a silvered insulating material to help the baby to retain heat.

We are all familiar with the use of radiant heat to cook food and to provide comfort in our homes, cars and work places, through heaters, fires, stoves, furnaces etc. It is also useful in helping to relieve discomfort, to dry wet or moist areas and to relieve some areas of congestion in the care of patients. This radiant energy is provided by heat lamps, infra-red lamps (which are utilised especially in physiotherapy treatments), and even light bulbs arranged on frames which can be set over areas like the abdomen or the perineal area.

The use of any of these devices on patients deserves the strong caution given in the previous section on conduction. It is very important here to know the correct quantity, strength and duration of heat to be applied and to ensure that exposure is never, under any circumstances, longer than the stipulated time. It can take only a few extra minutes for burns to occur with some patients. The distance of the heat source from the skin surface and the stability of the apparatus are also two items of concern in ensuring the patient's safety and promoting a positive effect of the treatment. Frequent checks on the patient and careful observation of the treated area cannot be overstressed.

EVAPORATION

Nurses are often requested to tepid-sponge a patient with an elevated temperature. The effectiveness of this treatment will depend, in a large measure, on the nurse's knowledge of what evaporation involves, and the various factors which can affect the process. Evaporation is one of the processes which causes heat loss during sweating (diaphoresis).

The evaporation process involves a change of state, since the substance being considered changes from a liquid state to a vapour state. For this to occur, the molecules of the substance (which are moving in a comparatively restricted fashion in the liquid state), take in a great deal of heat energy. This heat energy is then manifested as greater speed of movement of the molecules. Eventually, a situation arises in which the molecules are vibrating vigorously. This causes the molecules to overcome the attractive forces which had previously held them together, and break away from each other. The molecules now make up *a gas*. Note that this process occurs only at the *surface* of a liquid which is evaporating, in contrast to boiling which takes place throughout *all* of the liquid.

A liquid which is evaporating becomes cool because it is *supplying heat* to the molecules which are evaporating. If an alternate source can be used to supply the heat, e.g. a human body which requires cooling, then this requirement may be met. Thus, when we perspire and our perspiration evaporates, much of the heat energy required for evaporation is supplied by the body, which means that the body itself becomes cooler.

Factors Affecting Evaporation

The following factors affect evaporation:

Surface Area
The *larger* the surface area involved, the *greater* the rate of evaporation. With the body the same is true, although the need to expose as much skin area as possible does not outweigh the patient's need for modesty and privacy at all times during treatment.

Temperature of the Liquid
Warmer liquid will tend to *evaporate more rapidly* than cooler liquid, all other things being equal. However, the amount of heat absorbed by a warmer liquid is not as great (per mL) as that absorbed by a cooler liquid. Cooler liquid is thus more effective in cooling a patient, although some of this cooling is by conduction, by transferring body heat to the particles (molecules) of the liquid. However the problem of cooling the surface of the body too fast for the internal core, resulting in shivering should not be overlooked. Therefore, authorities recommend tepid to just cool fluid, at least in situations of moderate hyperthermia.

Type of Liquid
Some liquids evaporate much faster than others. Ether, petrol and alcohol are extremely volatile – they change state from liquid to vapour very rapidly. Since these liquids are also all highly flammable, great care must be exercised in their use. Water evaporates moderately quickly, while oils are very slow. It should be noted that mercury is a volatile and very toxic liquid, making

mercury poisoning an ever-present danger for people who are working with this liquid.

Ethyl chloride evaporates so rapidly that it numbs tissue and like other similar liquids is used as a local anaesthetic for minor surgery or preparation for injections. Once again, ethyl chloride and similar substances can be lethal and should always be handled with great care, because of both their toxicity and their highly flammable nature in some cases.

Ether and chloroform, which evaporate rapidly, were at one time used as anaesthetics, but they frequently caused shock because of their ability to condense and then vaporise in the lungs, causing the removal of large quantities of body heat! In fact, currently used anaesthetic gases such as nitrous oxide tend to do this to some extent.

Generally, water is the preferred liquid when sponging a patient in hyperthermia, An alcohol and water mixture can be used to increase the rate of heat removal but such a mixture often works too rapidly, causing shivering or even a shock-like condition.

Convection Currents

As molecules of a liquid on the surface of the patient's body evaporate, they will tend to move away only slowly, thus building up a 'cloud' of molecules around the body surface. This tends to slow down the process of evaporation, since other molecules then find it more difficult to break out of the liquid into the cloud, and some others will condense back on to the surface. Some means of keeping the molecules moving is then required and this is usually achieved by utilising natural air movement, breezes or fans.

Atmospheric Humidity

This is an *expression of the concentration of water in the atmosphere.* When the atmosphere is saturated, the humidity is 100 per cent, and rain will probably follow. However, rain can fall when the atmosphere at ground level is well below saturation.

When humidity is very high, *evaporation slows down* or ceases and perspiration becomes less effective as a cooling mechanism. The reason is simply that evaporation is not likely to occur if the atmosphere is already nearly saturated with water. The individual then feels very uncomfortable.

In these conditions patients should always be checked at intervals for wet or damp clothes or bed linen as the perspiration collects on them and increases discomfort. It is particularly important to check patients in the evening and during the night as both air and body temperatures tend to be lower then.

A patient lying in wet clothes or linen will feel or become

colder as heat loss is increased, and may develop chills. Also, damp material next to skin surfaces can increase the risk of tissue damage, especially in patients who are relatively immobile.

LATENT HEAT

This may be regarded simply as 'hidden heat'. It is hidden because we do not see evidence of its existence with a thermometer. Just as we have considered increased temperature to be indicated by more rapid movement of molecules, latent heat is indicated by a *rearrangement of molecules*.

Consider the arrangement shown in Fig. 2.8. Some pure ice, at say −10° Celsius, is gently heated while being stirred. The temperature rises steadily as time passes until 0° Celsius is reached (line AB in Fig. 2.9).

For a period of time, no further increase of temperature occurs, although heat is still being applied (line BC in Fig. 2.9).

This heat is used to break the bonds which hold the molecules of water together in relatively fixed positions in ice. The molecules are then able to move about more freely as liquid water. The heat required to rearrange the molecular state of ice in this way is called **the latent heat of fusion**.

Once all the ice has melted, the temperature begins to rise once more and increases steadily as time passes until 100° Celsius is reached (line CD in Fig. 2.9). Once again it is observed that the temperature remains steady, no matter how much heat is applied, as long as boiling water remains (line DE in Fig. 2.9).

The heat energy involved here is being used to rearrange the molecular state of the boiling water so that it becomes *steam*. This heat energy is called **the latent heat of vaporisation**.

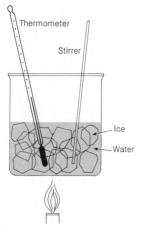

Figure 2.8.

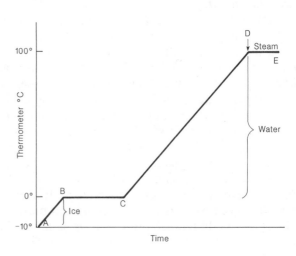

Figure 2.9. Temperature of ice (originally at − 10 °C) which is steadily heated over time, until it becomes water, and finally steam.

A comparison of the quantity of heat involved for 1 kg of water is most informative.

Step	Line	Heat Involved
1. Heating ice from $-10°C$ to $0°$	(AB)	42 kJ
2. Latent heat of fusion	(BC)	336 kJ
3. Heating water from $0°C$ to $100°C$	(CD)	420 kJ
4. Latent heat of vaporisation	(DE)	2260 kJ

It may be readily seen that the quantity of heat required in the last step is very much larger than the others. *All* of this heat is given out when 1 kg of steam condenses back to boiling water – this is the opposite of evaporation. This accounts for the devastating effect of steam on human skin and flesh. All of this heat is given out even before boiling water is formed. This boiling water in turn, adds to the severity of the burn.

Safety Note

Steam is invisible. The 'steam' which we see issuing from a kettle or boiler has already condensed into water droplets as a result of contact with cooler air in the same way that we see our own exhaled air in very cold conditions. What we are then seeing is condensed water droplets. If we don't see these droplets, *it does not mean that steam is not present.*

HEAT EXCHANGE AND ITS PREVENTION

Some examples of the exchange of heat in the body are:

1. Heat is often required to warm inspired air to 37°C, and this may be effected by an exchange of heat between *inspired and expired gases* within the respiratory tract. It should also be noted that a proportion of the heat of gases being expired is returned to the mucosa of the upper respiratory tract by condensation.

2. The heat content of saturated gases may be used as a central warming device in the treatment of hypothermia. Delivery is effected through assisted or full-control breathing devices, such as respirators or ventilators.

Vacuum, Thermos or Dewar Flasks

These are designed to maintain the temperature of liquids for example, by preventing transfer of heat – hot liquids are kept hot and cold liquids are kept cold.

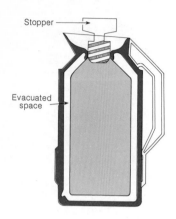

Stopper

Evacuated
space

Figure 2.10. A vacuum flask.

In a vacuum flask:

- heat transfer by *conduction* is minimised by having two glass walls with a vacuum between them. as seen in Fig. 2.10. The only contact between the inside and outside walls is at the join at the neck and even this may be insulated;
- heat transfer by *convection*, by movement of heated air around the container, is also minimised by the vacuum;
- heat transfer by *radiation* is minimised by having inside surfaces silvered to become very shiny.

Autoclaves

These appliances operate under high pressure and under such conditions water boils at temperatures very much higher than 100°C. Such temperatures will effectively coagulate protein including bacterial protein, so that their usefulness as sterilising devices is immediately apparent.

At the beginning of this chapter reference was made to the importance of developing a good general understanding of heat. It is hoped that the reader now shares this view!

REVIEW

1. If a neighbour tells you that she thinks her child may be sick because he 'feels' hot, why would the use of a clinical thermometer or one of the simpler temperature indicators be more satisfactory in determining the temperature of the child?
2. One contraceptive method involves measuring female body temperature. What does this achieve?
3. You have been asked to cease sponging a patient with an above normal temperature, because the patient is shivering. Why would such a request be given when the patient still has a high temperature?
4. Why is it of value to obtain body temperature readings over a 24-hour period when someone is ill?
5. A patient with a high temperature has been asked to remain in bed. What is the reasoning behind this intervention in the patient's activities?
6. A water-bed is to be prepared for a newly-transferred patient who is 80 years of age. What precautions and preventative measures should you think about in relation to the patient's need for body-temperature maintenance?
7. A child has a bleeding nose which is proving difficult to stop. What measure other than pressure might help?
8. In a soccer game, a child twists his ankle; an ice pack is applied. What is the reasoning behind this treatment? What precautions should be taken and why?
9. A heat lamp is ordered for a man who has a perineal wound. Explain the effects of this treatment.
10. What advantages are gained by the use of hypothermia with surgery?

11. Identify the major causes of abnormal body temperature.
12. What is latent heat? Use this concept to explain why steam burns are so serious.
13. When visiting a new mother, she asks for your advice concerning her 4-month-old baby who has a runny nose, is crying more and feels hot. In relation to the report of the baby 'feeling hot', what simple measures might you advise the mother to take, besides calling her doctor? On what rationale would you base each of your recommendations? Would there be any adverse responses for which the mother should watch, what should she do in those cases and what would be the explanation(s) for any such reactions?

3

The human machine (forces and mechanics)

OBJECTIVES

After studying this chapter the student should be able to:

1. Define some basic physical quantities, including vector quantities.
2. Utilise these concepts in nursing applications.
3. State Newton's three Laws of Motion and describe their relevance to nursing.
4. Describe the function of levers and pulleys in nursing situations.
5. Relate the importance of body posture to work situations.

INTRODUCTION

Why the study of mechanics? What do things such as forces, levers, pulleys, centres of gravity, vectors, laws of motion and such have to do with nursing?

At any moment in time every nurse is making use of some aspect of mechanics. This may apply directly to the way in which the nurse uses her body in the course of her work or to applications relating to patients. For example, a man involved in a rear end car accident has been brought in to the accident and emergency department of a hospital complaining of severe neck pain and reduced mobility in his neck, as well as showing evidence of a fracture in his right leg. A whiplash injury is suspected. Why? What problems will the man have to cope with immediately and in the future?

What mechanical forces would have been involved at the time of the accident? Did the seat belt contribute to the injury in any way? A knowledge of the answers to these questions, together with appropriate anatomy and physiology, will allow the nurse to make a comprehensive and accurate assessment of the patient's needs. It will allow the nurse to anticipate not only patient needs and potential problems but forms of treatment which may be required. This in turn provides an opportunity for a quicker and more effective response by the nurse to the situation.

An industrial or occupational health nurse, for example, may be conducting an injury prevention programme and is very much aware of the number of injuries arising from a lack of understanding of body mechanics. One of the objectives of this programme is to reduce the number of injuries caused by poor lifting or moving techniques.

Another nurse may be teaching a patient the best method of lifting him or herself to a sitting or standing position. Elsewhere, another nurse could be receiving instruction and being told not to rest the weights of a traction system on the patient's bed. Why?

A study of some of the basic principles of mechanics will give the reader an insight into the nursing activities mentioned above as well as many others of importance to nurses.

We will start by considering some of the basic ideas and concepts which the student needs to grasp in order to understand this section of work and be able to appreciate the applications to nursing which will be discussed.

Speed

This is a measure of *how fast* something is travelling. The 'thing' may be a human body or it may be a rock or bullet flying through the air, or a motor car.

$$\text{speed} = \frac{\text{distance } (\textit{metres})}{\text{time } (\textit{seconds})}$$

The units of speed are therefore *metres per second*, that is, the number of metres travelled in every second. It is usually shown in the abbreviated form **ms**$^{-1}$.

Velocity

In many practical situations, velocity is often the same as speed, but not always. The difference arises because when we speak of velocity we speak of *motion in a straight line*. Thus we can speak of a speed of 60 km/h travelling around a curve in a motor car, but this cannot be a velocity, since the *direction is changing*. A rock being swung around one's head on the end of a piece of string may be travelling at a constant speed but because the direction is changing it is *not* moving with a constant velocity.

The units of velocity are the same as those for speed but the *direction* must also be specified. For instance, 'The car was travelling at 30 ms^{-1} in a north-easterly direction'.

Mass

The *mass* of an object is the amount of matter contained by the object. Note that this definition takes no account of the force of gravity (on which *weight* depends). This means that the mass of an object remains the same whether we are measuring it on the Earth, the moon or Mars.

Acceleration

When the velocity of an object is being changed, it is said to be **accelerated**. Since velocity possesses both size or magnitude and direction, this means that the velocity is being changed if either:

- The *magnitude* is changing – it is speeding up or slowing down; or
- The *direction* is changing.

In the example above, of the rock on the piece of string, the speed may be constant, but since the direction is changing all the time, the rock is said to be undergoing acceleration.

$$\text{acceleration} = \frac{\text{velocity } (ms^{-1})}{\text{time } (s)}$$

Let us now consider an object which is increasing its velocity by 10 ms^{-1} each second, for example. We say that we have an acceleration of 10 ms^{-1} in *every second*, that is, 10 metres per second per second; or 10 ms^{-2}. This is a *positive* acceleration. If the body were slowing down, the *negative* acceleration would be -10 ms^{-2}.

Note also that since a velocity is involved, a direction would have been specified. This direction would still apply to the acceleration in this case since only the *magnitude* of the velocity has been altered.

Force

A force is a *push* or a *pull*. A force may act on a body in a number of ways:

It may change the state of rest of an object. If an object is at rest, a force acting on the object may impart an acceleration to the object.

If a body is travelling in a state of uniform motion in a straight line, a force may cause the object to:

slow down
speed up
change direction (i.e. to accelerate).

This means that whenever we think of applying a force, as in traction, we need to think of both the direction and the size or magnitude of the force. Quantities such as these, in which both magnitude and direction are involved, are called **vector** quantities. They are discussed in greater detail on p. 58.

The unit of force is the **newton** (N). The newton is defined as that *force which when acting on a mass of 1 kg produces an acceleration of 1 ms^{-2}.*

What is a newton like? As an example, if a nurse adds a 1 kg mass to a traction arrangement, the force acting is increased by almost 10 newtons. The precise figure is actually 9.8 newtons, since the force of gravity produces an acceleration of 9.8 ms^{-2}.

The Force of Gravity
One special example of a force is the force of gravity.

We are all aware that gravity exists but are not always aware of the effects which gravity has on the human body, and therefore of its application to certain aspects of our care of people. It can sometimes be seen that our awareness of gravity does not extend to an understanding of it in such situations as the location of straight drainage bags collecting fluids from body cavities such as the bladder. Such bags have been found lying on top of a patient's bed instead of hanging below the body and mattress level. This must surely reflect a lack of understanding of the concept of gravity and its applications.

It is observed that any *two objects in space will attract each other.* The sun and the earth attract each other, the earth and the moon attract each other and so forth. These forces of gravitational attraction between bodies in space affect many things. As an example, the gravitational attraction of the sun and the moon on the earth gives rise to tides.

In the same way, a human being and the earth attract each other. Since the earth has an enormously greater mass than a human being, the human being does most of the moving if the two are apart, such as if the person jumps into the air. This force is most important since without it we would not be able to stay on the earth – we would 'fall off'. It is interesting to note that, since the mass of the moon is only about one-sixth of the mass of the earth, the pull of the moon is only approximately one-sixth of the earth's gravity. Thus, people who walk on the moon's surface experience great difficulty in trying to stay upright.

The phenomenon of *weightlessness* occurs because the individual is so far removed from the effects of earth's gravity. Of course, that individual and any other objects nearby exert a gravitational pull on each other, but their masses are so small that this effect is not noticed. It is the absence of the gravitational pull of large bodies such as the earth which gives rise to weightlessness, and all the human problems associated with this. The reader is invited to think about the unfortunate space traveller trying to carry out everyday functions such as drinking, eating, urinating etc., under these conditions. Life without gravity would be different, to say the least!

We observe gravity as always acting *downwards* or towards the centre of the earth. In terms of the body, if we wish to decrease the blood supply to a limb to lessen bleeding, we elevate that limb. This means that gravity is acting against the heart and so the blood supply to the affected limb is lessened. Alternatively, the head of an individual who has fainted is lowered to below heart level, to increase the blood supply to that area. The force of gravity is acting *with* the heart in this situation. Let us now look at the relationship between the body and gravity more closely.

When an individual is in a standing position, those regions of the body which are above the heart must have blood pumped to them against the force of gravity. To overcome the force of gravity the heart must increase its contractile force to push the blood upwards. If the pumping force of the heart is not great enough to do this, insufficient blood may reach the brain, sometimes causing fainting. This situation is called **postural hypotension**. The normal consequence of this, of course, is that the body then adopts a horizontal posture, which counteracts the action of gravity so that the brain is no longer starved of blood.

On the other hand, gravity promotes the downward flow of blood to those regions which are below the heart. The difficulty which arises in these regions is with *venous return*. The flow of blood back to the heart is normally assisted by a number of mechanisms, such as the squeezing of veins by muscles and the presence of 'non-return' valves in the veins which prevent back flow. Lack of movement tends to slow that return. In such circumstances even wriggling the toes and feet inside shoes can help, and soldiers are told to do this when on parade to lessen the possibility of fainting. This movement causes the muscles to alternately squeeze and release veins, pushing blood out of the feet and back towards the heart. If sufficient blood volume is not returned, output from the heart is reduced, which will affect areas such as the brain quite rapidly.

People who have to stand for long periods of time sometimes exhibit distended blood vessels in the lower extremities and oedema (swelling) can be seen. These problems are also caused by lack of movement resulting in slowing of the return flow and a backup of blood in the vessels. As the vessels become full of blood, pressure inside them increases, causing a shift of fluid from the vessels into the surrounding tissue spaces. This is seen as a swelling or oedema. The detrimental effects of gravity on the circulation of blood in the body is an important point in health education. It has particular relevance to certain occupations such as shop assistants and to people with established circulatory disorders, as well as those with a tendency to developing them, such as pregnant women and the elderly. The health teacher can emphasise the need for:

- changing position, raising legs above heart level, walking, flexing feet and legs;
- avoiding constrictive clothing or apparel such as garters or elastic, tight shoes, tight girdles or tight jeans;
- supporting the lower blood vessels, in the form of special support hose or bandages.

All of these measures will promote better venous return, reduce the workload on the heart and avoid a possible build-up of blood in the lower vessels. They may even avoid higher pressure in these vessels which the heart has to overcome in order to keep blood flowing.

The concepts mentioned above are also relevant to patients in horizontal positions in certain instances. Distended vessels in arms and hands have been seen in patients whose limbs are left hanging over the edges of beds and chairs, when the patients have been unable to move themselves because they are unconscious or paralysed.

Changing the posture of the body, particularly in a patient who is unable to move either his body, or parts of it, will result in changes in blood pressure distribution and changes in the amount of work the heart has to do to maintain normal blood flow in all parts of the body, thus promoting good circulation.

Advantage is taken of the 'downward' pull of gravity to drain fluid from a number of cavities in the body, such as from the pleural space of the chest, from the bladder and from the

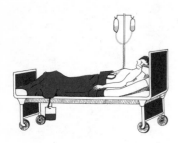

Figure 3.1. Peritoneal dialysis. Gravity is used to introduce fluids to the patient's body and to remove them from the body.

peritoneal space in the abdomen. The use of straight drainage can occur without the aid of suction apparatus, provided that the drainage collection bag is kept below the level of the cavity which is being drained. In some instances, unless the drainage tubing is clamped off, raising the bag can cause backflow of drainage into the cavity and possible contamination of the cavity, or damage to the tissues in that area.

A good example of the use of gravity in both *adding* fluids to a patient's body and removing them is seen in peritoneal dialysis (Fig. 3.1). In this treatment a solution which promotes diffusion is run into the peritoneal cavity under the influence of gravity. After a period of time, during which waste products and substances in excess, are removed from the circulation by diffusion, the fluid is drained out, once again under the influence of gravity. This type of treatment is sometimes used when a patient has a kidney disorder and is unable to pass sufficient water, wastes or other substances out in the urine.

Gravity is also employed in the use of *intravenous solutions*. These are solutions which are introduced into veins from suspended containers through tubes and needles. For example, five per cent glucose or dextrose/sodium chloride mixtures; blood transfusions – which may be whole blood, packed cells etc; and other solutions to provide the body with necessary nutrients (amino acids, fats, carbohydrates and vitamins) also follow the same concept.

It can be seen from the preceding examples that gravity plays a vital role in medical treatments. It allows us to easily add necessary substances to the body, to remove those which are building up to threatening levels, to support and maintain the body until such time as it can cope for itself and even to monitor changes within the body as in the measurement of central venous pressure. In turn, this becomes very significant for the nurse, since it is usually part of the nurse's role to check, maintain and monitor these treatments while ensuring that they do not contribute to the patient's physical or mental discomfort any more than is necessary.

Some treatment devices depend on gravity for their operation. These include electrical rocker beds, which tilt the patient's body up and down so as to improve circulation to and from the extremities (e.g. with premature babies), or to promote the rise and fall of the diaphragm to assist breathing (e.g. with polio victims).

The art of correctly positioning a patient, which is studied early in a nurse's training, takes advantage of gravity or may try to relieve the negative effects of gravity. A post-operative patient is usually placed in a position which promotes the flow of secretions or vomitus out of the mouth to avoid their aspiration.

Aspiration can occur if the patient is flat on his or her back –
perhaps unconscious or unable to swallow or cough. In prefer-
ence, the patient is positioned on his or her side or in a prone
position. Brain surgery may be performed with the patient in a
sitting position to decrease the danger of haemorrhage. The
patient may be tilted during abdominal surgery to facilitate
surgery on certain organs, as gravity helps to keep other organs
out of the way.

Centre of Gravity

The centre of gravity (C.G.) of a solid object may be defined as
*that point at which all the mass may be imagined to be
concentrated.* For our purposes, this may also be regarded as the
centre of mass. The *force of gravity* is then considered to act at
that point. Furthermore, if the object is suspended at that point
it will not display any tendency to rotate or to move.

This concept is perhaps better appreciated if it is borne in
mind that many of the objects with which we are familiar tend
to be uniform in shape and thus uniform in the distribution of
mass. Where a body is irregular, it behaves very differently, and
its centre of gravity tends to be located near the region of greatest
mass. The human body tends to be symmetrical on either side of
a line drawn from the top of the head to the crotch (the mid-
saggital plane), but is not symmetrical in most other respects.
Furthermore, human bodies vary from one individual to the
next; therefore the position of the centre of gravity will vary
between individuals. This will have obvious and very important
applications in any study of the art of lifting patients.

As an example of the concept of centre of gravity, consider
a typical sports car and a double-decker bus. The sports car is
very wide compared to its height, but the bus is the opposite.
Also, the weight of the passengers is located very close to the
ground and well down compared to the axles of the car. The
double-decker, however, has passengers located well above the
axles. This means that the centre of gravity of the bus will be very
high compared to the sports car. As a consequence, the bus will
be much less stable than the sports car and more susceptible to
being turned over, if not driven carefully (Fig. 3.2).

The practising nurse must apply the same principles in his or
her profession, particularly in lifting situations.

Centre of Gravity and The Nurse

In the human being, the centre of gravity is usually located in the
pelvic region near the base of the spinal column, at about the
second sacral vertebra. The centre of gravity is in line with the
spinal column and in the pelvic area when sitting or standing in
an erect posture. This location results in the *least strain on body*

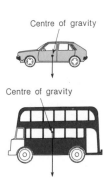

Centre of gravity

Centre of gravity

Figure 3.2. Centre of gravity. The bus, with its higher centre of gravity and narrow body, compared to its height, is more unstable than the car.

muscles and the lowest amount of energy to maintain the body in an upright position. In addition, the muscles of the thighs and spinal column in humans oppose the action of gravity.

The weight force which acts 'downwards' at the centre of gravity of a body is balanced by an equal and opposite 'upwards' force exerted on it by the earth, or any other object on which it rests. This 'upwards' force is necessary for the body to be able to maintain its position against the force of gravity; otherwise the body would simply sink lower and lower, as happens in quicksand.

The forces are then said to be in *equilibrium* with each other. The object will be stable if the weight acts through a line which falls well inside the base, as shown in Fig. 3.3(a). This is sometimes called *stable equilibrium*.

Note that the base in the diagram is that part which is in contact with the floor. The same is true of the human body. When standing, the base is that area occupied by the feet in contact with the ground. However, it is possible to increase the size of the human base by standing with the legs apart. This means that the centre of gravity of that body can be shifted as required, when lifting, without becoming unstable. The nurse then has a flexibility of postural changes while lifting, such as pivoting on the balls of his or her feet.

However, there are limits. If the distance between the feet is made too great, the opposite effect is achieved. The ideal distance will tend to depend on the height and build of the nurse, and is best determined by trial and error.

If the weight force acts near the edge of the base, as in Fig. 3.3(b), equilibrium does exist, but the body is not stable and would easily tip over. This is called *unstable equilibrium*.

In Fig. 3.3(c), the body cannot be in equilibrium, and is *unstable*, since the weight force acts outside the base, that is the weight is acting outside its base of support, and generates a turning force, causing the object to topple over.

It is important that the practising nurse understand the concept of stable equilibrium, both in relation to good posture

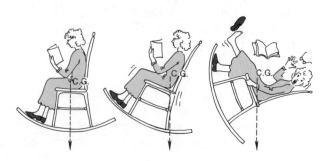

Figure 3.3. States of equilibrium and non-equilibrium.

and to proper methods of lifting both patients and objects. Fig. 3.4 illustrates the fact that a good posture ensures that one's centre of gravity rests directly over the centre of the feet area, enabling balance to be easily maintained and forces of gravity to be overcome.

The centre of gravity is altered by changes of posture. The slumping posture at the right shows that the centre of gravity has been shifted forward and the individual is not as stable. When bending forward or leaning backward or sideways, the centre of gravity shifts forward, backward or sideways according to the degree of body movement. This can put the centre of gravity either completely outside the base of support or toward the outer edges leaving the person in unstable equilibrium.

Furthermore, muscles have to compensate for this by increasing the number of muscles involved or the number of fibres within a muscle or by maintaining equilibrium of the body or by demanding larger quantities of energy – more oxygen, nutrients, and blood volume. While the person may not consciously be aware of the extra involvement of muscles in maintaining the body's position, *strain* is being placed on the muscles – particularly the back muscles, and is evident by fatigue, backaches or pain and the inability to maintain upright positions comfortably when standing or sitting for extended periods of time. In fact it has been found that this type of strain on the body can contribute to feelings of irritability, depression and other negative feelings which affect relationships with other people as well as attitudes.

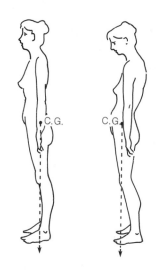

Figure 3.4. A slumping posture tends to shift the centre of gravity (C.G.) forward, causing a less stable equilibrium and abnormal muscle strain.

Posture is therefore a very important aspect of the health of a human being. This means special attention should be paid to those people who are likely to develop postural problems, such as those who lose a limb, pregnant women, people with ascites (accumulation of fluid in abdominal cavity), those carrying or lifting loads as part of their occupations and those using supportive devices such as crutches or braces.

The *lifting situation* is a good example to look at in detail. Nurses are particularly involved in lifting both heavy objects and patients. Sometimes the load involved approaches or exceeds the maximum levels advocated for many industrial workers. *Nurses are in a high risk occupational category for musculo-skeletal disorders.* Studies have shown that back disorders may account for a relatively high loss to the nursing profession, in terms of work capacities. It has also been shown that the frequency of back disorders is highest in those specialities where nursing staff frequently handle patients, e.g. in neurological units, intensive care, geriatric centres and orthopaedic units.

It is important to have the object being lifted *located directly over or under the centre of gravity* or as close to this as possible. Figure 3.5(a) shows a *correct* lifting technique. This means that

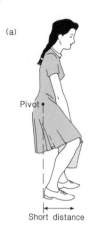

(a)

Pivot •

Short distance

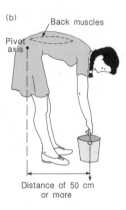

(b)   Back muscles

Pivot
axis •

Distance of 50 cm
or more

Figure 3.5.(a). Correct lifting technique. In this case the distance between the pivot and load is short and the back is not being used as a lever. Most of the lifting effort is achieved by the legs.
(b) Incorrect lifting technique. Strain is on back muscles from lifting objects which are far away from the body. Lifting should not be done this way, since the back is being used as a lever.

the centre of gravity will not shift far from the normal erect position. The powerful thigh muscles should be used to combat the increased effects of gravity due to the additional mass and not the weaker back muscles. Figure 3.5(b) illustrates how **NOT** to lift. In this case, the relatively weak back muscles are being used to oppose the effects of gravity on the object being lifted. The result here is back strain. If, however, the object had been lifted close to the body, with the back straight, feet spread and knees bent, then the thigh muscles would have been in a position to do most of the work in opposing gravity.

It is most important to recall at this stage that the actual location of *the centre of gravity* of an individual depends on such factors as *posture*, and the *position of the limbs* at that moment. It would be very useful for each nurse to test the concepts which have been discussed in this section to gain first-hand experience of the difference between stable and unstable equilibrium. It is suggested that you try standing with feet together, legs straight and then bend over from the waist and back up again, taking note of your sense of balance and equilibrium at all times. This should then be repeated with feet apart, then with knees bent as well, varying the distance between the feet and the angle at which the body is bent over. These simple procedures may prevent the reader from joining the long list of nurses who have become casualties of poor lifting techniques.

Mass and Weight

We have already defined mass as the *amount of matter contained by an object*. The weight of an object is a measure of the *force which gravity exerts on that object*. If we were to compare our mass and weight on the moon with that on the earth we would find that the mass was the same because the amount of matter in our bodies had not altered, but our weight would be only about a sixth of that observed on the earth, because the force of gravity on the moon is less. This arises because the mass of the moon is less. While most of our readers probably have little intention of ever nursing on the moon, it is hoped that this example will help to clarify these terms!

Mass is measured in *kilograms* (kg), and weight (being a force), is measured in *newtons* (N). When we speak of our 'weight' in everyday usage, we are really speaking of our *mass*.

Momentum

This is an expression of the product of mass and velocity of a moving object. Thus a bus has a greater momentum than a small car travelling at the same velocity, because the bus has the greater mass. Another identical bus which is moving faster, however, has a greater momentum than either because of its greater velocity. The small car could have a greater momentum than either bus if and only it, the product of its mass and velocity was larger than that for either bus.

Momentum is sometimes represented by the letter p and has the unit *newton second (Ns)*.

Since the unit of force is the newton and that of time is the second, it follows that the unit of p (momentum) is the newton second.

Inertia

This may be regarded as the *resistance to any change of the state of rest or motion of a body*. This is, in fact, another way of saying that a force is needed to bring about the change described. It follows that mass is a measurement of inertia. More will be said about this a little later.

NEWTON'S LAWS OF MOTION

These laws describe the behavior of objects or bodies in motion. In fact, the interpretation of the term 'bodies' will, in much of this work, be quite literal and apply to human bodies. Specific examples will be discussed under each law.

First Law – The Law of Inertia

This states that
a body at rest will continue at rest, and a body in motion will continue in motion with uniform velocity, unless acted upon by an unbalanced force.

This law is really quite simple. What it is saying is that an object will keep on doing the same thing unless there is some compelling reason to change. An object which is at rest will simply remain at rest unless an unbalanced force acts upon it, and an object moving along with uniform velocity will continue to do so unless an unbalanced force acts upon it. In the latter case, the force may cause the object to accelerate, that is, to speed up or slow down, or it may cause it to change direction, or cause a combination of these, for example to slow down and change direction.

Whiplash injuries are caused by the tendency of the human head to obey this law. If a vehicle is hit from the rear, the occupant's trunk is violently jerked forward, because it is in contact with the seat. The head, however, tends to remain at rest (in the absence of head restraints) and is snapped into an extension position. Since the head is attached to the trunk it is then 'whipped' forward violently, causing damage to the cervical spine.

Boxing and football injuries resulting in brain damage are caused in a similar manner. The brain tends to remain in a state of rest while the skull is snapped back. The resulting collision then damages the delicate brain tissue.

The tendency of a body to remain at rest is called its **inertia**. *Inertia may be regarded as the tendency of a body to resist a force which is applied to it.* If we consider a double-decker bus again, it requires a greater force to get it moving than does a small car, because of its greater mass and thus its greater inertia. Similarly, the same bus requires a greater force to stop it than does the small car.

Furthermore, a person standing in the bus while it is travelling, and not holding on, suffers an obvious fate if the brakes are suddenly applied. This person may well say, 'I was flung forward'. However, all that has happened is that the inertia of the person has caused his/her forward motion to continue, although the bus has stopped. This is another example of Newton's First Law. A patient in a wheelchair will suffer similar inconvenience if the wheelchair is stopped suddenly.

Second Law – Law of Acceleration

This law states that
the acceleration of a body is proportional to the applied force, provided that the mass remains constant.

If a force acts on a body having a fixed mass, it follows that a large force will produce a large acceleration and a small force will produce a small acceleration.

When we spoke of gravity, we spoke of a force of attraction between a person and the earth. This is a larger force than the force of attraction between a person on the moon and the moon, so that the force of gravity on the moon is much less than that on the earth, as previously discussed. This then means that the force of gravity which any person experiences on the earth, and thus the acceleration that this force produces, is greater than on the moon. Since most of us will probably never walk on the moon, what has all this to do with us? In practical terms it means

*that a larger force generates a greater acceleration on a given body
than a smaller force.*

Let us look at some other examples:

If a nurse has difficulty in moving a bed or a heavy trolley,
the aid of another nurse may be sought. The combined effort
means that a greater force is being applied, which in turn means
that a greater acceleration is then produced. This acceleration is
simply the change from a stationary position, of the bed or
trolley, to one of movement. Once the bed is moving at a
uniform rate it is no longer being accelerated, and the only force
required is that which is needed to overcome friction. This in
turn means that one nurse may now be able to manage
independently. When he or she comes to a corner, or has to go
through a doorway, a change of direction and thus an acceleration is involved, and once again the nurse may require assistance
to supply the necessary force to provide the bed with the
acceleration needed.

A larger child on a swing will require a bigger push than will
a smaller child, if the larger child is not to complain that he or
she is not swinging as high.

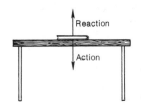

Figure 3.6. Static equilibrium. The force acting downwards (the action of the book on the table) is balanced by the force the table exerts upwards on the book (the reaction).

Third Law – Law of Reaction

This law states
that for every action there is an equal and opposite reaction.

If a book is resting on a table, it is exerting a downward force
on the table. The table must exert an identical upward force on
the book, to prevent it from going right through the table (Fig.
3.6). If the force exerted on the book were too great, the book
would be pushed upward. Thus the book and the table are in
equilibrium – the upward force is balanced by the downward
force.

Let us now consider some important examples. In walking,
the thrust of a foot or shoe on a floor surface normally means
that the person involved is pushing back on his foot with the
same force as the earth is exerting through the floor on the same
foot (Fig. 3.7). These forces are equal and opposite, but since the
earth is not likely to move backwards, the individual moves
forward by 'pushing' against the floor. If the floor has just been
waxed, however, the result could well be quite different.

Similarly, a patient who is trying to step or move from the
footrest of a wheelchair onto the floor or onto a bed, will surely
have an accident if the brake is not applied. As he pushes back
with his foot, the wheelchair will simply move backwards,
leaving him stranded. Many people come to grief in a similar

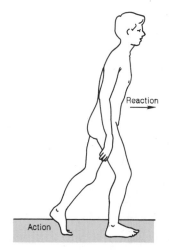

Figure 3.7. The backward push by the individual on his back foot (the action) generates a forward force (the reaction) which propels him forward.

manner when stepping from a small boat or canoe on to a wharf for the same reason.

FRICTION

The force of friction is called 'nature's brake'. This is the name given to a force which acts between any two surfaces which are not smooth. Even the wheels on a train and the rails on which the train travels are not perfectly smooth, since the train would not be able to move if they were. Car tyres need to provide good friction between the car and the road, if the car and its occupants are not to have an accident.

Friction has some disadvantages as it can chafe, remove or generally damage skin surfaces if care is not taken. Examples where friction is a problem are patients on bed rest and those with braces, crutches or immobilising devices – situations in which the skin is coming into contact with surfaces which are not perfectly smooth.

It should be noted that the force which enables us to walk is also the force of friction. Friction normally exists between the shoes that we wear and the surface on which we walk. If this friction is lowered because the soles of our shoes are smooth or the floor surface is too smooth or wet, then walking becomes difficult or even impossible, since the footwear cannot get a grip on the floor. The use of slippery quarry tiles and polished floors in some buildings and even some hospitals has led to some very bad falls. One hospital named a ward after a local shopping centre because it was kept filled with victims of the polished parquetry flooring in parts of that centre.

The force of friction is thus very important in our daily lives. If it did *not* exist, motor car engines would be much more efficient, but we would not be able to use motor cars! Friction is also very important in the body. Two examples will suffice:

- One of the very important functions of the pericardial sac surrounding the heart is to contain **pericardial fluid**, which keeps membranes apart and prevents them from chafing against each other as a result of friction from the beating of the heart.
- **Synovial fluid** reduces friction by acting as a lubricant or friction reducer between the cartilage-covered bone ends in synovial joints, e.g. knee joints.

When planning the daily care of many patients or clients, nurses often have cause to regret the effects of Newton's third law and the force of friction. Unfortunately, the two can (and do) combine to create a potentially devastating situation. Consider, for example, the patient on bed rest. Since he or she is not of a uniform shape, (e.g. a cube or sphere!), there are many curves and indentations. This means unequal weight distribution when the body is lying on the bed with the back surfaces in contact with the bed. The body tends to be supported by some of its curves, particularly on a firm surface, and at these points of contact the bed returns its reactive force.

The effect of this is **pressure** (discussed more fully in Chapter 7) being applied to these areas, which can lead to tissue damage and breakdown in that area. Friction between the body and the bed linen or clothes is also more likely to occur at these points, leading to abrasions or irritation and eventual wearing away of skin surfaces.

The effects of these two factors can be quite extensive. In fact, areas of breakdown of tissue in some patients have resulted in severe infections or exposure of bone and even such large and deep tissue loss that surgery was required.

The effects of friction combined with forces of weight and reaction are not confined to people in bed. They also apply to many other situations in which braces, crutches, tight clothing, or bandages are used, or any other situations where skin surfaces are rubbing or pressing against an object. A nurse with some knowledge of body mechanics can greatly assist a patient with musculoskeletal disorders by the skilful use of comfort and positioning devices. The nurse can relieve friction, pressure and discomfort and improve circulation through the use of padding, sheepskins and cushions. Relief can also be obtained by changing positions, giving skin care, using special support devices on wheelchairs and by the use of air or water beds.

Work

The **work** done on an object is given by *the force exerted on the object multiplied by the distance moved by the object in the direction of the force*, that is,

work done = force exerted × distance moved (in the
direction of the force)

Thus:

1. The body must move in the same direction as the force for this definition to be valid.

2. Note that if the body *does not move*, then *no work is done*. Anyone who has ever tried in vain to move a heavy object may

not agree with this, but this is the only way in which the term work may be used in science.

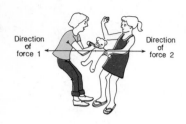

Figure 3.8. These forces are equal in magnitude and opposite in direction. Equilibrium is maintained until one force exceeds the other. The two vectors (Forces 1 & 2) are represented (to scale) by the arrows in magnitude and direction.

VECTORS

Vector quantities are those which *possess both magnitude and direction*. In nursing, we will be more interested in forces than in other vector quantities such as velocity and acceleration. The main areas of interest include forces as applied to the action of limbs and an understanding of the action of forces in traction arrangements.

A **vector** is normally represented by a straight line with an arrowhead at one end. This end is called the head and the other end the tail. The arrow then shows the *direction* of the vector force and its *length* may be used to represent its *size* or magnitude, by an appropriate scale. Alternatively, the size of the vector is sometimes written beside the arrow.

Addition

Frequently, *more than one force* may be acting on an object at any one time. These forces may be acting in different directions. For example, if we consider two children fighting over the same toy (Fig. 3.8), one will pull it in one direction (usually towards him/herself), and the other will pull it in another direction (usually the opposite of the first). It is thus necessary in such instances to consider the sum of all the forces acting on an object to find out what will happen to the object.

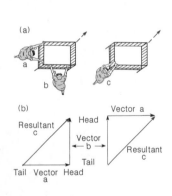

Figure 3.9. The addition method of vector forces. (a) illustrates one possible arrangement of two vectors, a and b, following the head-to-tail rule and (b) is an alternate arrangement of the vectors a, b. Both arrangements will produce the resultant c, which has the same direction and magnitude in each figure. The resultant thus represents the force produced by the two nurses. (Adapted from LeVeau: *Williams' & Lissner's Biomechanics of Human Motion.* 2nd Ed. Philadelphia. W.B. Saunders, 1977.)

In the example above, one has to consider the strength of each child as well as the directions in which they are pulling to work out what will happen to the toy. The toy may not move in any direction, if the two forces are equal in magnitude and opposite in direction. Should the force applied by one child be greater than and opposite to the force applied by the other child, the result will be a move in the direction of the stronger. The magnitude of this move will be the result of deducting the opposing force from the stronger. This is one of the simplest of vector situations since only two vectors are involved and they are opposite in direction. The *direction* and *size* or *magnitude* of each force can be represented diagrammatically as vectors.

Most situations involving vectors are more complex. Three or more forces may be acting on an object, they may be acting in a variety of directions, and the magnitudes may be quite different. To identify the overall result in these situations is not as straightforward as the toy one.

It is possible to *add vectors* in order to find a *single vector* which has the same effect as two or more others. This single vector is called the *resultant*. For example, in Fig. 3.9(b) the vector c̲ is the resultant of the two vectors a̲ and b̲ i.e. if a̲ and b̲ are forces, they can be replaced by the single force c̲ in both magnitude and direction. Thus the single force c̲ has exactly the same effect as the two forces a̲ and b̲ acting together.

The method of addition should be carefully noted. It is most important that the head-to-tail rule be used. In the example above, we start with one of the vectors (either one) and then put the tail of the second against the head of the first.

In Fig. 3.9(b1), the tail of b̲ is put against the head of a̲.

In Fig. 3.9(b2), the tail of a̲ is put against the head of b̲.

The resultant of the two vectors is then obtained by joining the tail of the first to the head of the second, and this is also the position of the head of the resultant.

In Fig. 3.9(b2), the tail of a̲ is joined to the head of b̲.

In Fig. 3.9(b1), the tail of b̲ is joined to the head of a̲.

In both cases note that the head of c̲ is pointing in the same direction and the length is the same.

An alternative method of finding a resultant of two vectors is the *parallelogram of forces* method. This involves placing the two vectors in a tail-to-tail position while maintaining the original directions of the vectors involved. A parallelogram is then completed and the resultant obtained by drawing in the diagonal from the tail-to-tail starting point to the opposite vertex. This is illustrated in Fig. 3.10.

In both cases it should be noted that the same answer is obtained, whichever method is used, as we would expect. It is quite useful for readers to be familiar with both methods, provided that this does not cause confusion.

If more vectors are involved the procedure is the same. Figure 3.11 shows a number of vectors acting at a point in (a), and two of the ways in which they may be **resolved**, or added together to find a resultant in (b) and (c).

Important Note: The vectors may be added in **any** order, provided that the head-to-tail rule is always followed.

Figure 3.12 illustrates this principle with three vectors, although the directions of two of these vectors are very similar.

This method of finding the single resultant force from the effects of several forces by addition is not the only method available. Resultant forces can be identified through the triangle method and the parallelogram method. However, the latter two approaches can be used only with two vectors at a time while the *addition method is applicable in all vector situations.*

In summary then, forces are vectors, with both magnitude and direction, which can be applied to an object to cause some

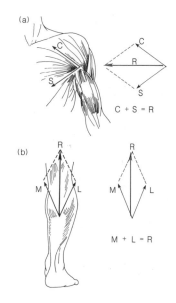

Figure 3.10. (a) Clavicular and sternal portions of pectoralis major together produce a single force acting horizontally across the chest (C ↔ S = R). (b) Medial, M, and lateral, L, heads of gastrocnemius together pull upward on the tendon of Achilles. (From LeVeau: *Williams' & Lissner's Biomechanics of Human Motion.* 2nd Ed. Philadelphia. W.B. Saunders, 1977.)

desired result or change such as a push or pull in a particular direction. A single resultant vector can be identified which has the same effect as two or more vectors in a given situation. The resultant vector can be altered by changing the magnitude and/or direction of any of the vectors involved.

It should be noted that for many movements in the human body, a number of muscles are involved, often acting in a number of different directions, but working together as a team, to achieve a particular result. Some examples are lifting an arm or leg, or grasping an object in the hand. This explains the fact that a *whole movement may be jeopardised* when only one muscle has been damaged. Since a change or loss of function in one muscle will change the direction and/or magnitude of one of the forces involved, the direction and/or magnitude of the resultant will also change. This also explains why it is sometimes necessary to immobilise a whole group of muscles when only one has been damaged or requires rest, since these muscles act as a 'team', although each muscle may act in a different direction.

Orthopaedic Applications of Vectors

The field of orthopaedics is one which bases a considerable number of treatments on the following concepts:

- the forces applied to an object can achieve certain desired results;
- these forces and their resultants can be manipulated, both in magnitude and direction;
- forces can be applied to the muscles and bones of the body.

The *main objectives in the use of forces* in the treatment and care of orthopaedic patients are:

- to reduce muscle spasms;
- to aid the healing of broken bones by pulling them into alignment and/or maintaining them in correct positions;
- to help relieve pain and discomfort from injured muscles or bones;
- to correct and prevent deformities;
- to stretch contractures;
- to immobilise or distract (pull apart) diseased or painful joints; and
- to allow patients greater mobility while still meeting previously stated objectives.

Forces are applied most frequently to stabilise injured extremities, necks, backs and pelvic areas. *Therapeutic traction is*

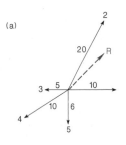

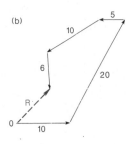

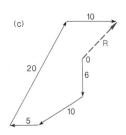

Figure 3.11. The graphical method for vector addition. (a) Forces acting at a point. (b) Illustration of graphical methods for vector addition. (c) Vector addition in reverse order. The vector sum is independent of the order in which the vectors were added. R = resultant, O = origin. The resultant obtained from (b) or (c) is shown in (a) for comparison purposes. (Adapted from Nave & Nave: *Physics For The Health Sciences*. 3rd Ed. Philadelphia. W.B. Saunders, 1985.)

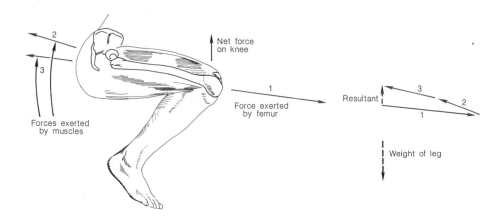

Figure 3.12. Vector sum of forces required to lift the knee (Adapted from Nave & Nave: *Physics For The Health Sciences*. 3rd. Ed. Philadelphia. W.B. Saunders, 1985.)

achieved by exerting a pull on the head, body or limbs in at least two directions, that is the pull of the traction and the pull of countertraction. The *traction force* usually consists of weights which may be of varying values to make up the force required to be applied to the area. The *counter-traction force* or second force is commonly provided by:

• the weight of the patient's body as it rests on, and tends to slide down, an inclined surface, such as a tilted bed; or
• other weights.

Whenever traction or pull is applied in one direction, an equal but opposite pull is also required in order to maintain stability and achieve the desired results. For example, if a force were applied without countertraction to a leg, the patient's body tends to continually slide in the direction of the force, lessening its magnitude and effect on the area being treated.

Traction Methods
Forces may be applied:

• manually, by pulling on an area with one's hands. This is sometimes used during the application of casts to position bone fragments or hold them in position prior to and/or during application, during transportation of a patient, or repositioning in bed; or during emergency care;
• mechanically, by exerting a pull on the injured area with a system of weights, ropes and pulleys applied to the skin or bones – skeletal traction;
• mechanically, using metal devices inserted in casts such as metal rods held in place by plaster;
• mechanically, using braces.

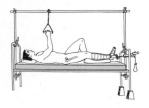

Figure 3.13. Buck's extension with overhead trapeze. (From Schmeisser, G. Jr.: *A Clinical Manual of Orthopedic Traction Techniques.* 1963.)

We will examine first a very simple form of mechanical skin traction apparatus in which the vectors can readily be identified. It will be seen that an understanding of vectors can be utilised to help a bone to heal in the best position, while helping to relieve the patient's discomfort (see Fig. 3.13 Buck's extension).

In this type of traction system, two forces are being applied to the broken bones in the patient's leg. These are out of place or out of alignment and must be brought into alignment so that the bone fragments or bone ends will heal together in a straight line. If the bones were left out of alignment the healing would be longer, the area would always be weak and prone to repeated fractures (breaks) and infections, and the leg, may have a more limited movement and less ability to bear weight.

One force, *a*, arises from the pull of the freely hanging weight which is attached to the patient's leg via rope and special adhesive-type bandages. In some cases, only bandages with no adhesive may be used. However, these tend to slip and the force may not then be applied where it is needed.

A *weight is not always necessary or available*, particularly during transportation of a patient. In these situations, some traction can be achieved by pulling firmly on the leg bandages attached to a rope and then quickly anchoring the rope to a fixed point such as the end of a bed or a special frame, while maintaining the pull.

The second force *b*, arises from the patient's weight. Note that the foot of the bed has been raised on blocks, thus slanting the bed and causing the patient to slide towards the head of the bed. This means that the patient's weight acts as a counter force pulling on the leg in the opposite direction to force *a*.

The anticipated result is the *gradual shifting of the bones* into the correct position for proper healing. The traction or pull on the leg also helps to reduce uncontrolled movement of the bones and thus relieves pain as well, but it is not as efficient in this respect as other forms of more locally restrictive traction. Patients must therefore understand what is being done and the importance of their positions in the bed, as well as the restrictions on their freedom of movement. Then they can make a positive contribution to their care and treatment by helping to keep the leg properly aligned with the weight and rope system, and by keeping the leg straight and at rest on the bed or surface support (pillow).

The nurse must obviously be aware of the importance of the forces involved and the factors which are creating these forces. If something *disrupts* the arrangement, then the forces may act in such a way as to be counterproductive. For example, if the weight was put on the bed or left resting on some object, then no pull would be exerted down the leg, and only one force would be acting – the weight of the patient down the bed. The result would be that the patient would slide down the bed and no forces would act on the fractured bone.

The same situation can occur, especially with children, if the bed is not inclined and the patient moves towards the weight. Then insufficient, or even no, counterforce exists to balance the applied weights.

Other factors which can disrupt traction are:

- slipping of the bandages or device holding the weight(s) to the leg;
- a rope which does not move freely because it is caught on something; this may alter the magnitude or direction of pull on the bone, causing sideways movement;
- the lifting or bending of the patient's leg, which will not only affect the forces being applied but also the position of the bone fragments.

In the above example a simple form of traction can be limiting in terms of the direction of applied forces – they can only be applied in two directions in a single plane. This means only uncomplicated, simple fractures could be treated in this way. It is used more to treat muscle spasm and immobilise a fracture in an emergency or prior to further treatment such as surgery or other traction forms. Furthermore, only small weights (2–3 kg) can be used with skin traction. This simple type of traction also limits patient movement (with the potential for associated complications to arise) and interferes with some aspects of nursing care. Hence, traction systems which permit greater patient movement, vector forces in more than one plane and direction, and can produce larger resultant forces if required, are more favoured. This is particularly true when fractures are complicated and require a longer period of treatment.

The Hamilton-Russell traction, which is used to treat fractures of the femur, is a type of skin traction which meets most of the characteristics listed above because it is a balanced or suspended traction system. Suspension or balanced traction can be used with either skin or skeletal traction. It performs two roles:

1. it exerts a pull on the affected part or area being treated; and
2. it supports the extremity in a hammock, sling or splint.

These roles are achieved through a system(s) of weights, pulleys and ropes.

Role 1: In Hamilton-Russell traction the patient's limb is suspended by a sling, as seen in Fig. 3.14.

Figure 3.14. Hamilton-Russell traction for immobilising femoral fractures. The resultant traction force applied to the femur is determined by the ropes, P, Q and S. Force $\tilde{R}$, acting on the limb, is obtained graphically by a vector diagram. (Redrawn from Flitter, 1948.) NOTES: 1. The arrows shown in the lower part of the diagram represents the vectors acting. In this case the vectors are forces, each of which is acting on the patient's leg. 2. Since each of the forces is acting through the same rope, they are equal in magnitude (or size), although the directions are different. 3. The only forces relevant to the patient's leg are those shown. The unlabelled force is merely a continuation of P and is not making any further contribution to the forces acting on the leg. 4. To find the resultant of these forces i.e. the single force which could replace these, the arrows are taken, head-to-tail in any order, maintaining the magnitudes and directions involved. 5. The resultant force is then represented (in both magnitude and direction) by the vector R.

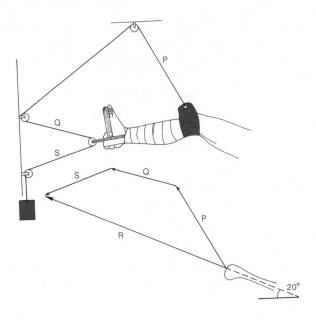

This allows the thigh to be maintained at an angle of approximately 20 degrees with the horizontal plane or with the bed, so that the *relation of the pulley ropes to the alignment of the limb remains constant*. The hanging weight(s) (4–5 kg) applies a load to the pulley-rope system which is distributed by the pulley arrangement in such a way that a number of vector forces are created. In other words, one force, the weight, is broken up into *multiple* forces to achieve a final specific resultant force on the fracture site.

The vector forces created can act only in the *direction of the ropes* and include (as shown in Fig. 3.14):

- an upward force P applied directly to the knee by means of the sling;
- two forces Q and S distal to the foot – whose combined effect reaches the femur through the leg.

The pulleys in the system act to establish the *direction* of the vectors (fixed pulleys) and to increase the *magnitude* of a force (movable pulley). The force distal to the foot, created by the arrangement of ropes Q and S, is nearly doubled by the use of the movable pulley.

The *resultant force* (R) of vectors P, Q and S can be found by the addition method previously explained and by the vector diagram (Fig. 3.14). R can be seen in line with the femur.

The patient's weight on an inclined surface (foot or bed raised) and the pull of thigh and leg muscles (Newton's Third Law) produces the necessary *counter-traction* force.

The resultant force can be potentially altered by:

- increasing or decreasing the weight or load, changing its magnitude;
- increasing the number of movable pulleys, also affecting magnitude;
- changing the numbers and/or positions of the pulleys, which alters direction.

Usually changes are made by altering the weight or the position of a pulley.

Role 2: The second role of this balanced traction is the supporting of the extremity. This is most important in carrying out nursing care and to the physical and mental comfort of the patient. The overall effect is to allow more movement of or by the patient while maintaining traction. The amount or range of movement will be governed by the amount of support and restraint the fractured limb is given.

The support in Hamilton-Russell traction is provided by the sling. Unfortunately this does not support the whole limb and movement is more restrictive than when a full splint (Thomas splint) is used. The sling is held in place by the arrangement of the weight(s), pulleys and ropes (see Fig. 3.14).

In this role, the *countertraction* or second force is not dependent on the patient's body, but is supplied by a system of ropes, pulleys and weights.

With balanced traction, *the pull of the system remains the same* even when the patient moves. The balanced or suspension apparatus supplies countertraction which takes up any slack in the ropes caused by the patient's movements, thus maintaining a continuous and even pull. This is the great advantage of balanced traction – it allows the patient to be lifted upwards, giving access to the lower back and buttocks, and relieving skin pressures. This not only makes nursing care easier but adds to the patient's comfort. However in Hamilton-Russell traction, the lower leg must be given support when the patient lifts, since the sling does not. The leg as a whole must rise as a single unit whenever the patient is lifted or lifts, in order for all forces and tension to remain stable. As the patient rises, usually with the help of an overhead trapeze bar, and with the leg supported by the sling and nurse, the traction system takes up the slack as the rope moves through the pulleys. However, this concept applies to raising and lowering the patient and does not necessarily apply when the patient is moved up and down the bed, as directions of pull can be altered.

One additional point: when splints are used for support, the splint itself has a system of ropes, pulleys and weights separate from the system which is applying the forces. The splint system only supports the splint and does *not* contribute any force to the fracture site.

Mechanical traction can offer a greater variety of methods and applications than those mentioned here. Our main objectives have been to explain vectors (mainly forces), and to show something of their important role on the healing of bones and muscles. Mechanical traction is the more useful method when pull is required over a period of time, and the forces involved need to be more exact in their direction and magnitude. The same concepts can be applied when only rest or immobilisation is required, or for dealing with muscle spasm.

Pulleys

A *pulley* is a grooved wheel on an axle which is used for changing the direction of the rope which passes over it. These simple devices or machines play a very important role in mechanical traction systems, and as such, they will influence the approach to and care of any patient undergoing such treatment.

Note: **A simple machine is a device which enables us to do certain work more conveniently**. It does not do the work for us, as do more sophisticated machines which use energy or fuel. As an example, four men may be required to lift a piano on to a truck. One man can do the same by using an inclined plane (a simple machine), but he will have to work four times as long as otherwise.

Similarly, one side of a car can be lifted quite easily by an average person with a lifting jack (another simple machine), but it would require a number of strong people to do the same job.

The Single Fixed Pulley
This device or simple machine (Fig. 3.15(a)) does not provide any *mechanical advantage* – i.e. a load of 200 newtons is lifted by an identical effort of 200 newtons (neglecting friction) – compared to systems described below where a load of 200 newtons is lifted by an effort of 100 newtons or 50 newtons or even less, depending on the number of pulleys involved.

The benefit arising from using a single fixed pulley is that *it changes the direction in which a force acts*. This means that an upward force, for example, can be achieved with a downward force acting on a rope which passes over a single fixed pulley.

(a)

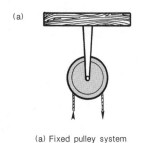

(a) Fixed pulley system

(b)

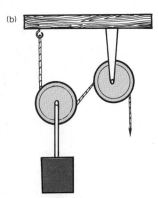

(b) Movable pulley system

Figure 3.15. Basic pulley systems.

The downward pull of gravity can also be changed to a horizontal or vertical direction with this device. Inspection of Fig. 3.16 will reveal the changes of direction achieved by each of the four pulleys.

The Single Movable Pulley

This is another simple machine (Fig. 3.15(b)) which enables one *to lift twice the load that would normally be possible.* If we overlook friction and the weight of the pulley itself it can be seen from the diagram that a force of 100 newtons is able to exert a force of 200 newtons through this system.

Thus we see that this pulley is not used to achieve a change in direction, but rather to obtain the advantage of being able to lift 200 N with a force of only 100 N. Thus, in a traction system we are able to exert very considerable forces to pull bones apart, etc. We are also able to arrange for a number of forces to act in such a way that the required resultant force is achieved, as in Fig. 3.16.

The nursing care of every patient in a therapeutic traction system involving pulleys includes at least daily checks of all pulleys to ensure that they are correctly positioned and that the pulleys are running freely. If this is not so, the resultant force on the patient's affected site may be greatly altered with negative consequences.

Other more complicated systems give an even greater *mechanical advantage.* In the example given above of shifting a

Figure 3.16. Traction apparatus involving vector addition of forces. (From Nave & Nave: *Physics For The Health Sciences.* 3rd Ed. Philadelphia. W.B. Saunders, 1985.)

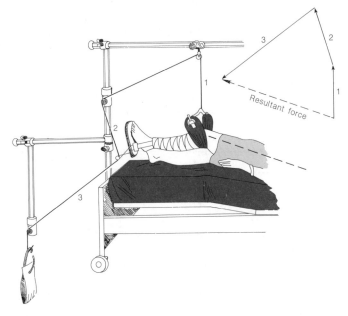

piano, because one man was doing the work of four, the mechanical advantage is four. A six-pulley block and tackle gives a mechanical advantage of six, i.e. a 100 newton force would be able to lift 600 newtons. While this is a most useful device, it should be noted that the 100 newton force would have to be applied for six times as long as it would be applied in a straight lift.

Levers

Examples of levers are given in Fig. 3.17 and Fig. 3.5.

When considered from the mechanical or functional view, the human body has some of the characteristics of simple or basic machines. It is possible to increase our understanding of the human body, particularly of its movements, by looking more closely at levers.

These are also simple machines. They consist of a rigid bar which is free to move about the point of suspension, which is called the *fulcrum* (F). A force which is applied at one point on the bar, called the *effort* (E), is used to overcome another force at another point, called the *load* (L). As with pulley systems, a large mechanical advantage can be obtained.

It is possible to make rough comparisons between levers and some aspects of the human body. For example:

- the bar can be thought of as a bone;
- the fulcrum as a joint;
- the effort force as a muscle or ligament;
- the load as parts of the body such as the hand or foot, or an external object to be moved.

With these thoughts in mind we can examine levers and lever systems found in the environment as well as in the body.

Levers are divided into three classes, as follows;

First Order Lever (seesaw type)
In this case, the *fulcrum is between the load and the effort* (LFE), as in a seesaw.

Examples are:

1. Movement of the head (see Fig. 3.17(a))
Load–head
Fulcrum – atlas/axis
Effort – sternocleidomastoid muscle
The result is that the muscle contracts to move the head.

2. Haemostats (see Fig. 3.18)

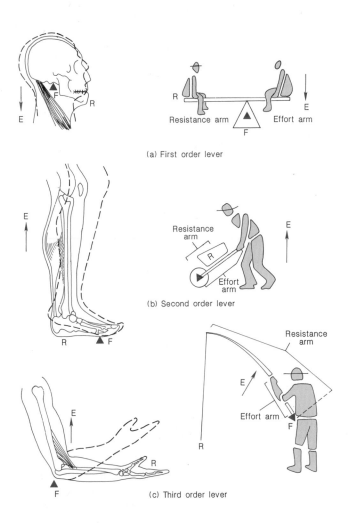

(a) First order lever

(b) Second order lever

(c) Third order lever

Figure 3.17 Orders of levers. Most levers in the human body belong to the third order, in which mechanical advantage is sacrificed in favour of greater distance of movement.

Second Order Lever (wheelbarrow type)
In this case, the *load is between the fulcrum and the effort* (FLE), as in a wheelbarrow, or a hand cart used for transporting gas cylinders.

Examples are:

1. Turning a mattress on a bed – one side of the mattress is kept on the bed to act as a fulcrum.

2. Standing on one's toes (see Fig. 3.17(b))

Fulcrum – ball of foot
Load – body weight acting through ankle bones
Effort – gastrocnemius muscle.

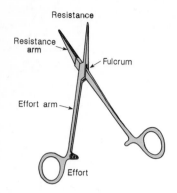

Resistance

Resistance arm

Fulcrum

Effort arm

Effort

Figure 3.18 Examples of a first order lever – a haemostat.

Third Order Lever (fishing-rod type)
In this case, the *effort is between the fulcrum and the load* (FEL), as in a fishing-rod.

Examples are:

1. Dressing forceps

2. Human forearm (see Fig. 3.17(c))

Load – lower arm
Fulcrum – elbow
Effort – biceps muscle

This type of lever has a number of *disadvantages*, the most important of which is the fact that the *effort exerted has to be greater than the load* since the turning effect about the fulcrum due to the load is greater than that due to the effort. On the other hand, this may be seen as an advantage, since the movement involved is magnified.

Sometimes it is necessary to make calculations concerning levers. For these purposes it is necessary to use a rule called the 'lever law' in some of the literature. This rule is really a special example of the **principle of moments**.

$$\text{force}_{\text{effort}} \times \text{distance}_{\text{effort}} = \text{force}_{\text{load}} \times \text{distance}_{\text{load}}$$

What this relationship tells us is simply that which was discussed earlier, i.e. levers, like any simple machines, make work easier but do not do the work for us. Thus, if one man lifts a log with a lever, he has avoided having to ask three of his friends to help. However, he will have to move the log four times further than if he had his friends assisting.

Another way of saying this is that the *work* done on the load of a lever system is the same as the work done by the effort of that system, assuming a perfect machine. This is a reasonable assumption for a lever system.

The work done is simply force × distance.
Let us now look at a typical problem.

A 5 kg object is to be lifted in the hand such that its distance from the elbow is 36 cm. How much upward force must be exerted by the biceps to lift the object? Into which of the lever systems could this movement be classed? It can be assumed that the biceps brachii muscle has an insertion point 2.5 cm from the elbow joint (ignore the weight of the arm itself).

Here is the solution to that problem.
1. Look again at Fig. 3.17. Note that the load is called the resistance in this case (both terms are common). We see that we are dealing with a third class lever.
2. Organise data:
   Force (load) [F_1]: 5 kg = 5 × 10 newtons = 50 newtons (using the approximation g = 10 m/s²)
   Force distance (load) [D_1]: 36 cm. (Since both distances are given in cm, we will use this unit.)
   Force (effort) [F_e]: to be determined.
   Force distance (effort) [D_e]: 2.5 cm.
3. Write down rule and perform calculation.

$$F_e × D_e × F_1 × D_1$$
$$∴ F_e × 2.5 = 0 × 36$$
$$∴ F_e × 2.5 = 1800$$
$$∴ Fe = \frac{1800}{2.5}$$
$$∴ F_e = 720 \text{ newtons}$$

4. Therefore the upward force exerted by the biceps brachii is 720 newtons.
   We have now looked at many of the very important and relevant applications of forces, levers, etc. to nursing and their importance in terms of efficient and effective care. It is equally important that the nurse understands the application of these principles to lifting procedures as a matter of simple survival.

REVIEW

1. What is the difference between speed and acceleration?
2. (a) What is the force of gravity?
   (b) In what way does gravity influence blood circulation?
   (c) How can gravity be utilised in adding fluids to the body and removing other fluids from the body?
3. If you are setting up a safety programme to prevent back injuries, what would the concept of 'centre of gravity' have to do with the rationale behind your safety measures?
4. Discuss inertia and Newton's First Law of Motion with respect to whiplash injuries.
5. Discuss Newton's Second Law of Motion in relation to steering a heavy bed around a corner.
6. Describe walking in terms of Newton's Third Law.
7. Give two examples where the body uses fluid to overcome the force of friction.
8. Take a diagram of Buck's Extension. By using vector diagrams, show all the forces which are acting and demonstrate that the result of adding all these vectors is zero.
9. What is the chief function of: (a) a single fixed pulley?
   (b) a single movable pulley?

10. Explain why each of the following is important in a traction system:
    (a) pulleys are functioning
    (b) ropes are intact and movable
    (c) weights are hanging freely

11. Using examples from medical instruments or the musculoskeletal system, describe the three orders of levers.

12. A 10 kg object is to be lifted in the hand such that its distance from the elbow is 38 cm. How much upward force must be exerted by the biceps brachii muscle to lift the object? Into which of the lever systems could this movement be classed? It can be taken that the biceps muscle has an insertion point 2.5 cm distal to the elbow joint.

13. While pushing a patient in a wheelchair, the front wheels hit a low obstacle on the pathway. Which lever system could you use to get the wheelchair and patient over the obstacle?

Atoms, ions and molecules in the body (atomic theory)

OBJECTIVES

After studying this chapter, the student should be able to:

1. Define fundamental terms such as atom, element, molecule, compound, mixture, atomic number, mass number, atomic mass and isotope and be able to distinguish between them.
2. Identify the four elements which together comprise over 95 per cent of the human body.
3. Describe the basic structure of the atom in terms of the position and properties of three of its main constituents.
4. Describe the arrangement of electrons around atoms and relate this to various types of chemical bonding.
5. Describe the formation of polar bonds and relate this to the properties of some substances.
6. Explain the formation of both positively and negatively charged ions.
7. Define the term 'electrolyte' and identify some of the electrolytes which exist in the body.

INTRODUCTION

'Is it of any real value for a nurse to study the structure and behaviour of the atom?' This question is frequently asked by student nurses and sometimes by nurse educators as well. It certainly does require a great stretch of the imagination to see how the atom and its characteristics, learned in a classroom, are of any use when one is out there in the 'real' working world. When actively nursing a patient who has just returned from abdominal surgery, for example, the nurse is working to relieve pain, measure blood pressure etc. The nurse is interested in doing all that can be done to make the patient as comfortable as possible and to monitor that patient's recovery. To do this as effectively as possible the professional nurse needs to understand the highly complex processes which are taking place within that person who is being nursed. After all, that person essentially consists of a collection of atoms! A truly magnificent, highly organised and very efficient collection of atoms, indeed, but atoms nevertheless.

As we shall soon see, the actual number of different types of atoms is quite small, but they interact, alter and combine together in specific ways to form this fantastic creature. How can we as nurses give high quality and truly comprehensive care without some knowledge of the atoms which make up this being for whom we care?

As an example, consider electrolytes, which are frequently discussed, particularly in states of emergency such as cardiac arrest. Imbalances of electrolytes can be fatal, so samples of blood are taken to test for them. What are they? What is their relationship with that other formidable group of substances which also cause us so much concern – the acids and bases? Once again, imbalances of these substances within the body can lead to death.

In recent years, attention has focused dramatically on the question of diet. It has come to be the answer to many problems. Do you know what the term 'polyunsaturated fats' really means? These may be recommended as part of a patient's diet. A nurse is often asked for advice or direction in these matters and must be equipped for the task. Read on and *you*, the nurse of the future, will find that an understanding of the humble atom will help you to answer these and many other questions.

ATOMS AND THE BODY

The body, like all other matter, is composed of **atoms**. Atoms are the building blocks of matter, and are so incredibly small that millions of them are able to fit on the head of a pin. The hydrogen atom, for example, has a diameter of about 6×10^{-11} m.

Let us illustrate this further by considering molecules of water, each of which is made up of three atoms – two hydrogen atoms and one oxygen atom. Imagine taking a glass of water and emptying that water into the Pacific Ocean. Let us further imagine that that water is completely mixed with all of the other water in the whole of the Pacific Ocean, so that our original glass of water is spread from Russia to Antarctica and from Australia to South America. If we were now to take a glass of water from the Pacific Ocean at any one of these points we would find several hundred of the molecules from that original glass of water present in our new glass! Each of these molecules is made up of the three atoms, as described above.

An atom is the smallest part of an element which retains the chemical properties of that element. If all the atoms in a particular piece of matter are identical, then that matter is described as being composed of a single chemical element.

An element may then be defined as a substance which cannot be broken down into simpler substances by any known means.

Over one hundred chemical elements are known to exist, and scientists have arranged these into a convenient 'filing system' or box-like arrangement called the **Periodic Table** (see Appendix VII). It is called this because the elements are arranged in 'periods', which essentially make up the rows. The use of the term 'period' arises from the fact that the eight elements which comprise each of the first two rows, for example, *repeat some characteristics* of their structure in a *periodic* fashion. As an example, each element in the second row has exactly the same number of electrons in its outermost shell as the element above it. Beyond the second row, the same principle applies, but other complications arise which are satisfactorily understood only after a detailed study of the electronic arrangement of atoms, which is not called for here.

The term 'groups' is also used to describe *those elements which occur under each other in vertical columns* in the Periodic Table, and which are found to have similar chemical properties.

Similarly, within each row a regular pattern is observed whereby the **valency** (or combining power) of elements tends to rise towards the centre of the row and then decrease towards the end.

CHEMICAL ELEMENTS IN THE BODY

The number of elements which occur in the human body is limited and our attention will now be confined to these (Table 4.1). It will be noted that the chemical symbols for a number of atoms have been given. Chemical symbols are a convenient notation for all of us to use (not just chemists!). Some originate from the Latin name for the element. For example, the Latin name for sodium is natrium, hence the symbol Na; that for potassium is kalium, hence the symbol K.

TABLE 4.1 Elements that make up the human body

Name	Chemical Symbol	Approximate Composition by Weight (%)	Importance or Function
Oxygen	O	65	Required for cellular respiration; present in most organic compounds, e.g. foodstuffs.
Carbon	C	18	Forms backbone of organic molecules; can form four bonds with other atoms.
Hydrogen	H	10	Present in all organic compounds: maintenance of acid-base balance.
Nitrogen	N	3	Component of all proteins and nucleic acids (genetic structure).
Calcium	Ca	1.5	Structural component of bones and teeth; important in muscle contraction, conduction of nerve impulses and blood clotting.
Phosphorus	P	1	Component of nucleic acids; structural component of bone and cell walls; important in energy transfer.
Potassium	K	0.4	Principal positive ion (cation) within cells; important in nerve function; affects muscle contraction and fluid and electrolyte balance.
Sulfur	S	0.3	A component of most proteins, activation of enzymes.
Sodium	Na	0.2	Principal positive ion in interstitial (tissue) fluid; important in fluid balance; essential for conduction of nerve impulses.
Magnesium	Mg	0.1	Needed in blood and other body tissues. The ion is important as a coenzyme.
Chlorine	Cl	0.1	Principal negative ion (anion) of interstitial fluid; important in fluid balance; component of sodium chloride and gastric acid.
Iron	Fe	trace amount	Component of haemoglobin and myoglobin; component of certain enzymes.
Iodine	I	trace amount	Component of thyroid hormones.

Other elements found in very small amounts in the body include manganese (Mn). copper (Cu), zinc (Zn), cobalt (Co), fluorine (F), molybdenum (Mo), selenium (Se), and a few others. They are referred to as trace elements.

Over 95 per cent of our bodies is made up from the elements O, C, H and N. The remaining 5 per cent is comprised of other elements in very small quantities, such as calcium, phosphorus, sodium, potassium and the others listed in Table 4.1.

As a comparison, the Earth's crust has over 90 per cent of its mass made up from the elements O, Si (silicon), Al (aluminium), Fe and Ca. The human body is thus quite different in composition to the earth on which it walks, consisting mainly of very complex compounds of the four elements O, C, H and N. The high percentages of O and H is largely due to the high water content of the human body.

Elements can be conveniently divided into two categories: *metals* and *non-metals*. (Some elements do not fit neatly into either category, e.g. silicon and germanium, but they will not concern us here). Table 4.2 shows a comparison of some of the properties of these (these are generalisations – some variations exist).

Trace Elements

Zinc: A component of a number of enzymes. Its presence is necessary in saliva for normal development of taste buds. It is important for growth, sexual development and taste acuity. Zinc plays an important role in protein synthesis and in cell division.

Copper: Occurs in several oxidative enzymes.

Selenium: Its only known function is as a constituent of glutathione peroxidase, which removes hydrogen peroxide and organic peroxides. Selenium is believed to be closely associated with Vitamin E in its functions.

Manganese: A co-factor for several enzymes. Manganese is concentrated in the liver and kidneys, particularly in the mitochondria.

Molybdenum: A constituent of some oxidases. It is also required for normal growth.

Cobalt: Its only known biological function is as a constituent of Vitamin B12 which is needed for maturation of erythrocytes.

Fluorine: Essential for dental health. Fluorine in the form of fluoride is incorporated into the hydroxyapatite crystals of the enamel, rendering them more resistant to the usual influences that lead to enamel dissolution and caries. Fluorine is also incorporated into bone structure.

TABLE 4.2 Properties of metals and non-metals

Property	Metals	Non-metals
Physical state	Usually solid, but mercury is a liquid	May be solid, gas or liquid
Lustre	Shiny	Normally dull
Conduction of heat and electricity	Good	Poor, i.e. good insulators
Oxide formed	Basic, i.e. turns red litmus blue	Acidic, i.e. turns blue litmus red

MOLECULES

The *smallest* part of an element or combination of elements which can have a *separate existence* (i.e. which is able to form a separate particle in the gaseous state, for example), is called a **molecule**. A molecule is made up of one or more atoms.

Some elements have only one atom per molecule, such as the metals and the rare gases helium, neon, argon, krypton and xenon, whereas others have two atoms per molecule, e.g. oxygen (O_2), nitrogen (N_2), and chlorine (Cl_2). A different form of oxygen, called ozone, has three atoms per molecule and has the formula O_3.

This latter substance is found in a layer in the upper atmosphere and has the capacity to absorb most of the ultraviolet light coming towards us from the sun. If this layer did not exist we would all be skin cancer cases overnight (or over a day!).

Molecules of substances are able to react together under certain conditions to form molecules of different substances. The reasons for this and, indeed, why elements and combinations of elements ever form molecules is explained later in the chapter.

Chemical and Physical Properties

Substances are sometimes identified on the basis of their *chemical properties*. Chemical properties describe the way in which any substance can **undergo change**, either on its own or in interactions with other substances to form *new* substances. Such changes are called **chemical reactions**.

We can list the chemical properties of any substance. For example, iron combines readily with oxygen to form rust. Gold does not react with nitric acid but copper does. Ether is no longer used as an anaesthetic because it undergoes a chemical change and forms peroxides, which renders it poisonous. Oxygen *supports combustion* of other substances, a reaction which involves a chemical change. This means that many precautions have to be taken in clinical situations where oxygen is being administered (see p. 207).

More frequently, however, elements or compounds (discussed below) are identified by measuring their *physical properties*. Such properties may be determined without changing the chemical nature of the substance and include:

- *melting point*, the temperature at which a substance changes from the solid to the liquid state. This is identical to the *freezing point*;
- *boiling point*, the temperature at which a liquid boils and changes into a gas;
- *density*, the mass of a fixed volume of a substance;
- *solubility*, the extent to which a substance dissolves in a particular solvent.

From such investigations, the identity of any element or compound may be uniquely determined.

MIXTURES

A **mixture** is made up of two or more elements taken together in any proportion. Elements which are present in a mixture still *retain their individual properties*. Thus sulfur remains yellow when mixed with iron filings and the iron still remains grey and magnetic. These two substances may readily be separated from the mixture, using a magnet. (The iron is attracted, but the sulfur is not.)

Mixtures can also consist of compounds mixed together in any proportion; or of elements and compounds mixed together in any proportion.

Air is a mixture of gases, petrol is a mixture of liquids, and soil is a mixture of solids (apart from some moisture, worms etc.!).

The term 'mixture' has pharmaceutical applications with which the reader will be or will become familiar. In the treatment of the common cold, for example, a number of substances known to have beneficial effects on the unfortunate sufferer, such as pseudoephedrine hydrochloride, atropine sulfate and scopolamine hydrobromide, are mixed together to form a single mixture. Each of these substances, once ingested, will perform its specific function; to dry up secretions, reduce coughing, and so on.

COMPOUNDS

Although most of the elements in the human body are found in various combinations with each other, they form substances known as **compounds** rather than mixtures. Examples are water, proteins, fats, carbohydrates etc. Some important exceptions are:

1. Oxygen, which exists as an element in the atmosphere and thus in the lungs, until it combines with haemoglobin (97%), or dissolves in the blood (3%).

2. Blood, which is a very complex mixture of solids (e.g. albumin), liquids (e.g. water) and gases (e.g. carbon dioxide and some oxygen).

3. Some elements such as sodium, potassium and calcium, which play very important roles in the body as *ions*. These will be discussed in detail a little later in this chapter.

A **compound** consists of two or more elements chemically combined together in fixed proportions by mass.

Note: We have made two very important distinctions between compounds and mixtures here:

1. The combination is in a fixed proportion by mass in a compound, whereas a mixture can have *any* proportion of the substances involved;

2. The combination in the case of a compound is *chemical*, giving rise to a substance(s) which usually has different chemical properties to those of the elements from which it formed. In a mixture however, the combination is purely physical, with no change in the chemical properties of the elements from which it formed, as we saw in the example of iron and sulfur.

When elements combine together to form a compound, a new substance is formed which may have properties similar to those of the elements of which it consists, but will more often have quite different properties. When sulfur and iron form a compound (iron sulfide), the yellow colour of sulfur no longer exists and the magnetism of the iron no longer exists.

When hydrogen (which burns explosively), combines with oxygen (which supports combustion), the compound water is formed, which is used to put out fires! This example illustrates very clearly that the properties of the resultant compound are quite different to those of the elements from which it was formed. In the form of an equation, this compound appears as:

$$2H_2 \quad + \quad O_2 \quad \longrightarrow \quad 2H_2O$$

an element	an element	a compound
(burns explosively)	(supports combustion)	(puts out fires)

and from above,

$$Fe \quad + \quad S \quad \longrightarrow \quad FeS$$

iron	sulfur	iron sulfide
(a grey magnetic element)	(a yellow powder)	(a grey non-magnetic compound)

These are examples of a 'shorthand' notation, called **chemical equations**, used to represent chemical changes.

It should be emphasised again that the proportions in which elements combine with each other to form a compound are *fixed* – the mass of one element which combines with a particular mass of another element is always the same. Thus, in the first equation above, we have:

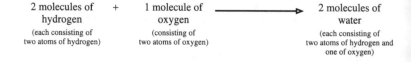

2 molecules of hydrogen	+	1 molecule of oxygen	⟶	2 molecules of water
(each consisting of two atoms of hydrogen)		(consisting of two atoms of oxygen)		(each consisting of two atoms of hydrogen and one of oxygen)

Similarly for the second equation:

| 1 molecule
of iron | + | 1 molecule
of sulfur | ⟶ | 1 molecule of
iron sulfide |

Remember that most of the substances which occur in the body do so as compounds – the exceptions have been discussed above. The chemical reactions above are shown as proceeding in one direction only. However, many chemical reactions (including most that occur in the body) are *reversible*. As we shall see later, one of the important factors involved in chemical reactions is *energy*.

In the reaction between hydrogen and oxygen above, it has been indicated that the reaction is explosive, i.e. a great deal of energy is released. However, it is possible to supply a great deal of energy and reverse the reaction. This can be done by the *electrolysis of water* in an apparatus called a *voltameter* (Fig. 4.1). (This is sometimes confused with a voltmeter, which has a quite different function.)

In the electrolysis of water, an electric current is passed through water which contains a small quantity of added electrolyte, such as common salt, to assist the conduction of an electric current. The current is passed through the water via two electrodes from an energy source, such as a battery of dry cells. Thus:

$$2H_2O_{(l)} \xrightarrow{\text{ENERGY}} 2H_{2\ (g)} + O_{2\ (g)}$$

water   hydrogen   oxygen

(l) means liquid   (g) means gas

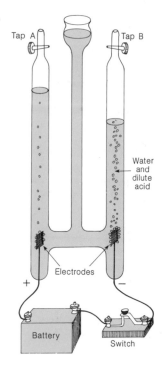

Figure 4.1. In this apparatus, an electric current is used to produce hydrogen and oxygen from water.

ANATOMY OF THE ATOM

Just as a proper understanding of the human body can be achieved only by looking at its structure, so it becomes necessary to look at the structure of the atom, in order to understand how the body builds up and breaks down various substances to maintain its physiological processes and thus the stability of the entire internal environment (homeostasis). This in turn will demonstrate how important it is for the body to be able to obtain the substances which it needs as sources of appropriate atoms.

Any atom consists of **protons**, **electrons** and **neutrons**. Other sub-atomic particles do exist but they will not be discussed here. A comparison of some of the properties of these interesting little fellows is given in Table 4.3.

TABLE 4.3 Properties of sub-atomic particles

Particle	Location	Mass (amu)	Charge
proton	inside nucleus	1	+1
electron	outside nucleus	$\dfrac{1}{1837}$	−1
neutron	inside nucleus	1	0

A charge of +1 means a positive charge of one unit and a charge of −1 means a negative charge of one unit. The atomic mass unit (amu) is defined as one-twelfth of the mass of a carbon-12 atom.

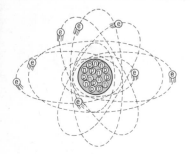

Figure 4.2. Simplified representation of the oxygen $^{16}_{8}O$ atom, showing a central nucleus with 8 protons and 8 neutrons, together with 8 orbiting electrons.

Figure 4.2 represents the atom as having a *central nucleus* containing particles such as protons and neutrons, around which the electrons move. For convenience, we have shown the electrons as moving in approximately elliptical orbits around the central nucleus, the orbits being at varying distances from the nucleus.

This is a convenient representation of the atom, but it must be emphasised that this is a highly simplified picture of the atom. Indeed, the very nature of electrons (not to mention other sub-atomic particles), as entities which have some of the properties of waves and some of the properties of particles, is not well understood. The way in which electrons move is equally not well understood, but is certainly much more complex than the movement of planets around the sun, for example.

Despite all this, some of the facts which *are* known give us greater insight which we can apply to our understanding of the body and to nursing practice.

Protons, Electrons and Neutrons

The number of each of these three major particles in any atom of a particular element may be determined as follows:

1. The number of protons is given by the **atomic number.** This number is an indication of the 'pecking order' of that element in the Periodic Table – the higher the atomic number, the higher that element is placed in the table and, of course, the greater the number of protons in any atom of that element. In other words:

the number of protons = atomic number.

The number of protons in an atom is relatively very *stable*. As we will see shortly, it is possible to change the number of electrons in some atoms very easily (when they form ions), but this does not happen with protons. This stability of the nucleus of an atom (and the particles such as protons within the nucleus) arises from the immensely powerful forces which hold a nucleus together. No ordinary chemical reaction is capable of breaking up a nucleus. Such powerful forces are unleashed only in a nuclear reaction – in a nuclear reactor or in a nuclear explosion. In such reactions, the products formed are different elements to those originally present.

Following on from this, as we have already seen, the number of protons in atoms of the same element is always the same. This provides each atom with a unique identity – while the number of electrons can change and the number of neutrons can change, the number of protons in atoms of a particular element *never changes*.

Another way of saying this is to point out that if a particular atom has six protons in its nucleus it *must* be carbon and no other element.

2. The number of electrons is *also* given by the atomic number. This is to be expected, since **an atom is electrically neutral** and thus the number of electrons (each with charge -1) must balance the number of protons (each with charge $+1$) to maintain this state.

Let us consider *carbon*, for example.

Carbon has six protons, each of which carries a charge of $+1$.

Therefore the total charge due to these protons is $+6$.

To balance this charge, a charge of -6 is required.

This is supplied by six electrons each with a charge of -1.

Thus carbon has six electrons. In other words,

the number of electrons = atomic number, and

the number of electrons = number of protons.

3. The number of neutrons is determined by subtraction. Looking at Table 4.3, it is observed that electrons have very insignificant masses compared to neutrons and protons. Thus, when the *total mass of the atom* is described by the **mass number**, electrons may be disregarded, for practical purposes. **The mass number tells us the total number of protons plus neutrons** *in an atom.* The mass number, by convention, is taken as the nearest whole number to the atomic mass. That is,

the mass number = number of protons + number of neutrons

or, mass number = atomic number + number of neutrons (since atomic number = number of protons)

and number of neutrons = mass number − atomic number.

Taking carbon as an example: atomic number is 6 and mass number is 12.

Therefore, number of protons is six,
number of electrons is six
and number of neutrons is $12 - 6 = 6$.

Note that it is only coincidence that all of these numbers are the same. This does not usually happen, as we shall soon see.

The mass number of an atom is often indicated by a superscript and the atomic number by a subscript. Carbon is then indicated by the symbol $^{12}_{6}C$.

Isotopes

The atoms of each element have the *same* atomic number (and thus the same number of protons and electrons), but some have *different* mass numbers. This means that the number of neutrons is different. These atoms are called **isotopes** of that element. Isotopes of an element have identical chemical properties to other atoms of that element, but have different masses to other atoms of that element. Thus oxygen atoms can have mass numbers of 16, 17 and 18 and these are represented as $^{16}_{8}O$, $^{17}_{8}O$ and $^{18}_{8}O$, respectively. Similarly carbon atoms can exist as $^{12}_{6}C$, $^{13}_{6}C$, $^{14}_{6}C$ and hydrogen as $^{1}_{1}H$, $^{2}_{1}H$ (known as deuterium), and $^{3}_{1}H$ (known as tritium). The diagnostic and therapeutic applications of isotopes will be discussed in considerable detail in Chapter 14.

Table 4.4 indicates the numbers of protons, electrons and neutrons in the atoms of several elements of importance in the human body. It is suggested that you practise determining the numbers of protons, electrons and neutrons of the elements from their mass number and their atomic number and then check your results against the table.

TABLE 4.4 Some important elements

Element	Mass Number	Atomic Number	Number of Protons	Number of Electrons	Number of Neutrons
hydrogen	1	1	1	1	0
carbon	12	6	6	6	6
oxygen	16	8	8	8	8
sodium	23	11	11	11	12
potassium	39	19	19	19	20
chlorine*	35	17	17	17	18

*Chlorine is a special case, in that it has two isotopes which are abundant. Note that while isotopes of oxygen, carbon and hydrogen exist, the frequency of isotopes other than the most abundant or common one (in each case, $^{16}_{8}O$, $^{12}_{6}C$, $^{1}_{1}H$) is very low. and their presence is not as significant as it is with chlorine, in terms of the **atomic mass** (defined below) of the element.

Atomic Mass
This is **the relative average mass** of the (naturally occurring) atoms of an element, compared to the mass of an atom of carbon. Thus the mass number gives us a definition of an atom (or a particular isotope if these exist), but the atomic mass defines the *average* mass of atoms of a particular element as they occur naturally.

In the case of chlorine, the *mass number* defines the mass of each of the isotopes of chlorine (i.e. 35 and 37), but the *atomic mass* defines the average mass of naturally occurring chlorine atoms as 35.453, chlorine being a mixture of these two isotopes. Thus, the atomic mass is not a whole number. This applies even to carbon because of the presence of isotopes other than carbon-12. Carbon's atomic mass is 12.011 (International Table of Atomic Weights, 1975).

It should be noted that the atomic mass is also called the **atomic weight**. This term is, in fact, more common, but since weight has units, and since we have defined atomic mass as a ratio (which cannot have units), the term atomic mass is, strictly speaking, more correct.

ELECTRONS AND ATOMS

We have already seen that some atoms keep together in pairs, and we know that atoms are able to react together to form compounds. We have also said that an understanding of the atom is important in studying the human body and the nursing process. The reason for this is that every cell of the body, and the structures within that cell, depend on the ability of atoms to *join together* to form compounds and radicals. These atoms are obtained from the food we eat and the air which we breathe.

Furthermore, it is this ability of atoms to join together in different ways which gives rise to the great complexity of matter in the body, and which allows structures such as cell membranes to be formed, electric currents to be conducted within the body, heart and skeletal muscles to contract and so forth.

The basis of the joining or bonding of atoms lies in the way in which electrons are arranged within an atom. It should be noted that the description which follows is a simplification, since electrons behave in a very complex fashion. Indeed, the very nature of electrons is very complex, as we have previously pointed out.

Electrons may be removed from an atom. It should be noted that the electrons involved are usually the outermost electrons or **valence electrons**, which are not held to the nucleus as strongly as others.

The orbits to which we have previously referred may be regarded as *energy levels*, which may be further subdivided into energy sub-levels. For convenience, we will refer to these levels and sub-levels simply as energy levels. These terms refer to the fact that the levels increase in energy as they increase in distance from the nucleus. The nearer an electron is to the nucleus, the less energy it has, and the farther away it is, the more energy it has.

An atom is described as being in its '*ground state*' when all of its electrons are in their lowest energy states. This means that each electron in the atom is occupying its 'normal' energy level.

If we look at chlorine in Fig. 4.3, we see that this means that an atom of chlorine has two electrons in the lowest energy level, eight electrons in the next lowest level and seven electrons in the next lowest level. Any electron which occupies any energy level *above its normal level* is said to be in an 'excited' state.

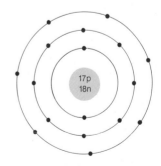

Figure 4.3. Chlorine.

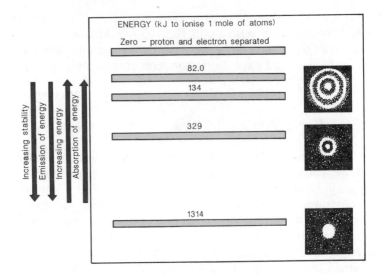

Figure 4.4 (Not to scale) Energy level diagram of the hydrogen atom. The energy is expressed as the work required to remove the electron from the hydrogen atom against the attractive force of the nucleus. Zero energy means that no further work is required to remove the electron; the removal has been completed. (Modified after Brescia, et al.)

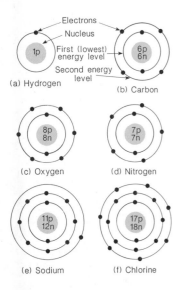

Figure 4.5. Bohr models of some biologically important atoms. *(a)* Hydrogen. *(b)* Carbon. *(c)* Oxygen. *(d)* Nitrogen. *(e)* Sodium. *(f)* Chlorine. Each circle represents an electron shell or energy level. Electrons are represented by dots on the circles. *p*, proton; *n*, neutron. (From Solomon & Davis: *Human Anatomy & Physiology*. Philadelphia. Saunders College Publishing, 1983.)

An electron can be 'promoted' from a lower energy state to a higher energy state by a number of different means, all of which involve providing additional, external sources of energy, such as by heating or by electrical means.

When the electron returns to its original state it will give out the same amount of energy that was used to promote it to the higher level (see Fig. 4.4). This amount of emitted energy is fixed for particular electrons, which in turn fixes the wavelength. If the wavelength is such that it falls within the visible light spectrum, the light emitted will have a particular colour. The light emitted by a hot sodium street lamp, for example, is always yellow while that from a mercury street lamp is always blue.

In Chapter 12 this knowledge will be applied to advantage when we discuss light and vision.

The elements have their electrons arranged so that the maximum numbers of electrons which can be accommodated in the first three energy levels or 'shells' are:

2 in the first energy level,

8 in the second energy level

and 8 in the third energy level.

We are also concerned with the elements potassium and calcium which have respectively one and two electrons in the fourth energy level.

Let us look at a few examples of atoms with which we will be concerned (see Fig. 4.5).

Hydrogen has *one* electron, which may be considered to be moving around a central nucleus in an elliptical orbit; and the next atom in the Periodic Table, helium, has *two* electrons moving in this orbit. This orbit is able to accommodate two electrons only, so that helium represents a situation in which the outside orbit has its maximum number of electrons. This confers a great degree of stability on this element, making it *extremely unreactive*. This means that atoms of this element are less likely to participate in chemical reactions, i.e. less likely to chemically combine with atoms of other elements to form compounds.

It is most important that the reader understand that: **any atom which has a complete outer shell of electrons** (such as the inert gases) **will be very stable, and thus much less likely to enter into chemical combination to form compounds than those atoms or ions which have an incomplete outer shell of electrons.**

As a consequence, and as a most important general rule, **atoms tend to lose or gain electrons, or share electrons with other atoms so that each atom or ion ends up with a complete outer shell of electrons**. By doing so, the atom or ion has conferred upon it the same degree of stability which the inert gases have.

This concept is fundamental to an understanding of the way in which atoms behave, ions are formed and new substances are made by the body.

Note that an 'ion' is formed when any atom loses or gains electrons.

Carbon (the sixth element), has two electrons in the innermost orbit (or shell) and the remaining four in the outermost shell. It will then tend to acquire four more electrons to make its outer orbit of electrons complete and thus become very stable. As we shall soon see, it does this by sharing electrons with other elements.

Oxygen has six electrons in its outermost shell and it can share two more electrons with other atoms to give it great stability. It is thus a very reactive gas.

Sodium has one electron in its outermost shell and seeks to lose it to give it the same arrangement of electrons as neon, which is very stable. By losing that one electron it forms a positive ion. Because it has a great tendency to do this, this element is very reactive – so much so that it needs to be stored under kerosene to prevent it from catching fire!

Chlorine, with an arrangement of 2, 8, 7, has seven electrons in the third shell. This element will then seek to gain one electron to give it a complete outermost shell and thus the same arrangement of electrons as the element argon (which is very stable because the third shell can accommodate eight electrons only). Chlorine is thus also very reactive because of its strong tendency to gain that one electron.

We have merely scratched the surface of the complex arrangement of electrons in an atom. If we proceed much beyond the element argon (that is, beyond potassium and calcium), we need to delve into the energy sub-levels which exist within the orbits which we have described in this simple model of the atom (called the Bohr model). This model is adequate for our purposes here, but the more advanced student will need to examine other models (such as the quantum-mechanical model) to achieve greater understanding of (or degree of confusion about!) the arrangement of electrons in an atom.

Why should we be concerned with all this structural detail?

The answer is very simple. Herein lies the key to understanding why sodium and potassium exist as stable ions in the body, why other gases are inert (or unreactive) and why oxygen is so reactive. Indeed, if oxygen were not so reactive as to readily combine with haemoglobin, what future would we all have?

BONDING

The existence of most molecules of elements and compounds depends upon the formation of some type of bond which is able to hold the atoms or ions together. Such bonds are called **chemical bonds**, the different types of which will be discussed shortly.

We have said that atoms tend to adopt the structure of the inert gases by completing the outermost shell of electrons. Thus electrons are gained, lost or shared in such a way as to ensure that each atom is surrounded by a complete outermost shell of electrons. The maximum number of electrons which the first shell can hold is two, and that for the second and third shells is eight.

The reasons for this, and for that which happens in the fourth and higher shells, is beyond the scope of this book.

The ways in which atoms can undergo changes to end up with a complete outermost shell of electrons are as follows:

1. By *sharing* electrons to form *covalent* bonds, as described below.

2. By *losing* one or more outermost electrons. When this happens, a *positive* ion is formed. This ion will have one positive charge if one electron has been lost, two positive charges if two electrons have been lost, etc.

3. By *gaining* one or more electrons to form a *negative* ion. This ion will have one negative charge if one electron has been gained, two negative charges if two electrons have been gained, etc.

Other types of bonding exist, such as those bonds which hold metals or ice together, but we will discuss only the major bond types.

The Sharing of Electrons (Covalent Bonds)

We can now apply our knowledge of the arrangement of electrons in atoms to understand why some gases are diatomic, i.e. have two atoms per molecule. Oxygen, for example, behaves as illustrated in Fig. 4.6.

In Fig. 4.6, Part (a) shows two oxygen atoms making up one molecule of oxygen. The following points should be noted:

1. The electrons in one atom are shown as dots, whereas the electrons of the other atom are shown as crosses. This is done to show from which atom each electron has come. All electrons are identical, however, whatever their source. Remember – if you've seen one electron, you've seen them all!

2. It is important to observe that the only electrons involved in the joining or bonding of the two atoms are those in the *outermost* shell. The other electrons are shown for the sake of completeness.

Part (b) shows the more common way of representing the formation of a chemical bond. Note:

1. In this case, only those electrons in the outermost shell are shown.

2. If the total number of electrons in the outermost shell of each oxygen atom is counted, it is found that each atom is surrounded by eight electrons, i.e. the number required (see above) to make each atom stable. This is achieved by a *sharing* process – although each atom is able to supply *six* electrons only, each atom ends up being surrounded by *eight* electrons and thus is stable.

3. It should always be remembered that this is a diagrammatic representation only – the actual situation is considerably more complicated than this.

Part (c) shows another common way of representing chemical bonds. In this case each dash represents a chemical bond, which is, in fact, **a sharing of a pair of electrons**. Since two dashes are involved, each representing a pair of electrons, *four* electrons are involved in this bond.

The vast majority of compounds found in the body are bonded through the sharing of electrons – for example, fats and carbohydrates.

Note: Remember that covalent bonds involve the sharing of electrons to form molecules of compounds or elements. When these bonds break, either new compounds or atoms (or both) are formed.

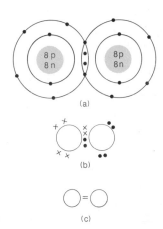

Figure 4.6. A molecule of oxygen. Part (a) shows the arrangement of electrons in the two oxygen atoms making up the molecule. Part (b) also shows the arrangement of electrons – but only those electrons involved in bonding – those electrons in the outermost shells. Each chemical bond consists of an eletron pair **shared** between the two atoms. Part (c) shows the most common way of representing a double bond – in this case between oxygen atoms.

Covalent Bonds and Energy

The formation of chemical bonds represents a *transfer of energy*. In any chemical reaction, some chemical bonds are broken and other chemical bonds are formed, with resultant energy changes:

1. The breaking of an existing chemical bond or bonds involves an energy change.

2. The formation of new chemical bonds involves an energy change.

3. The net result of the breaking of existing bonds and the formation of new ones depends on the relative amounts of energy involved. Let us look at an example and we will then apply this to the human body.

Let us consider the reaction between hydrogen gas and chlorine gas to give hydrogen chloride gas (note that this hydrogen chloride is a gas and is *not* hydrochloric acid – hydrochloric acid exists only when hydrogen chloride gas is dissolved in water, in which it is extremely soluble).

$$H_2 \quad + \quad Cl_2 \quad \longrightarrow \quad 2HCl$$
hydrogen   chlorine   hydrogen chloride

Thus:

Bonds broken: One $H-H$ bond and one $Cl-Cl$ bond.

Bonds formed: Two $H-Cl$ bonds.

Since this reaction gives out a great deal of energy (in fact it is explosive), it follows that the energy released by the formation of the new $H-Cl$ bonds is much greater than that which was used to break the old $H-H$ and $Cl-Cl$ bonds. Furthermore, we can now regard hydrogen and chlorine as *high energy* substances compared to hydrogen chloride.

What does all this have to do with the body? The point here is that the body is able to utilise the energy stored in chemical bonds to supply the energy which it needs for metabolism, and to store this energy in other chemical bonds so that it is readily available when required.

This whole subject is dealt with in Chapter 9.

Multiple Bonds

We have now come across single bonds such as $H-H$ and $Cl-Cl$ in which one pair of electrons is shared in each case; and double bonds such as $O=O$ in which two pairs of electrons are shared.

The element carbon is able to form each of the following: a

single bond (C—C) in which ONE pair of electrons is shared; a double bond (C=C) in which TWO pairs of electrons are shared; a triple bond (C≡C) in which THREE pairs of electrons are shared.

Compounds containing only single bonds between carbon atoms are said to be *saturated*. Compounds which contain double or triple bonds between carbon atoms are said to be *unsaturated*. Thus:

```
   H  H  H                                H  H  H
   |  |  |      O                         |  |  |      O
H—C—C=C—C                              H—C—C—C—C
   |          OH                         |  |  |      OH
   H                                     H  H  H
```

An UNSATURATED fatty acid   a SATURATED fatty acid

Here it may be seen that the saturated fatty acid has only *single* bonds between carbon atoms, but the unsaturated fatty acid has one double bond between two of the carbon atoms.

The word 'unsaturated' is an immediate indication that the compound is capable of accepting more hydrogen (or other) atoms by chemical combination, than it has at the moment.

Unsaturated fatty acids may be converted to saturated fatty acids by chemically combining with hydrogen (i.e. by hydrogenation):

```
   H  H  H                                            H  H  H
   |  |  |      O                                     |  |  |      O
H—C—C=C—C            +        H₂          ⟶        H—C—C—C—C
   |          OH             (hydrogen)              |  |  |      OH
   H                                                 H  H  H
```

(an unsaturated fatty acid)   (a saturated fatty acid)

Also, some compounds have more than one multiple bond between carbon atoms. Such compounds are called *polyunsaturated* compounds. Thus we have the term polyunsaturated fatty acids. There are many different fatty acids in the body, having differing numbers of carbon atoms (i.e. length of the fatty acid chain), and differing numbers and location of double bonds within that chain.

Trading in Electrons (Ionic or Electrovalent Bonds)

These types of bonds are formed by the active metallic elements such as sodium, potassium and calcium when they lose electrons, on the one hand; and the active non-metallic elements such as chlorine and fluorine, when they gain electrons, on the other. The reason is that this is the bond formation process which requires the least energy for these elements.

Let us now return to sodium, which has an arrangement of electrons of (2, 8, 1) (see Fig. 4.7). This element is in the position of having one electron in its outermost shell. If each atom of this element were able to gain seven electrons, it would then have the same electronic structure as argon and be very stable. This however is most unlikely, because very large quantities of energy would be required.

The alternative would be for each atom of the element to *lose* one electron, which requires little energy. If it were able to do this, it would then have the structure of neon (2, 8) and once again be very stable, but would no longer be an atom, since it would no longer be electrically neutral. In fact, it would form an *ion*, i.e. a charged particle. A sodium atom has 11 protons in the nucleus and 11 electrons outside the nucleus. If one electron is given up, it would have 10 electrons only:

$$\text{So that 11 protons} = 11 \times (+1) = +11$$
$$10 \text{ electrons} = 10 \times (-1) = -10$$
$$\overline{+1}$$

Thus we now have a resultant charge of + 1 and the sodium ion is represented by the symbol Na^+.

This is fine, but how can a sodium atom simply give up an electron?

To answer this question, let us look at another element, chlorine. Chlorine has an arrangement of electrons of (2, 8, 7) (see Fig. 4.7). By losing seven electrons, chlorine could then have the same electronic configuration as neon and form a stable ion. Once again, this is not easily achieved and the obvious alternative occurs, with chlorine forming an ion by *gaining* one electron, forming the chloride ion Cl^-. This ion then has the structure of argon and is thus very stable.

(This assumes that an electron is available for the chlorine to gain, of course.)

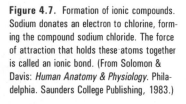

Figure 4.7. Formation of ionic compounds. Sodium donates an electron to chlorine, forming the compound sodium chloride. The force of attraction that holds these atoms together is called an ionic bond. (From Solomon & Davis: *Human Anatomy & Physiology*. Philadelphia. Saunders College Publishing, 1983.)

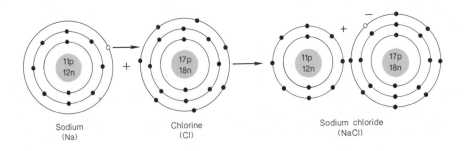

Sodium
(Na)

Chlorine
(Cl)

Sodium chloride
(NaCl)

That is:

    17 protons $= 17 \times (+1)$ $= +17$
    18 electrons $= 18 \times (-1)$ $= \underline{-18}$
                                        -1

We now have a situation where one element (sodium) is very anxious to lose one electron so that it can form a stable ion and another element (chlorine), is equally anxious to gain one electron so that it can form a stable ion. All that remains is for these two elements to get together and all will be well!

These two elements do in fact do this by reacting chemically. If clean sodium metal is placed into a container of chlorine it will catch fire spontaneously and form the compound sodium chloride or common salt ($NaCl$).

WARNING: Do not, under any circumstances, try this – your eyes, limbs and indeed your life, are at risk.

This compound then exists as a **crystal lattice** of sodium ions and chloride ions (note – NOT molecules) arranged in a geometrical array to form a cubic crystal. This is similar to the 'monkey bars' in many children's playgrounds, with the chloride ions and sodium ions at the junctions of the bars.

In forming this compound, the positively charged Na^+ ions are attracted to the negatively charged Cl^- ions and the compound is held together by an electrical force of attraction – the chemical bonds which are formed are purely *electrostatic*. Such bonds are called **ionic bonds**. Positive ions are called **cations** and negative ions are called **anions**.

Cation formation may be represented thus:

$$Na \longrightarrow Na^+ + e^- \quad (e^- \text{ is used to represent an electron})$$

Also:

$$K \longrightarrow K^+ + e^-$$

Elements which have two electrons in their outermost shells are usually able to lose two electrons to form cations with a charge of +2:

$$Ca \longrightarrow Ca^{2+} + 2e^-$$

The ions formed from sodium, potassium and calcium are all most important for such vital body functions as maintaining fluid balance and nerve and muscle activity.

Similarly, the formation of anions may be represented as:

$$Cl_2 + 2e^- \longrightarrow 2Cl^-$$

Note: Any one atom can only gain an electron if another atom has lost it. Thus the total number of electrons gained in the formation of negative ions must equal the number of electrons lost in the formation of positive ions.

What is the point of atoms losing or gaining electrons? We have already said that the ion which is formed by this process then has the same electronic configuration (arrangement of electrons) as one of the inert gases and is thus very stable. But why should stability be so important?

The answer is to reach a lower energy state and thus a more stable state. In looking at any chemical process such as a chemical reaction or the formation of an ion, it is important to be aware that everything works towards achieving the lowest possible energy state. Until that state is reached, various processes will occur which work towards achieving that state.

To Remove an Electron, or Not to Remove an Electron – That is the Question!

Electrons are kept in position around the nucleus by electrostatic forces of attraction between the negatively charged electrons and the positively charged protons. However, factors exist which tend to modify this force of attraction:

1. As the distance between the protons (in the nucleus) and the electrons increases, the force of attraction decreases very rapidly. In fact, the force of attraction is governed by an inverse square law. This means that if the distance is doubled, the force of attraction is only one quarter as strong and if the distance is tripled, the force of attraction is only one-ninth as strong, etc. (see Fig. 4.8).

2. The electrons closest to the nucleus tend to form a 'shield' against the penetration of electrostatic forces of attraction to the outermost electrons, thus weakening these forces and allowing electrons to be removed more readily. This is called a 'screening' effect.

These factors contribute to the greater mobility of the outermost electrons in an atom compared to the inner electrons. Thus the outer electrons in an atom are the ones normally likely to be involved in chemical reactions and are often called valence electrons for this reason. The greater the influence of these two factors above in lowering the amount of energy involved in losing or gaining electrons, the more likely it is that atoms of that element will form ions.

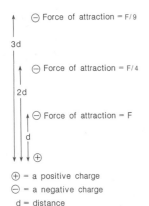

Figure 4.8. Diagram showing the relationship between force of attraction and distance – known as the inverse square law.

Therefore some elements readily form ions but others don't. Why?

The answer is once again a question of energy. If we consider carbon, for example, we find that it has three options:

1. To *gain* four electrons and form an ion with the same number of electrons as neon, and thus the same stability as neon.

2. To *lose* four electrons and form an ion with the same number of electrons as helium.

3. To *share* electrons with other atoms so as to have the same electronic arrangement as neon and, once again, the same stability as neon.

It is found that *much* less energy is required for option 3 than for either of the other two alternatives. Hence it is not surprising that carbon tends to bond this way.

If we now look at the Periodic Table, the following generalisations can be made:

1. Elements in Group IA and IIA tend to form Positive ions by *losing* electrons.

2. Elements in Group VIIA tend to form Negative ions by *gaining* electrons,

3. Elements in other groups show a greater tendency to form *covalent bonds* as the centre of the Periodic Table is approached from either end.

Note: The differences between ionic and covalent bonds are listed in summary form at the end of this chapter.

Polar Molecules and Solvents

We have so far dealt with ionic and covalent bonding separately, but at this stage it is appropriate to point out that most bonds are in fact a mixture of both ionic and covalent bonding.

This idea in turn gives rise to the phenomenon of **polarity**, which is a most important concept in understanding the behaviour of all cells in the body, particularly in such areas as transmission of impulses in nerves, the electrical behaviour of cardiac muscle cells and digestive processes.

Let us first consider hydrogen chloride (Fig. 4.9). Here we have a bond formed between an atom (hydrogen) which 'likes' to dispense with the only electron it ever had (it is thus *electropositive*) and an element (chlorine) which 'loves' electrons (and is thus *electronegative*). We have already seen that, given the slightest opportunity, an electron will be transferred from the hydrogen atom to the chlorine atom, to form ions. However, in

(a)

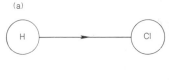

(b)

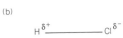

Figure 4.9. In (a) the arrow represents the direction in which electrons tend to move to create a greater electron density around the chlorine atom, as shown in (b) by the symbol $\delta-$. This creates a lower electron density around the hydrogen atom and is represented by the symbol $\delta+$.

the absence of water, this cannot happen with this compound. Since the electron transfer option is not available, sharing is the next best option, and a covalent bond is formed, with the sharing of an electron pair between the two atoms.

Nevertheless, hydrogen is still electropositive and chlorine is still electronegative. This means that the electron pair which is shared in the bond between them tends to move towards the chlorine end of the molecule, as shown by the arrow on the bond in the diagram.

This molecule is then described as a *polar* molecule, because it tends to have a negative end or 'pole' (the chlorine end because of the greater electron density there) and a positive end or 'pole' (the hydrogen end, because of the lower electron density there). This is often represented (as shown in the diagram) by the lower case Greek letter delta (δ).

Water, which is a *bent* molecule, is also polar because the oxygen atom tends to behave in the same way as chlorine. This means that the electrons in the two bonds are attracted towards the oxygen end of the molecule, as shown in Fig. 4.10.

Note: The slight redistribution of electrical charge in covalently bonded polar molecules, which has been described above, is very minor indeed compared to the total movement of one or more electrons which occurs when an ionic bond is formed and so should not in any way be confused with this.

In fact, if the bonds in water are broken, atoms are formed, not ions. Hydrogen chloride *appears* to be an exception to this, but is not, since all that happens in this case is that water can be regarded as assisting the complete transfer of an electron to form the very stable aquated hydrogen ion and aquated chloride ion.

Polar molecules, such as water, tend to be very good solvents for ionic substances such as sodium chloride and sodium bicarbonate, both of which are taken into the body and form very important ions, Na^+, Cl^- and HCO_3^-. The reason for this is that the polar water molecules are able to pluck ions out of the crystal lattice of the solid substance. In sodium chloride, for example, the hydrogen or positive end of the water molecule is able to pluck the negatively charged chloride ions out of the crystal lattice, and the negative end of other water molecules is able to pluck the positively charged sodium ions out of the crystal lattice.

It is immediately apparent that this process will occur more rapidly if more water molecules are brought into the vicinity of the sodium chloride crystals. This is what we are doing when we stir the mixture or heat it.

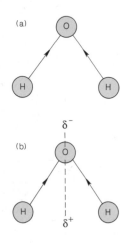

Figure 4.10. In this case, the tendency of electrons to move away from the hydrogen atoms towards the oxygen atom, as shown in (a), gives rise to a negative 'end' and a positive 'end' of the molecule, as shown in (b).

In general, polar solvents such as water are not good solvents of many covalently bonded substances such as starches, fats and proteins. Simple sugars and sucrose are obvious exceptions since these compounds readily dissolve in water. Note that it is just as well that the protein materials of our own bodies do not dissolve in water! If we want to dissolve non-polar, covalently bonded substances, we normally use *non-polar* substances such as alcohol or ether.

It is also noteworthy that most of the cell membranes in the body tend to be polarised with the negative charge on the outside. Bacteria and dead tissue, on the other hand, tend to be polarised with the negative charge on the inside of the cell. This facilitates the recognition of unwanted cells by the defence cells of our bodies.

Students will further utilise their understanding of the polar nature of some molecules in such fields as immunology.

Ions and Electrolytes

The behaviour of sodium chloride in solution (in water or body fluids) has just been described. Substances which behave in this way, i.e. dissolve in water to form separate ions, are called **electrolytes**. It should be noted here that in such substances as sodium chloride, the ions are already formed – they are simply removed from the electrostatic attraction which holds the crystal lattice together. We will be discussing electrolytes in more detail in later chapters.

Table 4.5 lists a number of body electrolytes and the 'normal' concentrations of various ions within these.

TABLE 4.5 Electrolyte composition of body fluids

Electrolyte	Plasma	Interstitial Fluid	Intracellular Fluid
Cations			
Na^+	136–145 mmol/L	142 mmol/L	10 mmol/L
K^+	3.5–5.0 mmol/L	4 mmol/L	140 mmol/L
Ca^{2+}	2.25–2.75 mmol/L	2.5 mmol/L	<0.5 mmol/L
Mg^{2+}	0.75–1.25 mmol/L	1.5 mmol/L	29 mmol/L
Anions			
Cl^-	96–106 mmol/L	103 mmol/L	4 mmol/L
HCO_3^-	23–29 mmol/L	28 mmol/L	10 mmol/L
Protein	60–80 g/L	20 g/L	160 g/L
Phosphate	1.0–1.5 mmol/L	2 mmol/L	38 mmol/L
Others	8–16 mmol/L	12 mmol/L	120 mmol/L

Note: 1. The values given in the literature are variable. The values given for blood are taken from Miller and Keane: *Encyclopedia and Dictionary of Medicine, Nursing, etc.*, and the others essentially from Guyton: *Textbook of Medical Physiology*. 2. Note that because proteins have different molecular weights, values given have to have units other than mmol/L. 3. We would have liked to represent these values diagrammatically. However, because protein values cannot be quoted in mmol/L, any such diagram could be misleading and would certainly be inaccurate.

*Inorganic salts, acids and alkalis are all examples of electro-
lytes.* Only some of each of these large classes of compounds exist
in the body: many of these are vital to our survival. The heart,
nerves, muscles, kidney function and in fact all cells of the body
involve electrolytes in one way or another.

The fact that *ions* are charged carriers and thus able to
conduct electric currents is one reason why we are so easily able
to be electrocuted. In this situation, the current conducted by the
body is much greater than the currents on which we depend, for
normal body function in the heart, for example. The result is that
these electrical impulses overcome the normal electrical impulses which cause the heart to beat, resulting in cessation of the
heartbeat altogether, or else abnormal beating of the heart (called
ventricular fibrillation).

We are thus able to make use of these facts in attempting to
revive a patient whose heart is beating abnormally or has stopped
altogether, by using equipment which passes a relatively large
current through the heart. This will be discussed in more detail
in Chapter 10.

Polyatomic Ions or Radicals

Sometimes, for complex chemical reasons, some atoms act
together as a group (poly = many), to form ions. Thus all of the
atoms in this ion are chemically bound together in such a way
that they may be regarded as acting as *one*, and behave as *one
entity*, carrying a charge.

As an example, the very physiologically important bicarbonate ion (more correctly known now as the hydrogen carbonate
ion), consists of one hydrogen atom, one carbon atom and three
oxygen atoms, all of which behave together as though they were
one entity, with a single negative charge.

Some examples of these, all of which are important in the
body are:

the ammonium ion	NH_4^+
the carbonate ion	CO_3^{2-}
the sulfate ion	SO_4^{2-}
the hydrogen phosphate ion	HPO_4^{2-}
the dihydrogen phosphate ion	$H_2PO_4^-$
the bicarbonate ion	HCO_3^-
(the hydrogen carbonate ion)	

These ions are held together by *covalent bonds*. One of the
less complicated of these structures is that of the ammonium ion

(as discussed on p. 241). The structure is best understood by considering its formation from the compound ammonia and a hydrogen ion:

$$H-N-H \quad + \quad H^+ \quad \longrightarrow \quad \left[\begin{array}{c} H \\ | \\ H-N-H \\ | \\ H \end{array}\right]^+$$

ammonia hydrogen   ammonium
(a compound) ion   (NH_4^+) ion

Here the pair of electrons in ammonia not involved in bonding are shown with crosses rather than dots for convenience, *but of course they are no different to the other electrons.* Now a hydrogen ion has *no* electrons around it, so that it is able to form a bond with the two 'spare' electrons in ammonia, and have a complete first shell of two electrons. When it does so, however, it brings its positive charge with it and this positive charge is spread over the whole ammonium ion. Furthermore, the new bond is formed by a *sharing* of electrons, so that this new bond is *no different* to the other three bonds, which are also formed by a sharing of electrons. That is, they are all *covalent* bonds.

The other polyatomic ions also have atoms which share electrons and form covalent bonds, but for various reasons are more complex.

Valence

When elements or radicals combine together to form compounds in chemical reactions, the ratio of the elements involved is determined by the **valence** (or **valency**). The valency of an atom or radical is the *combining power* of that element or radical.

In Fig. 4.11(a), for example, hydrogen has a valency of one and chlorine has a valency of one, so that these are able to combine together to form an electrically neutral compound.

In Fig. 4.11(b), oxygen has a valency of two and thus requires two hydrogen atoms, each with a valency of one, to form water.

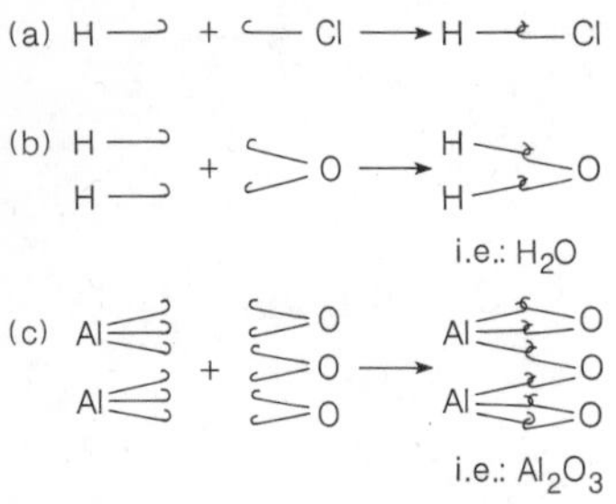

Figure 4.11. Valency diagrams for (a) hydrogen chloride, (b) water (c) aluminium oxide.

In Fig. 4.11(c), two aluminium atoms, each with a valency of three, require three oxygen atoms, each with a valency of two, to form aluminium oxide. This is the only way in which a compound can be formed between these two elements so that the final result is an electrically neutral compound.

The valency really represents the number of electrons which:

(a) an element (such as oxygen or chlorine in the examples above) *needs* to complete its outer orbit, to give it its full complement of eight electrons; OR

(b) an element *has available* for bonding purposes so that, when bonding has occurred, an outermost orbit of electrons is complete (two electrons in the case of hydrogen, but otherwise eight electrons).

However, the reader is reminded that the formation of chemical bonds, as previously described, may be effected either by a transfer process, as in ionic bonds; or by sharing as in covalent bonds.

Note: This model is useful for our purposes here but is inadequate to explain all bonding phenomena.

Table 4.6 lists the valences of some elements and radicals which are of interest to nurses.

CHEMICAL REACTIONS

A chemical reaction involves a *chemical change*, which means that the chemical composition of a substance has been altered by the loss or gain of one or more atoms, or both, or the re-arrangement of the atoms within the substance, or even all of these. In some cases, merely the rearrangement of electrons constitutes a chemical reaction, for example, electron transfer reactions. It follows then that the basis of all chemical reactions is a *rearrangement of electrons.*

During any such reaction, **energy** is invariably involved – an idea which we will pursue further because of its overwhelming importance in the human body. In fact, all of Chapter 10 is devoted to this subject.

Chemical Equations

We do not need to go into the mechanics of writing chemical equations. However, some important points need to be made about chemical equations.

TABLE 4.6 Common valences of some elements and groups

Valence	Name	Ion	Illustrative	Compounds
1				
Metals and	ammonium	$NH_4{}^+$	NH_4Cl	$(NH_4)_2SO_4$
positive ions	potassium	K^+	KBr	K_2SO_4
	silver	Ag^+	$AgNO_3$	AgI
	sodium	Na^+	$NaCl$	Na_2O
Nonmetals and	chloride	Cl^-	$NaCl$	HCl
negative ions	fluoride	F^-	KF	HF
	hydrogen carbonate*	$HCO_3{}^-$	$NaHCO_3$	$Ca(HCO_3)_2$
	hydroxide	OH^-	$NaOH$	$Al(OH)_3$
	nitrate	$NO_3{}^-$	KNO_3	HNO_3
2				
Metals and	barium	Ba^{2+}	$BaSO_4$	BaF_2
positive ions	calcium	Ca^{2+}	CaO	$CaCl_2$
	copper(II)	Cu^{2+}	CuF_2	$CuCO_3$
	iron(II)	Fe^{2+}	$FeSO_4$	$FeBr_2$
	lead(II)	Pb^{2+}	PbF_2	$Pb(CH_3COO)_2$
	magnesium	Mg^{2+}	MgF_2	MgS
Nonmetals and	carbonate	$CO_3{}^{2-}$	$CaCO_3$	H_2CO_3
negative ions	oxygen (in oxides)	O^{2-}	Na_2O_2	H_2O_2
	oxygen (in peroxides)	$O_2{}^{2-}$	Na_2SO_4	H_2O_2
	sulfate	$SO_4{}^{2-}$	Na_2SO_4	H_2SO_4
3				
Metals and	aluminum	Al^{3+}	Al_2O_3	AlH_3
positive ions	iron(lll)	Fe^{3+}	Fe_2O_3	$FeBr_3$
Nonmetals and	arsenate	$AsO_4{}^{3-}$	K_3AsO_3	H_3AsO_4
negative ions	phosphate	$PO_4{}^{3-}$	Na_3PO_4	H_3PO_4

*Common name, bicarbonate. (Adapted from Brescia: *Chemistry – A Modern Introduction*. W.B. Saunders, Philadelphia. 1978.)

1. Because some chemical bonds are being broken and others are being formed, energy will always be involved – either taken in or given out.

2. The number of atoms of a particular element *must be the same on both sides of the equation*. Note however, that the atom may be changed into an ion without affecting the count, providing that ions are counted as being equivalent for these purposes.

3. In counting atoms, a numerical subscript after an atom refers *only* to that atom. Thus, the chemical formula for sulfuric acid, H_2SO_4, shows that the molecules of this substance each consists of two atoms of hydrogen, one atom of sulfur and four atoms of oxygen.

In a chemical equation, if a numeral is placed in front of the formula, for example 2, the number of all the atoms in that formula is doubled. Thus $2H_2SO_4$ means that we have two molecules of sulfuric acid, giving a total of four atoms of hydrogen, two atoms of sulfur and eight atoms of oxygen.

4. A single arrow in one direction means that, under normal conditions, the reaction will proceed in *one* direction only. If arrows are shown going in *both* directions this is an *equilibrium* reaction, as will be discussed in Chapter 10. Most reactions in the body are of this type.

5. The subscripts (s), (1) and (g) stand for solid, liquid and gas, respectively.

Summary of Ionic and Covalent Bond Characteristics

IONIC BONDS

Formed by electron transfer. Atoms may gain or lose electrons.
Ions are formed and are bonded by electrostatic attraction.

COVALENT BONDS

Formed by electron sharing. Electrons may come from one or both atoms.
Each shared pair of electrons forms a chemical bond.

IONIC COMPOUNDS

Tend to have high melting points.
Tend to dissolve in polar solvents such as water and not in non-polar solvents such as alcohol.

COVALENT COMPOUNDS

Tend to have low melting points.
Tend to dissolve in non-polar solvents such as alcohol and not in polar solvents such as water.

In conclusion, our bodies are in fact a collection of atoms, ions and molecules and the beginning nurse becomes increasingly aware of this as she or he begins to look at blood test results where mention may be made of various electrolytes, of different serum proteins, of glucose, triglycerides, cholesterol, creatinine, bilirubin etc. (see Appendix III). Similarly, Appendix IV lists many of the components of urine which may be detected by such simple means as Clinistix.

It is hoped that this chapter has given the reader the insight necessary to begin to recognise the importance of atoms in the formation of substances and their properties. Only then will their vital role in body chemistry be appreciated and their relevance to our very survival be recognised.

REVIEW

1. What is an atom? Describe the composition of an atom in terms of the three major particles of which it consists.
2. Some physiology textbooks show Na^+ and Cl^- combining in the blood to form NaCl.

(a) What are species such as Na^+ and Cl^- called?

(b) What is the term for the smallest portion of NaCl which can exist separately?

(c) What is the difference between a sodium atom and a sodium ion?

(d) The textbooks referred to above are *wrong* in showing this recombination in a diagram. Why?

3. Is blood a mixture or a compound? Give full reasons for your answer.

4. What is the difference between atomic number and atomic mass? Illustrate by referring to oxygen.

5. Define the term 'isotope', giving examples.

6. The potassium ion (K^+), a common ion in the body, is much more stable than the element potassium. Fully explain why this is so, in terms of the arrangement of electrons in both.

7. Contrast the formation of covalent and ionic bonds, using examples. Contrast the behaviour of a covalent and an ionic compound when each is dissolved in water.

8. Many of the compounds found in the body are covalently bonded. Explain why this is the case, carefully drawing the distinction between ionic and covalent bonding in your answer. What advantage(s) would covalent bonding lend to these compounds in the body?

9. Many of the properties of membranes, especially their ability to allow the passage of some substances, can be explained in terms of the 'polarity' of these substances. Explain what is meant by the term 'polar compound' and describe how this polarity arises.

10. Define the term 'electrolyte' as it is used clinically, giving examples.

11. Carefully outline the difference in bonding exhibited by the chlorine atom in forming the following two substances:

(a) sodium chloride

(b) chlorine (as molecules).

5

Water in the body

OBJECTIVES

After studying this chapter the student should be able to:

1. Define terms such as kinetic energy, solids, liquid, gas, absorption, adsorption, density, cohesion and adhesion.
2. Outline the functions performed by water in the body.
3. Describe the differences in ionic composition between the intracellular and the extracellular fluid compartments of the body.
4. List the main fluid cavities in the body.
5. Distinguish between the processes of adsorption and absorption, giving examples of each from the human body.
6. Describe how the density of urine is measured to provide useful information.

INTRODUCTION

An eight-week old infant, who was admitted in an unconscious state to an emergency department of a hospital, died shortly thereafter. She had been vomiting and suffering from diarrhoea for at least three days prior to admission. Unfortunately, because the infant had continued to take normal feeds in the first day or two, and only a few feeds were vomited, the parents had not been unduly concerned. She had been passing frequent watery stools, some of which were very large.

When the infant began to refuse feeds, some home remedies were tried, such as heavily sugared water and flat lemonade. Other home remedies were tried on the continuing diarrhoea without success and at least 12–14 episodes of watery stools occurred in the 12 hours prior to admission. This situation conveys several important points about the importance of water to the human body and the fact that water does not always receive the respect it deserves for the powerful role which it plays in the life of the human being.

Most people are well aware that one can perish in the desert from lack of water. However, many do not realise that one can die *anywhere* from a lack and/or loss of water. We are aware of the need to take in liquids because of our very active thirst mechanisms, which may cause us to drop other activities and satisfy this drive. We are also sensitive to the need to eliminate some liquid from the body as urine – a drive so strong that we cannot refuse it.

However, many of us do not think beyond these fundamental drives about the nature and role of water as it relates to the human being. Therefore, we are unaware of the extent and powerful effect of water losses in the body which can lead to the unfortunate scenario described above. Even small changes in the water content of the body can cause alterations in the physiological state of numerous entities in the body, such as neurones, muscles and the whole circulatory system. Such alterations can compromise the integrity of the whole body and endanger life. In the case above, the parents were also unaware that some age groups (for example, the very young and very old) are very much more susceptible to small changes in water balance; otherwise they may have sought help much sooner and saved the life of their child.

The significant role of liquids in the body is going to be impressed on you even further in your nursing practice. For people whom you are nursing, you will be measuring the input and output of liquids, recording these, reporting, assessing, observing and testing them. In fact, a very large proportion of your bedside nursing care may involve some aspect of liquid management and maintenance. The fact that 60–70 per cent of the weight of the 'average' man and 50–54 per cent of the weight of the 'average' woman is water, will give you some idea of why you will be very much involved with this important constituent of the human body.

Homeostasis of liquids in the body is a matter of survival. In this chapter and following chapters we will be examining body fluids – liquids and gases – and various constituents of these. With electrolytes, for example, we will be examining these in terms of their influence on the body and each other and their importance to human physiology.

By the end of Chapter 6, the reader should have gained sufficient knowledge to understand many of the physiological changes which took place in the eight-week old infant; the importance of water balance in the body, particularly those of infants, and thus why the parents involved should have sought professional help sooner.

How does the patient fare in all of this? While an understanding of the role and functioning of water and other fluids is important to the care and monitoring of a patient's state of homeostasis, it must be stressed that *this is only one aspect of the total care of a patient's state with respect to liquid balance.*

This area, in particular, demands some understanding of the social, cultural, psychological and emotional aspects of the patient as an individual. Patients' preferences for different types of drinking fluids, their attitudes towards passing urine in the presence of another or by using bedpans etc., will heavily influence their responses. A knowledge of physiology plus an awareness of patient needs is the best combination for providing professional care to patients regarding their liquid intake and output.

THE STATES OF MATTER

In the last chapter we discussed the formation of compounds, but we have not said very much about the states in which they exist – although we did discuss the transformation of a solid to a liquid and then to a gas when we discussed latent heat in Chapter 2.

All substances (or matter) can exist as *solids, liquids and gases* (Fig. 5.1). The state in which a particular substance exists at room temperature depends on a number of factors which we will now examine. It should be noted that, in the body, we will be concerned with solids when we discuss the behaviour of muscles, with gases when we discuss breathing and with liquids in many applications which follow. It is with liquids that we are chiefly concerned in this chapter.

It is most important to realise at this stage that the whole question of states of matter is very much a question of **energy** – in this case *energy of movement* or **kinetic energy**.

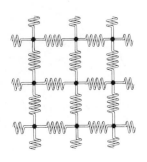

(a) solid

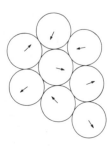

(b) liquid

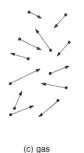

(c) gas

Figure 5.1. Simplified models of the three states of matter (From Nave & Nave: *Physics for the Health Sciences*. 3rd Ed. Philadelphia. W.B. Saunders, 1985.)

Solids

These consist of particles, which may be atoms, molecules or ions, held together in a fairly rigid arrangement by chemical bonds. The types of chemical bond depend on the particles involved and need not concern us here. However, the fact that solids are *not completely rigid* does concern us when we consider the elasticity of muscle fibres or the difference in bone rigidity of an infantile patient compared to a geriatric one, and the consequent implications in handling the latter.

The particles in a solid occupy mean or average positions about which they vibrate at all temperatures above absolute zero ($-273°C$). Thus they do possess kinetic energy, but less than particles of the same substance in the liquid state and less again than particles in the gaseous state.

When a solid is heated, the kinetic energy of the particles increases, the particles vibrate more rapidly and the kinetic energy keeps on increasing until the melting point is reached. At this particular temperature, which is very sharp and clearly defined in pure substances, the bonds holding the components of the substance together are broken and separate particles exist. As an example of this, let us consider ice. When ice melts, individual molecules of water can exist separately and no rigid structure is present, as is the case with ice. This rigid structure is often observed in snowflake crystals.

Thus a solid has *its own shape and does not adopt the shape of the container* in which it finds itself.

There are many different types of solids. As an example, both sodium chloride (common salt) and sugar (sucrose) are solids, and both dissolve in water. Common salt dissolves to form discrete Na^+ and Cl^- ions, producing a solution which conducts an electric current, but sugar breaks up to form a solution of sucrose molecules which does not conduct an electric current. Common salt is an example of an *ionic* solid; sucrose is an example of a *molecular* solid.

Another important type of solid is that illustrated by graphite and diamond (which are chemically identical, since both are pure carbon) and all metals. These substances are all covalently bonded together and are known as *atomic* or *polyatomic* solids.

Liquids

As observed above, these do not have a rigid structure like solids. The particles which make up a liquid are able to move relatively freely without the restraints of chemical bonds. However, the particles are not entirely free of each other's influence and so tend to hang together rather like dancers on a crowded dance floor – free to move to some extent and changing positions with respect to each other, but with no one moving very far.

In some of the later work in this book we will see that some of the 'dancers' in liquids in the body are in fact electrolytes, ions and other dissolved substances. When a liquid, which is just a state of matter and is thus distinguished from solids and gases, contains other substances dissolved in it, it is then called a solution. The two components of any solution are the *solute*, the substance(s) which is dissolved; and the *solvent*, the component in which substances are being dissolved. It should be mentioned here that while it is common to have a solution which consists of a solid dissolved in a liquid, this is not the only type of solution. Other types include liquid in liquid (e.g. alcohol in water) solid in solid (e.g. metal alloys such as brass) and gas in liquid (e.g. aerated soft drinks).

Liquids *have no fixed shape* and are able to *adopt the shape of the container* in which they are placed.

Gases

When the molecules of a liquid are heated, once again the kinetic energy increases, and keeps on doing so until some molecules gain sufficient energy to break away from the liquid state. Often this occurs at the bottom of a container, and many of these molecules with very high energy group together to form a bubble. In turn, this bubble can rise up through the liquid, because of its lower density and leave the liquid completely, thus allowing the gas molecules to become completely *independent*.

Gases occupy the whole of the container in which they exist. The molecules move around at very high speeds, colliding with each other and with the walls of the container. In fact, the collisions of these particles with the walls of the container give rise to the *pressure* which the gas exerts.

All of the changes which we have described above are purely changes of state or physical changes – the molecules which make up the substances described still have the same chemical structure. Furthermore, the changes are reversible.

It should also be noted that sometimes some substances take 'short cuts'. For example, carbon dioxide changes directly from the solid state (as dry ice) to the gaseous state. Ammonium chloride, sometimes known as sal ammoniac, changes directly from the vapour or gaseous state to the solid state, in a process called sublimation.

WATER

We stated earlier that our main concern in this chapter was with liquids, and since water is the solvent and chief constituent of the

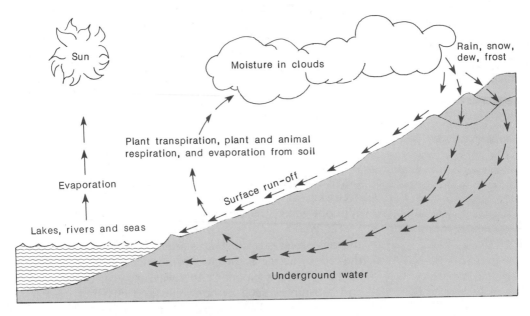

Figure 5.2. The water cycle.

various liquids which are found in the body, a closer examination of this most remarkable substance is now appropriate.

Each molecule of water consists of *two atoms of hydrogen and one atom of oxygen*, so that it is represented by the formula H_2O. By weight, however, it consists of eight-ninths oxygen and one-ninth hydrogen, because an atom of oxygen weighs 16 times as much as an atom of hydrogen. Some two-thirds of the human body consists of water.

When pure, water is transparent and almost tasteless. Most of the taste of tap water is due to dissolved substances, including oxygen and carbon dioxide.

The Water Cycle In Nature

We obtain water by precipitation, that is as rain, dew, frost, snow etc. Some of this water will evaporate, some will soak into the soil, and some will pass through the soil to form an underground flow which can then end up in lakes, rivers and oceans, as it does by surface run-off.

Water is then returned to the atmosphere by evaporation and by plants and animals, including humans. See Fig. 5.2.

As a health professional, a nurse should be aware of the issue of pollution and of its effect on the water cycle and the consequent effect on the quality of life and health of the community.

Water in the Body

Let us now consider some of the important roles which water plays in the body.

1. Water is not a universal solvent, but it does *dissolve more substances than any other liquid*. The substance which dissolves in a solvent such as water is called the *solute*, and this forms a solution. Within all of the cells of the body substances are kept in solution and an ideal medium is thus provided in which chemical reactions can occur. This could be called the very essence of life – the sum total of thousands of chemical reactions occurring at every moment of our lives (i.e. metabolism). Without water, the whole system fails very rapidly.

2. Water provides a means by which the correct concentrations of various substances are maintained inside and outside the cell, by acting as the chief component of the transport system of the body, the blood. In this way, oxygen, essential nutrients and substances such as hormones and enzymes are carried to cells and particular sites. Also, waste products such as carbon dioxide and urea are carried from cells to the lungs, kidneys and sweat glands, so that they may be excreted.

Water also provides the means by which the correct concentrations of electrolytes (such as Na^+, K^+, Cl^- and HCO_3^-) are maintained. Indeed, as we shall see later, the reverse is also true – the water requirements of cells of the body are maintained by differences in the concentrations of some of these ions inside and outside the cell.

3. We have already discussed the importance of water as a *cooling agent of the body*.

4. Water also acts as a lubricant, since it is the major constituent of mucous and other fluids which act in this way – the *synovial* fluid which lubricates joints such as the knee, and *pericardial* fluid which occupies the pericardial cavity around the heart and prevents the heart from chafing against its outer protective covering, the parietal pericardium (or pericardial sac), as it beats.

5. Water also acts as a *chemical reagent* in such processes as hydrolysis of some food materials. In this way it assists digestive processes.

6. Water is also a component of blood and as such it is one of the chief substances involved in maintaining vascular or blood volume. The maintenance of blood volume is one of the factors which determines blood pressure.

Thus water relates very closely to many aspects of nursing – and the responsibility which the nurse assumes in the course of his or her work. Examples include blood pressure measurement, fluid intake and output measurement, assessing for fluid imbalance in dialysis and post-operative care. Of particular relevance is the possibility of a crisis developing – a crisis which the well-informed nurse may be able to rectify by initiating early treatment.

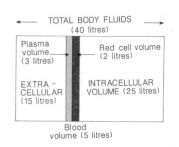

Figure 5.3. Diagrammatic representation of the body fluids, showing the extracellular fluid volume, blood volume and total body fluids. (From Guyton: *Physiology of the Human Body*. 5th Ed. Philadelphia. W.B. Saunders, 1979.)

Body fluids

An 'average' 70 kg man has a total water content of about 40 litres – about 60 per cent of his body mass. About 25 litres of this is fluid inside the cell or *intracellular fluid*. This is sometimes described as being in the intracellular compartment of the body. The remaining 15 litres or so of fluid is outside the cell or *extracellular fluid*. This is described as being in the extracellular compartment (as shown in Fig. 5.3). We will compare these fluids a little later. However it must be emphasised that the maintenance of the chemical and fluid environment inside and outside the cell (so that the cell may receive nutrients and remove wastes) is critical for survival and embraces the concept which we have described as homeostasis.

The Extracellular Fluid Compartment
This consists of the interstitial fluid compartment and the plasma.

The interstitial fluid compartment
This contains the fluid (approx. 12 L) which surrounds the cells outside the *vascular compartment* (the blood vessels and the heart). It includes *lymph fluid* and *transcellular fluid*, which consists of secretions and excretions of the body such as urine and perspiration together with those fluids listed under Fluid Cavities of the Body. It is essentially formed from substances passing through either capillaries or cell membranes.

Under normal circumstances, the interstitial fluid contains:

- only small quantities of proteins and blood cells;
- electrolytes in the form of large quantities of Na^+ and Cl^- ions, a reasonable quantity of HCO_3^- ion, but small quantities of K^+, Ca^{2+}, Mg^{2+}, HPO_4^{2-}, SO_4^{2-} and organic acid ions;
- dissolved gases such as oxygen and carbon dioxide; and
- nutrients (such as glucose and amino acids) and waste products.

This fluid *aids the movement of various substances* to and from the cells.

The plasma

This is the fluid found within the vascular compartment. It is very similar in composition to interstitial fluid, but contains approximately *four times* the quantity of *proteins*. This fluid acts as a *medium for circulation of blood cells* – a general transport system which carries nutrients and oxygen to the cells, carbon dioxide and waste products from the cells and other substances such as hormones to their target organs.

It is formed from substances which originate in the gastro-intestinal tract, bone marrow, interstitial fluid (lymph in particular), the lungs and endocrine glands.

The Intracellular Fluid Compartment

Under normal circumstances, the intracellular fluid (about 25 L) contains:

- electrolytes in the form of large quantities of K^+ and HPO_4^{2-} ions and a moderate quantity of Mg^{2+} ion;
- *small* quantities of Na^+, HCO_3^- and Cl^- ions; and
- a large quantity of proteins – approximately four times as much as plasma.

This fluid is contained in the billions of cells in the body, and although some variation of cell constituents can occur, the overall concentration of these ions etc. is much the same from one cell to another. It is thus convenient to speak of all of these as one compartment.

It is this compartment which must be kept supplied with oxygen and nutrients and have carbon dioxide and other waste products removed – these functions being performed by the extracellular fluid. Table 5.1 illustrates compositional variations between the fluids discussed.

Body Water Content

It was previously stated that the normal total body water content for an 'average' 70 kg man is about 60 per cent of his body mass. However, variation does occur because of:

- *Age* – a most important factor of which nurses should be well aware. Infants, for example, have a water content which is very high indeed – as much as 77 per cent in the newborn. Even the smallest imbalance therefore immediately becomes evident and can have serious and rapidly developing conse-

TABLE 5.1 Chemical composition of body fluids

	Extracellular Fluid	Intracellular Fluid
Na^+	142 mmol/L	10 mmol/L
K^+	4 mmol/L	140 mmol/L
Ca^{2+}	2.5 mmol/L	<0.5 mmol/L
Mg^{2+}	1.5 mmol/L	29 mmol/L
Cl^-	103 mmol/L	4 mmol/L
HCO_3^-	28 mmol/L	10 mmol/L
Phosphates	1.3 mmol/L	2.5mmol/L
SO_4^{2-}	0.3 mmol/L	0.7 mmol/L
Glucose	5 mmol/L	0 to 1 mmol/L
Cholesterol	ca 5 ⎫	Variable – up to 200 ×
Phospholipids	ca 3 ⎬	the extracellular fluid
Neutral Fat	ca 10 ⎭	values
pO_2	35 mmHg	20 mmHg(?)
pCO_2	46 mmHg	50 mmHg(?)
pH	7.4	7.0
Protein	ca 70 g/L	ca 550 g/L

Note that these compositions are illustrated in Fig. 5.8. (Modified after Guyton A.C., *Textbook of Medical Physiology*, 6th Ed., Philadelphia, W.B. Saunders, 1981.)

quences. This is seen commonly in an infant or young child who is vomiting or suffering from diarrhoea. Thus the accuracy of fluid observations is vital for all sick children.

In Table 5.2 it may be seen that the percentage of water content in a body *decreases with age* to remarkably low levels. Any decrease in this already diminished water volume will obviously lead to problems. Diminished water content is reflected in old people in their skin, muscle tone and hair.

- *Individual differences* – variations in this case are due to the proportion of body fat present in the adult, since fat is essentially water-free. The obese individual will then have less fluid per kilogram than the thin individual, all other factors being equal.
- *Sex* – women tend to have a larger proportion of body fat than men, so that women will have a lower proportion of fluid per kilogram of body mass.

TABLE 5.2 Body water at various ages as a percentage of body weight

Age	Newborn	6 months	2 yr	16 yr	20–39 M F	40–49 M F
Total body water (%)	77	72	60	60	60 50	55 47

Fluid (i.e. Liquid) Cavities in the Body

Apart from the general distribution of liquids throughout the body, particularly in blood and in lymph tissue there are a number of localities or *cavities* in which fluid is retained for various reasons. We will now look at some of these.

1. The Gastrointestinal Tract
A number of liquids are important in the digestive system of the body. These include:

- *Saliva* – a liquid secreted into the mouth by the salivary glands. It is more than 99 per cent water, and contains a number of inorganic salts and other compounds, including salivary amylase, an enzyme which assists the chemical breakdown of starch and complex sugars into more simple sugars. Saliva is produced in sufficient quantities to also act as a lubricant, a stimulant to taste buds and a tooth cleanser.

Along the rest of the gastrointestinal tract, proteins called *mucins* are released by small gland cells to form mucous when mixed with water. Mucous serves to moisten and lubricate food particles to enable them to slide easily through the digestive system (imagine the effect of a dry biscuit or potato chip on the walls of the oesophagus if this were not so!).

- *Gastric juice* – this most important liquid is secreted by the glands of the stomach and contains a number of substances.
- *Other liquid substances* including pancreatic juice (which contains important enzymes and substances which assist these, called co-enzymes), bile (which is important in the digestion of fats); and intestinal juice (which contains a number of digestive enzymes).

These fluids of the gastrointestinal tract deserve special attention during such medical procedures as suctioning or drainage of liquids from parts of the tract, and during disturbances such as vomiting and diarrhoea. All of these factors can disrupt the balance of fluid in the tract and possibly lead to a general fluid imbalance in the body as a whole, including an imbalance in the various constituents of these liquids, especially the electrolytes.

This is almost predictable if we consider that about 8 litres of liquid per day is poured into the gut and under normal conditions all of this except about 100 mL should be reabsorbed to maintain liquid balance within the body.

2. The Brain and Spinal Cord

These are covered by a layer of tissues called the **meninges**. The inner layer is the **pia mater**, the middle layer the **arachnoid** and the outer layer is the **dura mater. Cerebrospinal fluid** (CSF) circulates in the sub-arachnoid space between the pia mater and the arachnoid and through the ventricles of the brain. The ventricles are cavities in the brain which are linked to each other and to the sub-arachnoid space in the brain and spinal cord. The total volume involved is about 135 mL. It is secreted by cauliflower-like capillary networks in the ventricles called **choroid plexuses** and is a clear, colourless liquid. Its essential function is to offer protection to the delicate tissues of the brain and spinal cord. In fact, the brain tends to float in the CSF, thus offering excellent cushioning against sharp blows to the head.

If too much CSF is produced or a blockage occurs, **hydrocephalus** (commonly referred to as 'water on the brain' or, more accurately 'water on the head') can result. This, in turn, causes increased pressure to be exerted on the brain, which may result in swelling of the head in children and then brain damage. In severe cases mental retardation can result. It is most common as a congenital condition in children and infants.

Cerebrospinal fluid may be removed for *diagnostic* purposes. When this occurs it is most important that the patient be kept lying down for several hours afterwards until the normal volume of CSF has been restored. Any attempt to move the patient, to turn his head or to sit him up may cause jolting of the brain, resulting in severe pain or headache.

3. The Pericardial Sac

This contains a very small volume of fluid contained between the heart and a loose-fitting sac called the *pericardium*, which surrounds the heart and the origins of the great blood vessels. It is a watery fluid which provides lubrication between the membranes surrounding the heart and prevents friction from occurring.

4. The Pleural Cavity

This is a space between the lungs and the chest wall which also contains a very small quantity of fluid for the same reason as the pericardial sac.

5. Articular or Joint Capsules

These structures contain **synovial fluid** and the joints involved are thus referred to as synovial joints. The majority of the joints of the body are synovial – the knees, elbows, wrists, ankles and lower jaw or mandible. The fluid itself is rather like the white of egg in consistency and serves to lubricate cartilages at the ends of bones, cushion shocks and provide a source of nutrients. As a lubricating agent, synovial fluid apparently has no peer and is the envy of mechanical engineers for its efficiency. It appears that a type of squeezing action operates to immediately provide fluid where it is needed most, which results in an almost friction-free system.

6. The Semi-Circular Canals
These contain fluid which is most important for the maintenance of *posture*.

There are numerous other cavities in the body which contain liquids, usually in quite small quantities, for example in the eyes and glands.

It can readily be seen from all that has been said about water and liquids in the body that they have a comprehensive and vital role in all aspects of body function. However, we will be concentrating on the fluids of the intracellular, interstitial and vascular spaces since these are the liquids which are most mobile and thus have the greatest influence on fluid homeostasis in general. In addition, these fluids are the ones which are most frequently altered by disorders or disturbances to the body's physiology.

Water Intake and Loss

Homeostasis involves, among other things, maintaining a delicate balance between water gain and loss. The 'normal' intake and loss is shown in Table 5.3

It is important to point out that we are not aware of this water loss at the time, compared to perspiration, for example, of which we are aware – hence the term 'insensible'. People living in hot, dry climates can lose enormous quantities of water in this

TABLE 5.3 Daily water intake and loss in adults

Intake	Millilitres per Day	Loss	Millilitres per Day
By drinking	1200	Insensible loss†	
By eating	1000	Skin	400
By metabolic processes*	200	Respiratory tract	400
TOTAL	2400	Perspiration	100
		Urine	1400
		Faeces	100
		TOTAL	2400

* *Metabolic processes* refers to all the chemical processes which occur in a living cell, including the breakdown of food.
† *Insensible water loss* is the loss of water by diffusion through the skin and by evaporation from the respiratory tract.

way and certainly not be conscious of having perspired. A mirror held in front of the mouth will soon indicate water loss through the respiratory tract.

Insensible loss is greatly altered by disease (fevers and acute bronchitis); disorders such as burns and eczema; climate and exercise. It follows that it must also be taken into account when caring for a patient in fluid imbalance. For example, accurate counting of the rate of respiration and careful observation of the depth of respiration, as well as loss from the skin surface is necessary, especially if the body is not coping well with fluids, as occurs in kidney failure.

From Table 5.3 two facts are well worth noting.

1. It should be emphasised that in actual nursing practice, account must be taken of fluids ingested as food as well as those ingested directly as fluids, in any attempts to accurately monitor fluid intake. This is particularly important when a patient is in crisis, such as when the kidneys cease functioning;

2. Urine output from the kidneys is the largest loss of fluid from the body. This then provides a good indication of overall fluid loss from the body in each 24 hour period, compared to intake.

Note: It must be appreciated that these figures are intended as a guide only, and the actual figures will vary not only from one individual to the next, but for any one individual from one day to the next, depending on how hot the particular day is and the extent of physical activity. For example, the perspiration loss on a hot day may be well over 1000 mL, and during prolonged heavy work or exercise, may well be closer to 5000 mL.

Oedema

This condition reflects a breakdown of the normal fluid distribution of the body, in which excess interstitial (i.e. extracellular) fluid is present in the tissues (Fig. 5.4). This leads to an abnormal swelling of the tissues, which may be just local – e.g. swollen ankles as a result of a long flight in which the passenger has little opportunity to walk around and allow lymph fluid to circulate – or else a general swelling of the whole body. The most important causes are usually due to circulatory disturbances or the retention of excess salt as a result of kidney, heart or adrenal cortex disease.

Various types of oedema exist, depending on the cause and location of the build-up of fluid. In postural oedema, for example, the excess fluid shifts to the lowest part of the body –

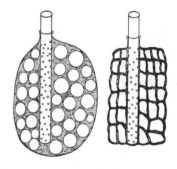

Figure 5.4. A physical model of a rubber bag with a perforated tube to simulate a capillary, balloons filled with water to simulate cells and cotton between balloons to simulate intercellular elements. The diagram on the right shows the non-oedema state and that on the left, the state described as oedema. (From Guyton: *Textbook of Medical Physiology.* 6th Ed. Philadelphia. W.B. Saunders, 1981.)

to the feet if standing or to the back of the lungs and the lower back (sacral) area if supine, in response to the effects of gravity.

SOME SPECIAL PROPERTIES OF MATTER

Absorption and Adsorption

Table 5.3 described the normal ingestion of fluids (in whatever form) through the mouth. Water will then be absorbed from the gastrointestinal tract into the blood and lymph. It should be noted that water and other liquids can be absorbed directly from a tube which has been passed up through the anal sphincter into the lower end of the bowel. However, this method is used only rarely in present day medicine.

The following two terms are sometimes confused with reference to the movement of substances in the body.

Absorption is the 'taking-in' of a substance by another. Thus we make use of the properties of sponge rubber in wiping up a spill of water. We say that the sponge absorbs the water. Similarly the small intestine absorbs water and dissolved materials into the blood and lymph through villi.

Adsorption, however, is the adhesion of a substance to the surface of a solid. Poisonous gases such as chlorine can be adsorbed by 'activated' charcoal, charcoal which has been specially prepared for this purpose.

Activated charcoal is one of a number of substances used to help neutralise and remove toxic substances from the body by adsorption during emergency treatment for poisoning.

A number of drugs act as adsorbers. One example is aluminium silicate, which is found in Kaolin and Kaoexpectate. This acts as an adsorber, binding with irritating substances so as to relieve diarrhoea.

Cohesion and Adhesion

The molecules of solids and liquids exert strong forces of attraction on each other and these strong forces tend to keep the solid or liquid together. Such forces, involving *like* molecules, are called forces of **cohesion**. One obvious example is the invisible 'skin' which appears to exist on the surface of water, and which tends to cause water to form into droplets rather than to spread out evenly.

However, *unlike* molecules tend to attract each other also, for example, water molecules and glass molecules – these forces are forces of **adhesion**.

Meniscus Formation

Forces of cohesion and adhesion give rise to the formation of a **meniscus** on the surface of liquids.

If the forces of adhesion are greater than those of cohesion, the meniscus will be as shown in Fig. 5.5a (as in water). In this case measurements are taken from the bottom of the meniscus.

If the forces of cohesion are greater than those of adhesion, the meniscus will be as shown in Fig. 5.5b (as in mercury). In this case, all measurements are taken from the *top* of the meniscus.

Surface Tension

This is the tendency of a liquid to draw the surface molecules into the body of the liquid and therefore to reduce the surface area to a minimum. This results from the *cohesive forces* between molecules and is the name given to the phenomenon which causes the formation of the skin or film on the surface of water.

In the body of a liquid, any one molecule is surrounded by other molecules and is attracted equally in all directions by these molecules. However, molecules at the surface are unbalanced because they do not have other 'like' molecules on all sides. As a result they cohere more strongly to those directly associated with them on the surface and below. Those molecules beneath them exert an unbalanced downward force which tends to draw surface molecules into the body of the liquid, minimising the surface area. These strong cohesive forces being exerted on surface molecules, cause tension to develop at the surface of the liquid and a 'film' to form. The 'film' on the surface makes it more difficult to move an object through the surface than it is to move the object once it is immersed in the body of the liquid.

The surface tension can be strong enough in some liquids to support the weight of such things as very small insects (e.g. water spiders). *Surface tension varies between liquids.* The surface tension of mercury is greater than water, although water does have a relatively high tension as well. Alcohol has a low surface tension as do many antiseptics and disinfectants.

The effectiveness of solutions appears to be related to their surface tension levels. Those with lower levels, other factors being equal, are usually more effective. They spread out more and wet the surface of the area to be treated more thoroughly. This means for example, greater contact between the antiseptic or disinfectant and the area to be treated.

Since low surface tension liquids tend to spread out more and have lower cohesive forces they evaporate more quickly (e.g. alcohol). Higher tension liquids, such as water, tend to form droplets (due to stronger forces), not spreading out as well and

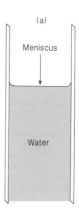

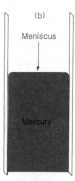

Figure 5.5 The shape of the meniscus depends upon the relative forces of adhesion and cohesion. (a) Water-adhesion stronger than cohesion. (b) Mercury-cohesion stronger than adhesion.

thus not evaporating as quickly. This does have an advantage, in that they can be used in an aerosol form or in a nebuliser to greater effect.

Most liquid surfaces have a constant tension, i.e. there is no change in tension with a change in area. The cohesive forces between surface molecules are not dependent on the total surface area. Regardless of size, all bubbles formed from water have a constant tension. However, some liquids do have a *variable tension*. One example is the material in the lungs – as the area increases, so does the surface tension. Therefore the surface tension of the liquid on lung surfaces rises during expansion and decreases during compression. (A specific discussion of lung surface tension, its effects and the substance (surfactant) used to decrease it, will be found in Chapter 7.)

The surface tension of a liquid can be lowered by various means:

- mechanical – such as agitation;
- thermal – by raising the temperature; and
- chemical – by adding a substance which interferes with or alters the tension forces.

The function of soaps and detergents (the two terms are synonymous) is to act as 'wetting agents' – to lower the surface tension of water so that cohesive forces are reduced and the water is able to penetrate the pores of the skin, dirty clothes or the dirt on one's car.

It should be noted that the mechanical action of washing is important. The nurse who simply wets her hands with water and detergent may end up with hands which are not really clean.

Capillarity

Capillarity results from forces of adhesion and surface tension and is most effective in very fine tubes. The liquid tends to 'crawl up' the sides of the tube due to the forces of adhesion between the sides of the tube and the liquid. The upward force at the edges of the liquid caused by the adhesive forces, results in an upwardly turned meniscus. The presence of surface tension, which tends to keep the surface intact, means the whole surface of the liquid is pulled upward as well, This is limited by the weight of the water lifted. As long as it is less than the net upward force, the water will continue to be pulled upward (Fig. 5.6).

Absorbent cotton or gauze, paper towelling and wick-type surgical drains depend on capillarity for their action. A much more significant application, however, is the fact that capillary

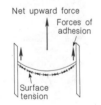

(a) Adhesion and surface tension contribute to capillarity

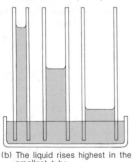

(b) The liquid rises highest in the smallest tube

Figure 5.6. The basis of capillary action.

action assists the heart in moving blood through very fine capillary networks. In these capillaries, the normal pressure of the blood would be insufficient without this assistance from capillary action.

Density

This is defined as *mass per unit volume*. The mass of an object is simply the amount of matter which it contains. The volume is the amount of space occupied by the body.

To make this idea clearer, let us draw a comparison with common usage. When we speak of a dense crowd, we refer to the fact that people are packed tightly together – we have a large number of people in a small area, for example. If we now consider particles instead of people and a volume instead of an area, when we have a dense substance, we have a large number of particles and thus a large mass in a small volume. Thus if we have a one centimetre cube made from lead, it will have a much larger mass than a one centimetre cube made from sponge rubber or polystyrene foam or balsa wood. The particles in the cube of lead will then be packed much more tightly and there will be more of them present than in the cube of sponge rubber which is loosely packed and does not contain as many particles. Of course, the same applies to the polystyrene foam and balsa wood – they are also loosely packed and thus the number of particles present is smaller than is the case with lead. This indicates to us that lead has a much greater density than sponge rubber, polystyrene foam and balsa wood.

The correct SI unit for density is kilogram per cubic metre (kg/m^3). However, everyday usage tends to maintain the old unit of grams per cubic centimetre (g/cm^3). This is no doubt connected to the fact that it is simply more convenient to talk about the density of water as $1 \ g/cm^3$ than $1000 \ kg/m^3$. Table 5.4 lists the densities of a number of common substances.

TABLE 5.4 Densities (g/cm^3)

Item	Density
air	1.3×10^{-3}
ice	0.92
water	1.0
aluminium	2.7
iron	7.8
lead	11.0
mercury	13.6
gold	19.0

ARCHIMEDES' PRINCIPLE

Archimedes was the early Greek whose king gave him the task of finding out whether the gold, which the king was buying, was really pure gold, since the king suspected foul play. It is said that Archimedes discovered the solution to the problem while he was in the bath and ran down the street stark naked yelling 'eureka', meaning 'I have found it'. We are not concerned with the king's gold, but we are now going to see how Archimedes' Principle can be applied to an important measurement which is frequently made in nursing.

Before we state Archimedes' Principle, we will revise some background points which we hope will make it easier to understand.

- If we place an object of known volume into some water which is in a measuring cylinder, the reading of the water level will increase by that volume. For example, if we take an object of volume 6.0 mL and place it in some water in a measuring cylinder which is reading, say, 56.0 mL, the new reading on the measuring cylinder will be:

$$56.0 + 6.0 = 62.0 \text{ mL}$$

that is, *the volume of water displaced is equal to the volume of the object.*

- If we weigh an object on a spring balance while it is suspended in the air and then weigh the same object while it is immersed in a liquid, our second reading is lower. This is because of the upthrust or *buoyancy* of the water. It is this upthrust or buoyancy which enables us to float in water.

It follows, then, that the object weighs less in water than in air, that is, there has been an apparent loss in weight of the object while it is immersed in water or another liquid.

- The observation above holds true whether the object is wholly or partially immersed in the water.
- At the beginning we discussed the volume of the fluid which had been displaced. If we now look at the *weight* of that displaced fluid, we find that this weight *is equal to the apparent loss of weight* if that same object is immersed in the fluid, whether wholly or partially.

Archimedes' Principle can then be stated: **the apparent loss of weight of a body which is immersed (wholly or partially) in a liquid**

is equal to the weight of liquid displaced.

We can now apply this principle to the urinometer.

The Urinometer

This is a special kind of hydrometer, which is rather like a fishing float, in that it has a weight in the lower end and a thinner 'stalk' section on the upper end, as can be seen from Fig. 5.7. The upper section has markings and values of *specific gravity* or *relative density*, defined as follows:

The specific gravity (relative density) is the ratio of the density of a substance (at a particular temperature) to the density of water.

$$\text{S.G. (R.D.)} = \frac{\text{density of substance}}{\text{density of water}}$$

Since this is a ratio, it has *no units* and is stated simply as a number. Furthermore, it doesn't matter which of the units we use for density, provided we use the same units for both the substance and the water. Since the relative density or specific gravity is a *ratio*, it will not be altered by units. For example, the density of water in the old units is 1 g/cm^3 and in SI units is 1000 kg/m^3, but *the relative density* or *specific gravity* is simply 1. Thus by using the ratio specific gravity or relative density, complication with units is avoided.

A mixture, such as urine, has a number of constituents, and thus its density will change as the composition varies. By measuring the density we are then able to determine if any marked change of urine composition has occurred, which can be very useful for diagnostic purposes.
Also:

1. If the concentration of dissolved substances increases, the density will increase and the urinometer will float higher. Since the instrument is graduated to reflect this, a higher reading will be indicated.

2. If the concentration of dissolved substances decreases, the density will decrease, the urinometer will float lower in the urine and a lower reading will be obtained.

Figure 5.7 shows the normal value of 1.025, although the specific gravity of urine can range from 1.001 to 1.035.

The advances of technology are such that urinometers are becoming things of the past. It is now possible to obtain reagent strips which indicate specific gravity.

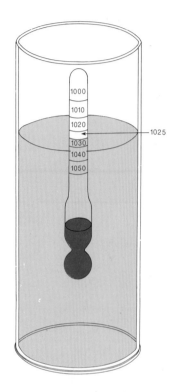

Figure 5.7. A hydrometer used to measure the specific gravity of a urine specimen. The narrow tubing is calibrated so that the specific gravity (1.025) can be read from the tube.

ELECTROLYTES

These are a major constituent of *all* body fluids. It is most important for the nurse to fully understand their roles in the body since they affect the functioning of many physiological processes and to recognise the signs and symptoms of any imbalances (Table 5.5).

Electrolytes are chemical substances which, when dissolved in water (or melted), dissociate into ions and can conduct an electric current. They are ionically bonded compounds and do not conduct electric current in the solid state. There are two types of ions.

1. **Cations**, *which are positively charged*, the most important of which are sodium (Na^+), potassium (K^+), calcium (Ca^{2+}) and magnesium (Mg^{2+}).

2. **Anions**, *which are negatively charged*, the most important of which are chloride (Cl^-), bicarbonate (HCO_3^-) and phosphate (PO_4^{3-}).

It should be noted that the ions in any part of the body at any time will consist of an *equal number* of anions and cations, but they may not be evenly distributed in a local area, such as on a cell membrane.

These ions, which are themselves often referred to as 'electrolytes' in medical practice, are *essential* to the normal function of all cells and:

- are involved in metabolic activities;
- are involved in creating charge differences on which the functioning of nerves and muscles depend;
- are involved in fluid homeostasis.

The concentration of these ions (electrolytes) is maintained in the body within a very narrow range for each ion (Table 5.6). How-ever, the optimum concentrations in the extracellular fluid differ from those in the intracellular fluid. For example, the concentration of potassium ions is about 30 times higher inside the cell than outside the cell, but the situation with sodium is opposite, there being about 15 times the concentration of sodium ions outside the cell than inside, as seen in Fig. 5.8, Table 5.1 and Table 4.5.

The terms used to describe the imbalance of these ions are made up from three terms:

1. a prefix, either *hypo*, meaning under, or *hyper*, meaning over (as in 'a hyperactive child');
2. a term involving either the Latin or English name for the *element* from which the ion is derived and
3. the Latin suffix *-emia* (blood).

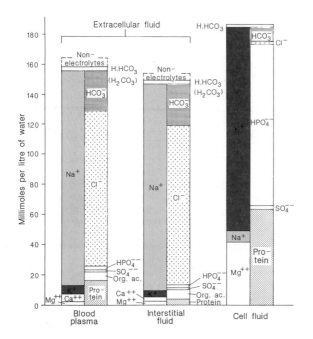

Figure 5.8. The compositions of plasma, interstitial fluid, and intracellular fluid. (From Guyton: *Textbook of Medical Physiology*. 6th Ed. Philadelphia. W.B. Saunders, 1981.)

Thus *hypernatremia* means an excess of sodium (Latin: *natrium*) ions in the blood; and *hyponatremia* refers to a shortage of sodium ions.

The maintenance of correct electrolyte balance in the body depends upon homeostatic mechanisms which regulate the absorption, distribution and excretion of water and the solutes dissolved in it. These processes depend upon:

1. The individual ingesting normal amounts of water and electrolytes. These normal amounts can be disrupted by certain foods, such as those with a high salt content; medications, such as intravenous solutions; vitamin pills; and home remedies such as sodium bicarbonate or salt tablets.

2. The amount of each ion ingested compared to the amount of that ion lost by urination, defaecation and perspiration. Some medications give rise to abnormal losses of particular ions. For example, some diuretics cause excessive loss of potassium ions.

TABLE 5.5 Common electrolytes

Ion	Requirement	Sources	Main Functions	Homeostatic Regulation	Loss
Sodium (Na^+)	Approximately 40–100 mmol (920–2300 mg)* daily. An average Western diet normally contains well over this amount.	Very high in processed and preserved foods; it is also found in unprocessed foods – milk, meat, eggs and some vegetables; table salt.	1. Principal agent in the regulation of fluid volume within body fluid compartments, particularly that of the ECF in which it is the major ion. 2. Maintains blood volume and controls size of the vascular compartment. 3. Helps control muscular contractibility, especially heart muscle. 4. Increases cell membrane permeability. 5. Acts as a buffer base (sodium bicarbonate) and thus helps to regulate H^+ concentration. 6. Controls body water distribution through the maintenance of an osmotic equilibrium between ICF and ECF. 7. Assists in maintenance of neuromuscular irritability. 8. Stimulates conduction of nerve impulses.	Hormonal: a) aldostcrone (secreted by the adrenal glands): controls Na^+ excretion and retention; corticosteroids (secreted by the adrenal glands): promote Na^+ reabsorption by kidney tubules. Gastrointestinal tract: controls Na^+ excretion in presence of Na^+ depletion.	Urine, faeces, perspiration.
Potassium (K^+)	50–140 mmol (1950–5460 mg)* daily; average diet contains 2–4 g.	Meats; whole grains; fruits – for example, bananas, oranges, grapefruit, peaches, apricots, figs, prunes, tomatoes; vegetables – legumes, broccoli (high), cauliflower.	1. Aids in regulation of acid-base balance by cellular exchange with H^+. 2. Is involved in the transmission of nerve impulses. 3. Assists in the regulation of water and electrolyte content of cellular fluid. 4. Assists in skeletal muscle function. 5. Promotes cellular growth.	a) The kidneys conserve K^+ when cellular K^+ is depleted and excrete 90% of ingested K^+. b) The hormone aldosterone influences K^+ loss and gain. c) The sodium pump maintains high cellular $^+$ levels by actively excluding Na^+.	Urine, faeces, perspiration.

TABLE 5.5 Common electrolytes (cont.)

Ion	Requirement	Sources	Main Functions	Homeostatic Regulation	Loss
Calcium (Ca^{2+})	Adults – 800–1000 mg* Ca^{2+} daily. Children and infants – 300–1200 mg* daily, depending on age. Pregnant and lactating women – 1100–1600 mg* daily, depending on stage. Women in menopause – 1000 mg daily.	Major: dairy products. Others: egg yolks, nuts, green leafy vegetables, legumes, whole grains.	1. Building of bones and teeth. 2. Essential for blood clotting. 3. Promotes nerve impulse transmission. 4. Essential for normal muscle contractibility. 5. Promotes normal neuromuscular irritability. 6. Strengthens capillary membranes.	1. Controlled by parathyroid glands and hormone (parahormone [PTH]). 2. Absorption depends partly on presence of vitamin D. 3. Level of calcium is affected by an inverse relationship with phosphorus levels; i.e.: a) if blood level of phosphorus is increased, calcium level will be lower; b) if blood level of phosphorus is decreased, calcium level will be elevated. 4. To a lesser extent by calcitonin from the thyroid gland.	Urine and faeces.
Magnesium (Mg^{2+})	Approximately 270–320 mg* daily in adult. Lactating women 410 mg* daily.	Major: include nuts, soyabeans, seafood, whole grains, dried beans and peas.	1. Activates a number of enzyme reactions, particularly in carbohydrate metabolism. 2. Assists in regulation of serum phosphorus levels. 3. Essential for maintenance of neuromuscular system.	Absorption may be increased through influence of parathyroid hormone.	Primarily faeces, low in urine.

*National Health and Medical Research Council Values (1985).

TABLE 5.5 Common electrolytes (cont.)

Ion	Requirement	Sources	Main Functions	Homeostatic Regulation	Loss
Protein ions	Approximately one gram of protein daily per kg of body weight will provide sufficient for its various functions.	Major: meats and dairy foods. Others: grains and vegetables.	1. It provides the essential colloid osmotic pressure necessary to maintain blood volume. 2. As the second major anion of the cell, it contributes to the maintenance of the intracellular volume. 3. It is necessary for growth, maintenance and repair of tissues and cells. 4. Comprises bulk of muscular, visceral and epithelial tissue and is a constituent of haemoglobin, blood cells and antibodies. 5. It is the most basic and vital constituent of living cells, and forms enzymes and hormones.		Through catabolism and excretion into urine.

TABLE 5.6 Concentration in body fluids

Ion	Requirement	Sources	Main Functions	Homeostatic Regulation	Loss
Hydrogen Ion (H^+)	Normally about 0.00004 mmol/litre.	1. The largest number of H^+ ions are produced by the body's complex metabolic processses. 2. Ingested in medications containing ammonium or mineral salts. 3. A small amount is ingested in an average diet.	1. Essential for the binding of oxygen by haemoglobin. 2. The concentration determines the relative acidity or alkalinity of body fluids. 3. It promotes efficient functioning of enzyme systems.	1. Kidneys can excrete or retain H^+. 2. Lungs can excrete this ion in the form of CO_2 and water. 3. Dilution of H^+ excess by extracellular fluids. 4. Buffering of H^+ by the buffer systems in the blood.	Lungs, urine.

Treatments such as gastric suction can also cause excessive ion loss.

Many diseases and conditions can interfere with these processes and cause an imbalance. One example is renal disease, in which the filtering unit of the kidney, the nephron, is not able to function normally. This causes a retention of water, sodium chloride, hydrogen carbonate and calcium ions so that the glomerular filtration rate falls (i.e. the process of removal of ions etc. from the blood by the glomerulus in each nephron in the kidneys).

Similar effects occur if the blood supply to the kidney is inadequate or if there is an imbalance of renal regulatory hormones, such as aldosterone and ADH, an antidiuretic hormone.

The effects of an electrolyte imbalance are not isolated to a particular organ or system, but may cause changes and disturbances throughout the body.

Electrolytes and the Gastrointestinal Tract

The correct functioning of the gastrointestinal tract (GIT) depends upon secretion of a number of types of substances including various organic substances, mucus, water and electrolytes.

Without going into the rather complex details of the theories which have been postulated in regard to electrolyte activity, two points can be made:

1. The physical presence of water and electrolytes gives rise to a flushing effect on the secretory glands associated with the lining (epithelium) of the GIT, which washes organic substances into the lumen (hollow centre) of the tract.

2. The presence of these ions provides a means whereby the signals from nerve endings in the wall of the GIT, which control the release of organic substances, are transmitted through the cells involved. Unless these ions are present in appropriate concentration, the whole process of digestion is jeopardised.

REVIEW

1. (a) If you do not have access to test sticks, what instrument could you use to measure the specific gravity of urine?
    (b) Explain how this instrument works.
    (c) Why is the specific gravity measured?
2. Hydrotherapy is often used in the treatment of some physical disabilities such as partial paralysis. What advantage is provided by the use of a water medium?

3. Why would age be a factor to consider when anticipating a patient's fluid balance needs after surgery?
4. What consequences might follow from the loss of a large volume of water from the body?
5. Draw the meniscus produced by water and that produced by mercury. Explain the reasons for the difference between these two. What difference does a meniscus make to the reading of a fluid level?
6. A patient's fluid intake and output may be more carefully monitored in some situations than in others. An example would be the case of a patient with renal failure (i.e. kidneys not functioning). Identify the ways in which fluid may be gained or lost which are less obvious, but which should be taken into account in the above situation. Include the average volumes lost or gained.
7. Compare the extracellular and intracellular compartments in terms of solutes and solvents.
8. Identify the cavities in the body which contain fluids and list a few of the functions of those fluids.

6

Body fluids
(liquids and gases)

OBJECTIVES

After studying this chapter the student should be able to:

1. Explain the concept of the mole.
2. Distinguish between homogeneous and heterogeneous mixtures, solutions and suspensions; and also between emulsions and gels.
3. Describe, and distinguish between the various transport mechanisms in the body.
4. Give examples of the functioning of these mechanisms in the body.
5. Identify the importance of these mechanisms in the maintenance of homeostasis.
6. Distinguish between various types of dehydration.

INTRODUCTION

There are times in any profession when things do not go according to plan. This is never more true than in nursing. In nursing we are dealing with *people* – other staff, patients and visitors, all of whom make demands upon us and all of whom are individuals with varying needs. Thus, situations arise with the potential for disrupting even the best laid plans.

As an example, we may be working to a schedule involving the administration of 1000 mL of an intravenous solution to a patient in ten hours. Many things could happen to interfere with that plan – blockages or kinks in the tubing, poor communication of information during staff changeovers, or inadequate supervision. When you realise that only half of the correct quantity has been administered and less than two hours remain, it could be very tempting to open the controls and let the solution flow in as fast as possible.

In such a situation, *stop.* Do you know what the solution contains? Do you have any idea of the effects of that solution on the internal environment of the body and on the state of the patient's health? Could such an action cause a too rapid change which the body may not be able to handle at this time? Will the administration of the solution in this manner meet the objectives of the treatment, which may be supportive rather than replacement?

By such an action you may overload the patient with fluid with negative results. Let us look at the effects of fluids and their movements in and around cells and on the role which they and their components play in the circulatory system and other fluid spaces. You may then judge for yourself the wisdom of the procedure which may have occurred to you in this situation.

HOMOGENEOUS AND HETEROGENEOUS MIXTURES

Before proceeding to discuss solutions, we need to define some of the terms which we are going to use:

An **homogeneous** mixture is one which has
uniform composition throughout.
An **heterogeneous** mixture is one which has a
variable composition.

Let's consider some water to which common salt has been added. Some of the salt will immediately dissolve, but most will settle on the bottom, and the mixture will be heterogeneous. If we then stir this mixture until no visible trace of the salt remains and it has all dissolved, we then have an homogeneous mixture.

Many pharmaceutical mixtures are heterogeneous and will settle out even after shaking. Thus their labels carry an injunction to 'Shake the Bottle', so that the measured dose delivered to the patient will be homogeneous and contain the appropriate ingredients in their correct proportions.

Solutions

A solution consists of a **solute** – the substance(s) being dissolved and a **solvent** – the substance in which the solute is dissolved.

Solutions may be defined as *homogeneous mixtures of two or more substances with different molecular structures*. The term is most frequently applied to solutions of solids in liquids, but other types of solutions are important. One outstanding example is blood, which is a solution in which the gases oxygen and carbon dioxide are dissolved. However, before proceeding further, the point should be made that the situation with blood is far from simple, and the reader should not gain the impression that these gases are carried only in simple solution. More will be said of this later.

The other types of solution with which we will be chiefly concerned are *liquid in liquid*, such as a solution of alcohol in water; *solid in liquid*, for example, a sodium chloride (0.9%) solution; and *gases in liquid*, for example, liquid foam. Others which exist are *gases in solids*, such as in the manufacture of foam rubber; and *solid in solid*, as in alloys.

Solutions in which water is the solvent are described as *aqueous solutions*. Thus an aqueous solution of sodium chloride is one in which sodium chloride has been dissolved in water.

Some other terms are important and should be mentioned at this stage:

1. A *saturated solution* is one which contains all the solute which the solvent is capable of dissolving at a particular temperature.

2. An *unsaturated solution* is one which does *not* contain all the solute which the solvent is capable of dissolving at a particular temperature.

3. The solubility may be expressed in terms of: a) weight (w/w); e.g. a 10% aqueous solution of sucrose *by weight* is prepared by dissolving 10 g of sucrose in 100 g of water; b) volume (v/v); e.g. a 10% aqueous solution of alcohol *by volume* is prepared by dissolving 10 mL of alcohol in water and making the solution up to 100 mL; c) a combination of the two (w/v); a 10 g/100 mL aqueous solution of glucose is prepared by dissolving 10 g of glucose in water and making the solution up to 100 mL.

Note: If a solution strength is quoted as a percentage, it should always be specified whether this is by weight or volume.

It is important to note that temperature is significant. In cold climates, for example, it is not unusual to find that crystals may form from IVI (intravenous infusion) solutions after a period of time, as a result of a very low temperature.

4. A *supersaturated solution* is one which forms only under special circumstances, and for reasons which we will not go into here, contains *more* solute than a saturated solution.

This may lead to the formation of *renal calculi* (kidney stones) in the human body (as a result of a change in pH), dehydration, obstruction of urine flow; or kidney disease. If for example, the kidney is excreting an excess of a stone-forming substance such as uric acid, it is thought that a supersaturated solution of uric acid may then form stones under certain conditions, which in turn arise from such factors as high solute concentrations.

Other substances which form stones in the kidneys include urates (salts of uric acid) and calcium oxalate, which come from acidic urine; and calcium phosphate which forms from alkaline urine.

5. A *suspension* is similar to a solution but the important difference is that the particles in a suspension are finely divided but NOT dissolved. Blood is in some respects a suspension because blood cells are *suspended* in the liquid medium which we call plasma.

Penicillin is another example of a suspension, which the nurse may have to make up by adding water to the drug in the solid (powder) form.

6. A *colloid* is a special type of solution in which the molecules of the solute do not exist separately but tend to form solute particles. These particles cannot be detected as such with the naked eye, or even with a conventional microscope – an ultramicroscope is needed. However, these particles cannot pass through a semi-permeable membrane because of their larger sizes (Fig. 6.1).

Proteins of the blood, such as serum albumins, form colloidal solutions in the plasma of the blood. These large particles play a very important role in helping to maintain the level of water in the blood and in preventing constant leakage of liquid out into the interstitial spaces. Colloids are also formed as part of the *immune* or *defence systems* of the body when invading agents are neutralised by adsorption. Another common example is starch.

The size of a colloidal particle is approximately in the range 1 to 1000 nm (remember that a nanometre [nm] is 10^{-9} of a metre).

The most important colloids are *sols, emulsions, gels* and *aerosols*.

Sols consist of a solid dispersed in a liquid. 'Milk of magnesia' is solid particles of magnesium hydroxide dispersed in water.

Emulsions consist of a liquid dispersed in a liquid. Mayonnaise consists of oils dispersed in water and milk consists of

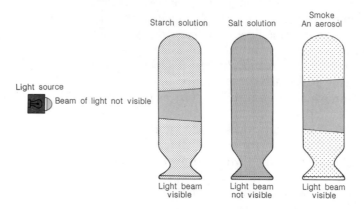

Figure 6.1. The presence of colloidal particles is easily detected with the aid of a light beam. Thus it may be seen that smoke and starch are colloids, but salt solution is not. (Adapted from Brescia: *Chemistry: A Modern Introduction.* W.B. Saunders. Philadelphia. 1978.)

butterfat dispersed in water. 'Vanishing cream' has a small quantity of oil dispersed in water, so that when the water 'vanishes' only a trace of oil remains.

Gels consist of liquid particles dispersed in a solid. Examples are jellies, gelatin and non-drip paint.

Aerosols consist of either solid particles or liquid particles, dispersed in a gas. Smoke is an example of the former; fog of the latter.

Aerosols are widely used in respiratory therapy in nebulisers. These are mechanical devices which force air and/or oxygen through a solution. The resulting aerosol consists of microscopic droplets of the substance which are delivered directly and deeply into the patient's airways. They may consist of sterile distilled water or 0.9% sodium chloride solution, which is used to humidify inspired gases and/or medications such as bronchodilators, mucolytic agents, pulmonary surfactants, antibiotics or corticosteroids. This type of therapy is frequently used in the treatment of patients suffering from cystic fibrosis, emphysema or chronic bronchitis.

Molar Solutions

Before explaining what these are, we need to explain the term **mole**. A strict definition of the mole is that *amount of a substance* which contains *Avogadro's number* of particles (be they atoms, molecules, ions, electrons etc). **Avogadro's number** is defined as the number of atoms in exactly 0.012 kg (12 g) of the ^{12}C isotope of carbon. It has the numerical value 6.022×10^{23}.

Note that a mole of oranges is Avogadro's number of oranges, a mole of peanuts is Avogadro's number of peanuts and a mole of books is Avogadro's number of books, etc (Fig. 6.2).

It has been calculated that 1 mole of oranges would form a sphere the size of the earth; and 1 mole of rice grains would cover Australia to a depth of approximately 1 km.

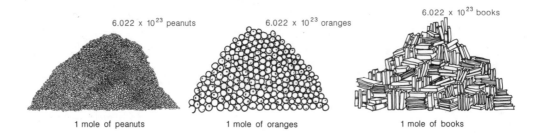

6.022 x 10^{23} peanuts   6.022 x 10^{23} oranges   6.022 x 10^{23} books

1 mole of peanuts   1 mole of oranges   1 mole of books

Figure 6.2. The mole. A mole of any entity or object would mean it comprised 6.022 × 10^{23} of those entities or objects. This unit is usually used for the measurement of very small entities such as ions or molecules.

As discussed in Chapter 4, the atomic mass of an element is based on a comparison of the mass of that element with that of carbon-l2, taken as 12.

Since the atomic mass of sodium is 23, it follows that 23 g (or, more precisely, 22.9877 g) or 0.023 kg of sodium atoms is one *mole* of sodium atoms and contains 6.022 × 10^{23} atoms of sodium.

Similarly, since the atomic mass of chlorine is 35.453, it follows that 35.453 g of chlorine atoms is one *mole* of chlorine atoms and contains 6.022 × 10^{23} atoms of chlorine.

Also, since the atomic mass of oxygen is 15.9994, it follows that 15.9994 g of oxygen atoms is one *mole* of oxygen atoms and contains 6.022 × 10^{23} atoms of oxygen.

In more practical terms, a **mole of an element is the atomic mass of that element expressed in grams** – 23 g of sodium, 16 g of oxygen (atoms) etc, (unless extreme precision is required).

A mole of a *compound* contains the *formula mass* (or *molecular mass*) of that compound expressed in grams. A mole of sodium chloride (NaCl) contains 58.5 (23 + 35.5) g of sodium chloride (since sodium, Na, is 23 and chlorine, Cl, is 35.5) and a mole of water (H_2O) contains 18 (2 × 1 + 16) g of water (since hydrogen, H, is 1 and oxygen, O, is 16). Remember that each contains 6.022 × 10^{23} molecules.

In passing, it should be noted that while we may speak of the molecular mass (it is better in this instance to speak of formula mass) of sodium chloride, this *does not* imply that sodium chloride exists as molecules. As previously explained, it exists as an arrangement of sodium ions and chloride ions.

For the benefit of any readers who may not be familiar with finding molecular masses, one further example is given. Bearing in mind that C = 12, H = 1 and O = 16, we can find the molecular mass of sucrose ($C_{12}H_{22}O_{11}$) by calculation:

(12 × 12) + (1 × 22) + (16 × 11), which is
144 + 22 + 176 = 342.

The mass of any molecule may be found in this way. The reader might like to work out the molecular masses of:

1. urea – formula $CO(NH_2)_2$; and

2. cholesterol – formula $C_{27}H_{45}OH$;

given that C = 12, O = 16, N = 14 and H = 1.
Answers may be compared to those given in Fig. 6.3.

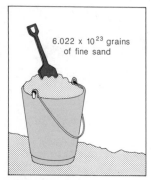

6.022 x 10²³ grains
of fine sand

1 mole of sand grains

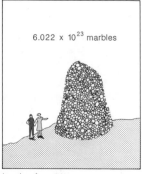

6.022 x 10²³ marbles

1 mole of marbles

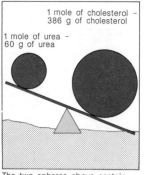

1 mole of cholesterol –
386 g of cholesterol

1 mole of urea –
60 g of urea

The two spheres above contain different weights of the substances urea and cholesterol – but each contains the same number of molecules, i.e. 6.022 x 10²³ molecules, and thus each is 1 mole.

Note: These diagrams are not drawn to scale, and should not be regarded as being so. If the middle one were to scale, for example, the humans would be so small as to be invisible.

Figure 6.3. Moles.

Furthermore, a mole of hydrogen *atoms* has a mass of 1 g, but a mole of hydrogen *molecules* has a mass of 2 g (since each hydrogen molecule contains 2 atoms). Similarly, a mole of oxygen *atoms* has a mass of 16 g, but a mole of oxygen *molecules* has a mass of 32 g.

Note: From the discussion above it may be seen that although one mole of different substances will have different masses, (e.g. one mole of sodium atoms has a mass of 23 g, one mole of oxygen atoms has a mass of 16 g, and one mole of marbles has a mass of ? g), and these different entities have very different properties, they all have *one thing in common* – one mole of each will contain the same number of basic entities:

1 mole of sodium atoms (23 g) contains
6.022×10^{23} atoms;
1 mole of oxygen atoms (16 g) contains
6.022×10^{23} atoms;
1 mole of oxygen molecules (32 g) contains
6.022×10^{23} molecules;
1 mole of marbles (? g) contains
6.022×10^{23} marbles.

A molar solution can then be defined as *1 mole of the solute dissolved in the solvent and made up to one litre of solution.* (Note that this is *not* the same as dissolving one mole of the solute in one litre of the solvent since the solute still accounts for some of the volume even when dissolved.)

Another way of expressing this is to say that a molar solution contains 1 mole of a substance in 1 litre of solution.

Similarly, a **millimolar solution** contains 1 millimole (one-thousandth of a mole) in one litre of solution.

Thus a 1 molar solution of sodium chloride will contain 1 mole (58.5 g) of sodium chloride in 1 litre of sodium chloride solution. A millimolar solution of sodium chloride will contain 0.0585 g of sodium chloride in one litre of solution.

Appendix III shows the concentrations of various solutions (such as the concentration of glucose in the blood) in both the correct SI units and the old units which are still found in some textbooks.

NEW UNITS – A HELP OR A HINDRANCE?

All change is not necessarily an improvement. Some of the readers of this book will be metric thinkers, but others will have had to convert to the metric system (i.e. SI units). One of the authors well remembers the complaints of a migrant from France when the metric system was introduced – he had spent years learning the Imperial system and now had to learn the metric system all over again!

What of the practising nurse? Two examples will highlight the differences between the old and the new – and these differences are more than cosmetic.

1. A laboratory report on the blood of a patient listed (among other things), two substances which are, in part, products of metabolism or the breakdown of some proteins and fats:

Cholesterol	*Urea*
250 mg/100 mL	73 mg/100 mL

It would appear from this information that the concentration of cholesterol in the blood of this patient is about three times that of the urea concentration. Remember that this way of expressing concentration (in the old system of units), puts the accent on the *mass* of the substance present in a specified volume – in these cases 100 mL.

The same values expressed as molar concentrations in the new system would read:

Cholesterol	*Urea*
6.46 mmol/L	12.2 mmol/L

Now since there are 6.022×10^{23} particles of a substance present in one mole of any substance, there will be 6.022×10^{23} divided by 1000, i.e. 6.022×10^{20} particles present in a millimole of any substance.

It then follows that the figures above give us a *direct comparison of the number of particles* present in a specified volume – in this case a litre.

Thus the concentration of cholesterol in our patient's blood is *not* about three times as great as urea but less – in fact only about half that of urea.

It may be seen then that the new units are more useful in making such comparisons and the student nurse will come across many of these, particularly in such areas as physiology.

2. In this second example, the question of drug dosage and accuracy, and the communication of that dosage arises.

Consider the situation where a doctor orders 10 mg of morphine for a patient. Does the doctor want 10 mg of active morphine or 10 mg of morphine sulfate which contains only 8 mg of active morphine? If the morphine is ordered in moles then the quantity given is the exact quantity of active morphine which the doctor has ordered. This follows since the molar unit would reflect only the number of active morphine molecules rather than the possible confusion which arose in the first instance.

This *usage of molar doses* will eventually allow a more *direct comparison* of drug potencies by dealing with the relative number of active drug particles involved. This occurs irrespective of whether the drug is in tablet, capsule or liquid form.

Sedatives, tranquilisers and relaxants will be used much more satisfactorily than in the past since many of these drugs are very similar but respond differently in different individuals, have fine differences in their potencies and are potentially dangerous if overdoses are administered

Molar measurement is restricted to substances and ions whose atomic, molecular or ionic masses are known. Some very complex compounds have structures which are not precisely known, such as some proteins – these must therefore still be measured in grams per litre or one of the other units.

OSMOLARITY

When we look more closely at *osmotic pressure*, we will see that the osmotic pressure exerted by a solute in solution, depends upon the number of molecules or ions of solute. To express the concentration of a solute in terms of its **number of particles**, a unit called the **osmole** is used in place of a gram, which measures mass. In the case of glucose, there is no difference between a mole and an osmole, because glucose does not break down into other particles in solution. However, since one mole of solid sodium chloride breaks up into one mole of sodium ions and one mole of chloride ions, thus producing two moles altogether in solution, one mole of sodium chloride will contain two osmoles of sodium chloride.

Similarly, since magnesium chloride breaks up into one magnesium ion and two chloride ions, a total of three ions in solution, a one molar solution of magnesium chloride will contain three osmoles of magnesium chloride.

Therefore:

no. of osmoles = no. of moles × no. of ions in each molecule

and

osmolarity = molarity × no. of ions in each molecule.

Any two solutions which have the same osmolarity are said to be *isosmotic*.

OSMOLALITY

A **molal** solution is one in which one mole of solute is contained in one kilogram of solvent. Note the difference to a **molar** solution in which one mole of solute is contained in **one litre** of solvent.

Thus the **osmolality** is then given by:

osmolality = molality × no. of ions in each molecule

This unit is used to express such quantities as serum osmolality, e.g. 289 mosm/kg H_2O. The nurse will find that, in most cases, *osmolarities* are used, as in Appendix III.

However, since the relative density of water is very close to 1,000 at ambient temperatures, a litre of water weighs very close to a kilogram, so that osmolality and osmolarity are virtually identical and may be regarded as identical for all practical purposes. In fact, some textbooks, including some highly regarded anatomy and physiology texts, use the two units interchangeably.

Osmolal Gap

For those students who come across this term, an osmolal gap is the mean (average) difference between the measured and the calculated osmolality for a particular solution, such as serum.

MEMBRANES

Since all of the cells of the body contain and are surrounded by solutions and mixtures, we will briefly examine the membranes through which these are continually moving. We will then better understand the reasons for the range of movement or transport mechanisms in the body and the obstacles presented to the movement of water, electrolytes, gases, nutrients and waste products in the body.

The **permeability** of a membrane is the tendency of the membrane to allow molecules to pass through it.

If a membrane is such that it permits the passage of some molecules and not of others, the membrane is described as *selectively permeable* or *semipermeable*, depending on which book one reads! Unfortunately, some discrepancies exist as to the precise meaning of these terms. To overcome this problem, we will define these terms in a particular way, without claiming that these are the most correct usages of the terms under all circumstances, and will consistently use these terms as defined.

A **semipermeable membrane** is defined as a *non-living membrane* such as cellophane and those used in dialysis (discussed later), where the function of the membrane is essentially to separate large and small molecules in solution.

A **selectively permeable membrane** is defined as a *living* membrane as in cells, where the membrane has the capacity to select which ions or molecules it will allow to pass and which it will not allow to pass. This implies that the membrane has the capacity to change its permeability when required and in fact does so in such cases as the transmission of a nerve impulse (Chapter 13).

A number of different membrane types exist in the body, since all of the physical structures in the cell are surrounded by membranes, as is the cell itself. The different membranes include the cell membrane, the nuclear membrane, the endoplasmic reticulum membrane and the membranes of the mitochondria, lysosomes, Golgi complexes and other organelles. They are all similar both in structure and in the properties which they possess in order to function efficiently. The common type of structure is called the unit membrane and will be discussed in the next section.

The Cell Membrane

Every living cell is surrounded by a very fine sheath or barrier, rather like a thin sheet of plastic, some 5 to 10 nm thick. It has to have certain properties, which include:

1. It must act as a *selectively permeable* structure and thus allow the passage of certain molecules or ions as required; these include metal ions, amino acids – the building blocks of protein molecules and sugars.

2. It must be an *electrical insulator*, since the charge held by ions on each side of the membrane is not always the same, as we shall soon see.

3. It must have considerable mechanical *strength* which must be retained throughout the life of the cell.

To meet all of these requirements, cell membrane structure is, to some extent, a compromise; it has to be fluid enough to

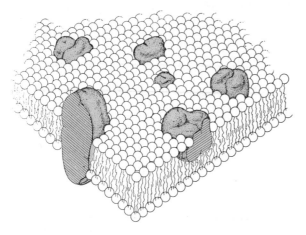

Figure 6.4. A lipid/protein model of a cell membrane. The lipid matrix consists of two layers of lipids with the hydrophilic (water-loving) spherical ends on the outside and the hydrophobic (water-fearing) ends on the inside. The solid bodies with stippled surfaces represent the globular proteins, which are randomly distributed throughout the lipid matrix. (From Giese: *Cell Physiology*. 5th Ed. New York. Holt, Rinehart & Winston. 1979.)

allow the passage of particular molecules, but not so fluid that the normal contents of the cell leak out. Furthermore, at various times the cell permeability with respect to some ions and molecules must be capable of alteration.

Membranes are composed of *proteins* and *lipids* in an approximately 2:1 ratio and although the precise structure is unknown, Fig. 6.4 gives some indication of it. A number of different structures have been proposed, but it is inappropriate to go into further detail here, although the presence of pores of about 1 nm diameter has been inferred, complete with linings of either positive or negative charges. Suffice it to say that the membranes around organelles within a cell and around the cells themselves effectively meet all the requirements listed.

TRANSPORT MECHANISMS

Having discussed solutions and some of the major constituents of solutions in the body, such as electrolytes, and having referred to others, it is appropriate to examine the mechanisms by which these substances move in and out of cells. It is also important to appreciate the relationships which these substances have with body fluids and their potential for altering fluid and component balance and thus for altering the homeostasis of the body.

The various transport mechanisms can be divided into 'passive' transport mechanisms and 'active' transport mechanisms. In passive processes, the substances move across the cell membrane without any need for cellular energy to drive the processes and usually without any assistance from the cell. In active processes energy is expended by the cell in order to move the substances into or out of the cell.

PASSIVE MECHANISMS

Diffusion

When we spoke of gases, we made reference to the fact that they consist of particles called molecules which are in a constant state of active motion. If we remove the barrier betwen two containers which are filled with different gases, we find that the gases soon become completely mixed. This mixing, which results from the random movement of molecules, is called **diffusion** (Fig. 6.5). Similarly, a bottle of ether opened at one end of a ward is soon noticed throughout the whole ward! Examples of gaseous diffusion are numerous.

However, diffusion is a characteristic of all fluids – liquids as well as gases. We can define diffusion as the **movement of molecules or ions from one region to another**, because of random molecular (or ionic) motion, until a dynamic equilibrium is reached.

We have already described the continuous but random motion of molecules in the liquid state (in Chapter 5). These molecules are constantly moving around and bumping into each other, so that over the course of time, the millions of collisions which take place each second result in thorough mixing of liquids, or of ions within a body of liquid. Normally, molecules will tend to move from a region of higher concentration to a region of lower concentration until a dynamic equilibrium is attained. That is, the molecules will continue to move primarily toward the region of lower concentration until the concentration is the same in both regions.

However it does not stop here, since molecules, because of their random movement, will continue to shift back and forth throughout the solution or between the regions. The difference now is that no primary direction exists, but movement in one direction is completely offset by an equal amount of movement in the other. Therefore the situation is in balance or equilibrium and is dynamic, not static. Sometimes this diffusion in fluids occurs through a membrane, as in the body. One example of this is the movement of oxygen from alveoli in the lungs through the fine capillary membrane into the blood stream within the capillary. It is important to note that quite often a substance that can diffuse in one direction may also diffuse in the opposite direction through a membrane. Therefore, the most important aspect of diffusion to the cell is the 'net quantity' of molecules diffusing, either in or out.

Many substances in the body diffuse, including electrolytes, amino acids, various gases and glucose.

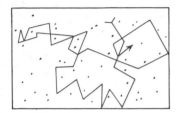

Figure 6.5. Diffusion of a gas molecule during a fraction of a second. (From Guyton: *Textbook of Medical Physiology.* 6th Ed. Philadelphia. W.B. Saunders. 1981.)

The rate at which diffusion occurs depends upon a number of factors which include:

1. **The size of the molecules**. Larger molecules move less rapidly, since more kinetic energy is required to move them about. It follows that the rate of diffusion will then be less rapid.

2. **Concentration**. Each ion or molecule will tend to 'do its own thing' – it will diffuse independently of other molecules or ions, and the extent and rate of its own movement will depend upon the size of its concentration difference between regions or across a membrane. The greater the difference in concentrations, the faster the rate of diffusion. The net movement of that ion or molecule will always be down a concentration gradient, from a region of high concentration to a region of low concentration (other factors being equal), until the concentration difference is eliminated or minimised. See Fig. 6.6A.

3. **Electrical Potential Difference**. A typical cell is normally maintained with an electrical charge difference (See Chapter 13) between one side of the membrane and the other – the outside of the membrane is more positive than the inside. This situation is made possible by the presence of ions (electrolytes) in the body fluids. If any disturbance occurs to the barrier (the cell membrane) which alters its permeability, thus allowing the charged ions to move, they will move along their 'electrical gradients'. No concentration difference for any specific ion need exist for this movement. Rather the ions respond to the unbalanced electrical charges present on either side of the membrane.

Alternatively it is possible to have a situation in which one type of charged ion (e.g. positive) has been moved across a membrane in large numbers, creating an electrical potential difference, due to the decrease of positive ions on one side of the membrane and an increase on the other. An example of this is the shifting of positive ions out of the kidney tubules during reabsorptive processes. This creates, as in the first situation, an imbalance of electrical forces on each side of the membrane.

In both situations ions will move, given the opportunity, in response to this imbalance along their electrical gradients. Therefore, as in Fig. 6.6B, negative ions will shift across the membrane, being attracted by the higher number of positive ions on the inside and being repelled by the increased concentration of negative ions on the outside, until the electrical balance is restored, if this is possible. However, it must be remembered that this movement of ions has not been caused by the nature of the ions but only by their electrical charges. Therefore a variety of types of negative or positive ions may be shifted in these situations, for example Na^+, K^+, and Mg^{2+} and/or Cl^-, HCO_3^- and SO_4^{2-}.

Some of the Factors Affecting Net Diffusion Rates

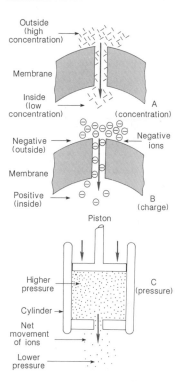

Figure 6.6 A) The higher concentration of molecules on the outside of the membrane compared to the inside, sets up a concentration gradient which drives molecules or ions through the membrane. B) The negative charge on the outside drives the negative ions into the cell. The positive charge on the inside of the cell also attracts the negative ions, assisting the inward movement of negative ions. In the same circumstances, positive ions would be driven outwards. If the polarity is reversed, the ions move in the opposite directions. C) The piston and cylinder represent the effect of pressure difference. Molecules and ions move in or out of the cell in response to such pressure differences. (Adapted from Guyton: *Textbook of Medical Physiology.* 6th Ed. Philadelphia. W.B. Saunders. 1981.)

Since little happens in isolation in the body, it follows that when a number of ions are being shifted, even in response to electrical differences, an eventual difference in concentration of specific types of ions will exist and a new situation develops to which the body must respond.

4. **Pressure Difference**. A difference in the amount of pressure on either side of a membrane may occur, which will also affect diffusion rates. Pressure here is a reflection of the sum of all the forces caused by the different ions and molecules in the fluid spaces striking a unit surface area of a membrane at a given instant. An example of this is found in the glomerulus of the kidneys.

This means that an increase in the number of ions and molecules or in their kinetic energy will cause more frequent striking of the membrane surface area resulting in an increase in the total force on that side of the membrane and therefore an increase in pressure. Since there is now an imbalance in pressure across the membrane, more molecules will tend to move down the developed pressure gradient from the higher pressure side to the lower pressure side, until a dynamic equilibrium is reached across the membrane. This effect is illustrated in Fig. 6.6C.

One example of this situation is found in the capillaries. Blood arriving in the capillaries is very high in nutrients creating a much higher pressure inside the arteriolar end of the capillary than outside. The net quantity of molecules diffusing is outward from the capillary.

Note that pressure is established by the presence of a variety of ions and molecules and may be altered by changes to one or more kinds of ions or molecules.

5. **Temperature**. The higher the temperature the faster the diffusion rate, due to an increase in the molecular movement.

6. **Surface Area**. The more extensive the surface area, the greater the number of molecules or ions can come into contact with it, particularly in the case of membranes, and thus diffusion will be faster.

7. **Other Factors**. These include agitation, size of the chamber or distance travelled and the thickness of the membrane.

As an example, the rate of diffusion of oxygen and carbon dioxide through the respiratory membrane depends upon the thickness of the membrane and its surface area, the diffusion coefficient of these gases in the tissue fluids and within the membrane, and the difference between the partial pressures of the gases in the alveoli and the blood.

The concept of passive transport forms the basis of three other types of associated diffusion mechanisms – facilitated diffusion and osmosis and filtration.

Facilitated Diffusion

Although insoluble in the lipid matrix of the cell membrane, some substances can pass through the matrix with the assistance of a **carrier**. This process occurs with some sugars, of which glucose is an outstanding example.

This is illustrated in Fig. 6.7. Glucose combines chemically with a carrier substance (C) at the point (1) to form a compound which is represented as CG1. This compound is soluble and diffuses to the point (2), where the compound breaks up. The glucose then passes into the cell and the carrier returns to pick up more glucose.

Remember that this process can occur only while the concentration of glucose outside the cell is higher than that inside the cell. The exact nature of the movement is still not fully understood and some substances may need not only a carrier but another substance to release the carrier or to assist it in some way.

Insulin, the primary hormone secreted in the pancreas, is involved in glucose transport and greatly increases (by up to ten times) the rate of movement of glucose into cells.

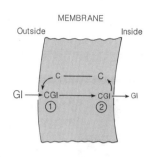

Figure 6.7. Facilitated diffusion of glucose (Gl) through the cell membrane. (From Guyton: *Textbook of Medical Physiology.* 6th Ed. Philadelphia. W.B. Saunders. 1981.)

Osmosis and Osmotic Pressure

Osmosis is the term usually used to describe the **diffusion of a solvent** across a membrane. In the cases which will be considered here, water is the solvent involved. In this process, the solute (the dissolved substance(s)) is left behind. If we consider Fig. 6.8(a), two solutions of different concentration (of sugar in this case) are separated by a membrane.

All of the molecules in each of the compartments A and B possess kinetic energy and are thus moving around within each compartment Only the presence of the membrane prevents the solute molecules from moving into compartment B and thus the two solutions from mixing completely. However, the membrane, being semipermeable, permits the passage of solvent molecules through it.

In a similar way, sodium ions and chloride ions are prevented from passing from one side of a membrane to the other side (in Fig. 6.9(a)) by the semipermeable membrane, which does, however, permit the passage of solvent (water) molecules.

Osmosis, like many other processes which occur in living tissue, is a dynamic process. Because of the kinetic energy of the particles involved, solvent molecules will diffuse in both directions simultaneously, but the net result is a movement of the solvent in the direction of its lowest concentration. Whenever

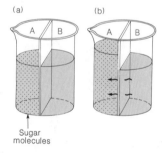

Figure 6.8. Osmosis. A semipermeable membrane is used to separate a container of water into two compartments. Water molecules can pass freely through the pores in the membrane, but most solute molecules are too large to pass through the membrane pores from one compartment to the other. (a) Sugar molecules (dots) are dropped into the water but cannot pass through the membrane. (b) Water molecules diffuse through the membrane by osmosis from compartment B, where they are more concentrated, to compartment A, where they are less concentrated. (Adapted from Solomon & Davis: *Human Anatomy & Physiology.* Philadelphia. Saunders College Publishing. 1983.)

solvent movement is being considered, it is the concentration of the *solvent itself* which is important, not the concentration of the solute.

In Fig. 6.8(a), for example, the concentration of the solvent (water) is higher in compartment B because nothing else is present, while the same volume of liquid in compartment A contains both solvent (water) molecules and solute (glucose) molecules. Therefore the concentration of water molecules is lower in this solution. The effect of the higher concentration of water molecules in compartment B will be a net movement of water molecules from B to A, from higher concentration of water molecules to lower concentration of water molecules, as in Fig. 6.8(b). That is, osmosis occurs from B to A.

This process would tend to continue until the concentrations of solvent on each side of the membrane are equal and no further net movement occurs.

In practice, of course, this cannot happen while ever the glucose molecules exist, since no matter how dilute A becomes, glucose molecules are still present in A, and not in B. Thus the water will keep 'trying' to create equal concentrations of water in both compartments by diffusing from B to A, but will never succeed.

In practice, osmosis is complicated by another factor, that of pressure. If pressure were to be applied to the non-diffusable solute/solvent solutions in our illustrations, the osmosis of water into these solutions could be slowed or stopped if the pressure were sufficient.

You will notice in Fig. 6.8(b) and Fig. 6.9(b) a change in the height of the solutions in compartment A. As osmosis occurs, the height of the solution in compartment A becomes higher than the water level in compartment B. This disparity between the two levels generates a fluid pressure difference across the membrane, being greater on that side of the membrane in compartment A. Compartment A now has a greater volume of fluid created by the increase in the number of water molecules in it due to osmosis. This increase is contributing to the increase in pressure on that side of the membrane. The higher pressure will tend to oppose the diffusion of more water molecules into compartment A.

Eventually an equilibrium is reached whereby the tendency of the water molecules to cause a net rate of diffusion is balanced by the fluid pressure or osmotic pressure. Note that diffusion has not ceased but it is occurring equally in each direction since the membrane remains permeable to water.

From the above we can conclude that the pressure that develops across a membrane can be created by the numbers of non-diffusible solute particles and water molecules on one side and the number of water molecules on the other. Osmosis would

(a)

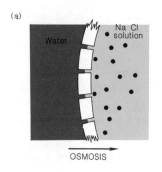

(b)

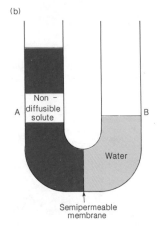

Figure 6.9. (a) Osmosis occurring at a hypothetical cellular membrane when a sodium chloride solution is placed on one side of the membrane and water on the other side. (b) Demonstration of osmotic pressure on the two sides of the semipermeable membrane. (From Guyton: *Physiology of the Human Body.* 5th Ed. Philadelphia. Saunders College Publishing. 1979.)

occur, reducing the numbers of H_2O molecules until the pressure became sufficiently great on the other side to slow or stop a net movement of solvent across the membrane. It can also be seen that the numbers of non-diffusible solute particles present have an extremely important effect. They not only contribute a potential pressure in the fluid, but it is their presence which can result in osmosis and the contribution to the fluid pressure of the new solvent molecules. The important factor here is that the numbers of solvent molecules moving is indirectly affected by the numbers of these solute particles, since it is their numbers that are resulting in the lower solvent concentration. Thus the number of solute particles has the potential to determine the extent of osmosis.

Any two solutions which have the same osmotic pressure are said to be *isosmotic*. If the two solutions are then separated by a membrane, solvent molecules will interchange, but *no net movement of solvent will occur*. It should be noted that no mention has been made of the nature of the solute particles, since osmotic pressure is a function only of the *number of solute particles present in a given volume, i.e. the concentration*. This has particular relevance to the body, since the concentration of particles in different internal environments will determine fluid movement in and out of all cells of the body as well as the kidneys, the bloodstream, the lymphatic system and so forth.

Measurement of Osmotic Pressure
The difference in height which exists at equilibrium between the two compartments labelled A and B (in both Figs 6.8(b) and 6.9(b)) can be measured. It is called the osmotic pressure. The osmotic pressure depends on the difference in concentration of the solvent in the two solutions.

Another way of measuring osmotic pressure is to consider the pressure needed to *stop* the net diffusion of the solvent. This leads to a common definition of osmotic pressure of a solution as the pressure required to prevent the diffusion from a pure solvent into that solution. The unit used should be that used in the SI system for any pressure (i.e. pascal (Pa)) but may be millimetres of mercury (mmHg) or similar. The difference in concentration of the solvent is often referred to as a concentration gradient. Just as water will tend to flow downhill (down an altitude gradient) so water will tend to diffuse down a concentration gradient. Also, since a hill can give rise to a water pressure, so a concentration gradient can give rise to an osmotic pressure.

It is interesting to observe that the osmotic pressure of the blood with respect to water is about 700 000 Pa or 700 kPa. This is equivalent to the pressure required to support a column of water about 67 metres high! However, blood is never interfaced

Figure 6.10. Osmosis and the living cell. (a) A cell is placed in an *isotonic* solution. Because the concentration of solutes (and water molecules) is the same in the solution as in the cell, the net movement of water molecules is zero. (b) A cell is placed in a *hypertonic* solution. The solution has a greater solute (and thus a lower water) concentration than in the cell. Therefore, it exerts an osmotic pressure on the cell. There is a net movement of water molecules out of the cell, and the cell becomes dehydrated, shrinks, and may die. (c) A cell is placed in a *hypotonic* solution. The solution has a lower solute (and thus a greater water) concentration than the cell. The cell contents therefore exert an osmotic pressure on the solution, drawing water molecules inward. There is a net diffusion of water molecules into the cell, and the cell swells and may burst. (Adapted from Solomon & Davis: *Human Anatomy & Physiology*. Philadelphia. Saunders College Publishing. 1983.)

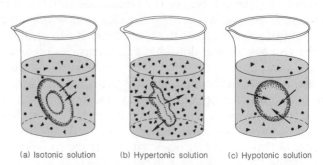

(a) Isotonic solution   (b) Hypertonic solution   (c) Hypotonic solution

with pure water in the body, and the osmotic pressures generated in the body are usually quite small.

The Importance of Osmosis in the Body – Tonicity

If we now refer to Fig. 6.10 and the explanation below the diagram, we see one example of the importance of osmosis in the body. In each of these three cases, just before, the solvent will flow down its concentration gradient. The normal sodium chloride concentration of the blood is 0.9% (0.9 g sodium chloride/100 mL water). Thus it follows that the normal sodium chloride concentration of an erythrocyte or red blood cell will also be 0.9%. A dynamic equilibrium then exists, with water molecules moving into the cell at exactly the same rate as water molecules are moving out of the cell. It is interesting to note that the volume of water moving into (and also out of) each red blood cell per second is approximately 100 times the volume of the cell itself. It then follows that the rates of movement of water molecules in and out of the cell must be precisely equal, otherwise the cell will either shrink to nothing or else burst.

The normal situation described above is one where the cell is said to be **isotonic** with the blood. This means that the cells have the same *tonicity*, i.e. they have *the same concentration of dissolved substances* as the blood.

In Fig. 6.10(a), a cell has been placed in an *isotonic* solution. The water concentration inside and outside the cell is equal, so that a dynamic equilibrium exists in which the rates of water movement into and out of the cell are equal. Thus the cell is not altered in any way.

A solution which causes the cell to shrink is said to be **hypertonic.** A solution with a sodium chloride content of more than 0.9% is hypertonic.

In Fig. 6.10(b), a cell has been placed in a *hypertonic* solution. This is a solution which has a *higher* solute concentration than the cell. This means that the water concentration in the solution is lower than the cell and thus *water will move out of the cell* into the solution by osmosis. The effect of this, as indicated in the diagram, is to shrink the cell. This is called *crenation*.

A solution which causes the cell to swell is said to be **hypotonic**. A solution with a sodium chloride content of less than 0.9% is hypotonic.

In Fig. 6.10(c), a cell has been placed in a *hypotonic* solution. This is a solution which has a *lower* solute concentration than the cell. This means that the water concentration is the solution is higher than the cell and thus *water will move into the cell* from the solution by osmosis. The effect of this, also indicated in the diagram, is to cause the cell to swell and perhaps burst. This is called *haemolysis*.

Thus the shifting of water in and out of the cells influences the state of tension or *tone* of the cells. It can be seen from these potential effects on cells how important it is to maintain body fluids in a relative state of balance or homeostasis with the cells they surround. Osmosis is a major mechanism in maintaining a state of fluid balance in the body. Through it water is able to shift across membranes in relation to changes in water concentrations within the cells and external fluid compartments. Hopefully this will not be as dramatic as in our examples, since in practice the movement of solutes and solvent is very small when all controlling mechanisms are operational.

It should be emphasised that hypertonic and hypotonic are *relative*, not absolute, terms. This means that each term has meaning only when expressed relative to another solution. Thus a 2% sodium chloride solution is hypertonic to plasma with a sodium chloride concentration of 0.9%, but hypotonic to a solution with a sodium chloride concentration of 5%. Note that a 0.9% sodium chloride solution is commonly used in intravenous infusions.

The term isosmotic refers to two solutions which exert the same osmotic pressure.

Most of the preceding information is summarised in Fig. 6.11.

As an example of some of the concepts which we have discussed so far, let us consider the drug mannitol, which is used in a number of clinical settings. This alcohol acts as an osmotic agent and, since it is not absorbed through the alimentary canal, it is administered parenterally. It then becomes widely distributed throughout the ECF (extra-cellular fluid, i.e. the fluid outside the cells) with very little entry into the cells themselves and is essentially excreted by the kidneys. If this drug is administered intravenously, the mannitol enters the bloodstream and hence the ECF, causing the number of particles in the ECF to increase. This means that the number of particles (or number of moles) per unit volume, i.e. the osmolarity of the ECF, has increased.

As a consequence of this, water will move from the ICF (the intracellular fluid) to the ECF, as shown in Fig. 6.12. The

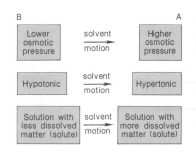

Figure 6.11. The direction of solvent motion in osmosis. (From Nave & Nave: *Physics for the Health Sciences*. 3rd Ed. Philadelphia. W.B. Saunders. 1985.)

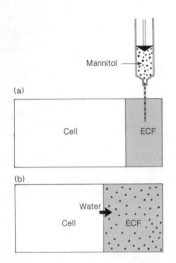

(a)

Mannitol

Cell   ECF

(b)

Water

Cell   ECF

Figure 6.12. Diagram showing the increase in osmolarity and consequent increase in volume of the extracellular fluid (ECF) after the intravenous administration of mannitol. *Note*: the increase in osmolarity of the extracellular fluid as a result of the addition of mannitol causes water to move from the cell into the extracellular fluid, thus increasing the volume of the ECF as shown.

solvent, water, is thus moving in the direction indicated in Fig. 6.11.

It is for this reason that mannitol is used in the treatment of cerebral oedema (a condition in which water accumulates in brain cells). The effect of the mannitol is to cause water to move from the cells of the brain into the ECF, thus relieving the oedema. Mannitol can relieve intraocular (within the eye) pressure by the same mechanism. Furthermore, mannitol acts as a diuretic, i.e. it increases urine output from the body. The reason that it acts as a diuretic is that the extra volume of ECF increases the intravascular pressure or blood pressure. This in turn causes a greater glomerular filtration pressure in the kidneys, which in turn leads to a greater urine output.

However, a word of caution. An increase in the volume of the ECF may be harmful to some people, such as those with congestive heart failure, because the extra fluid volume will increase blood pressure and thus the workload on the heart. In such cases, mannitol may be inappropriate.

Remember the situation which we described in the opening paragraphs of this chapter? If the patient has already lost fluid from the vascular compartment, resulting in high solute levels, the solvent level may then rise very rapidly if the solution is administered too quickly. This will then increase the volume of the blood, which in turn may give rise to a higher level of venous return. As we will see later, **Starling's Law of the Heart** tells us that venous return is the most important factor in determining cardiac output, so that our patient's heart may then become overloaded.

Filtration

The final type of passive transport is that of filtration. This involves the removal of particles from a solution by allowing the liquid to pass through a membrane or other partial barrier. In the body it involves hydrostatic pressure which forces liquid with ions and small molecules dissolved in it, through membranes, leaving behind large molecules (e.g. proteins) and other structures (blood cells). Filtration occurs in the capillaries when blood pressure forces some of its liquid plus small dissolved particles through the walls into the interstitial spaces. It also occurs in the glomerulus of the kidneys, where plasma is forced out and into other structures (Bowman's capsules). This is the beginning of the formation of urine and the substance pushed out is known as the filtrate or glomerular filtrate. It is a one-way process, unlike diffusion.

SUMMARY OF PASSIVE TRANSPORT

Passive transport mechanisms possess the following characteristics:

1. Energy for the process is provided by the kinetic energy of the molecules themselves, the membrane being passive. The membrane is able to control the rate of diffusion by virtue of its permeability, but supplies no energy for the transport process.

2. The tendency in such processes is to always proceed in such a direction as to equalise the differences of particular materials on each side of the membrane. Thus passive diffusion processes occur down a concentration, electrical or pressure gradient, e.g. from a region of high pressure to a region of low pressure. This normally occurs by one of two mechanisms:

(a) By substances or ions becoming dissolved in the lipid matrix or protein molecules of the cell membrane and then diffusing through it in the same way that diffusion occurs in water; or

(b) By diffusion through the pores in the membrane.

The first mechanism is utilised by some substances which can dissolve in the lipid matrix. These include oxygen, carbon dioxide, alcohols, fatty acids and many anaesthetic gases, etc. The diffusion is slower due to the nature of the lipid substances. Water and water-soluble substances may diffuse through the protein molecules present in the membrane but the molecules are selective or specific and the passage of ions and molecules is therefore restricted to specific ones or to certain conditions.

DIFFUSION THROUGH PORES

Some substances such as water, and the various ions dissolved in water, can pass directly through pores as well as through the proteins of the membrane, in some circumstances. The factors which are relevant in diffusion through pores are:

Permeability

A more precise definition of this factor is the rate of transport through the membrane for a given concentration difference. One of the most significant factors determining permeability is obviously pore size. Thus larger molecules such as glucose and plasma proteins are usually not able to pass through the pores.

Factors affecting pore permeability

Pore permeability is not necessarily fixed. The presence of calcium ions is able to alter the permeability of nerve fibres, for example, as we shall see in Chapter 11. Some pores of cells in the kidneys are also affected by antidiuretic hormone (which helps conserve water and reduce diuresis), an important hormone secreted by the posterior pituitary gland. Thus, ions and hormones and possibly other factors such as stimulation can affect pore permeability.

Electrical Charge

This will obviously affect ions, the nature of the charge in turn determining whether the rate of diffusion is impeded or enhanced. Pores are generally believed to be lined with charges, either positive or negative.

ACTIVE TRANSPORT MECHANISMS

Active Transport

This may be defined as the transfer of materials across a membrane against a concentration (or electrical or pressure) gradient. Such a process obviously requires energy and will occur only in living membranes which have a source of energy. There are many instances of active transport in the human body although much remains to be learnt about them.

Why is such a mechanism necessary? In a typical cell, the concentration of potassium ions outside the cell is low, whereas the concentration of potassium ions inside the cell is much higher. However, to maintain this higher concentration inside the cell, the cell has to do continuous work to move K^+ in. It has to expend energy because it is pushing 'uphill', as it were.

Similarly, but conversely, the cell has to maintain a low concentration of sodium ions inside the cell while a higher concentration of sodium ions exists outside the cell.

This mechanism is often referred to as the sodium-potassium pump, and is illustrated in Fig. 6.13.

Ions which are transported by this mechanism include sodium, potassium, hydrogen, calcium, iron, chloride, iodide and urate ions. Substances also transported in that way include several different sugars and amino acids.

The mechanism thought to be involved in active transport is similar to facilitated diffusion, in that it depends upon carriers (see Fig. 6.14). A carrier C combines with a substance S and

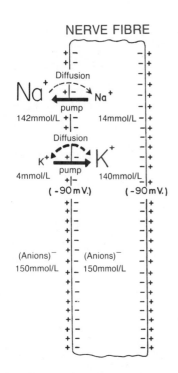

NERVE FIBRE

Figure 6.13. Establishment of a membrane potential of −90 millivolts in the normal resting nerve fibre and development of concentration differences of sodium and potassium ions between the two sides of the membrane. The dashed arrows represent diffusion and the solid arrows represent active transport (pumps). (Adapted from Guyton: *Textbook of Medical Physiology.* 6th Ed. Philadelphia. W.B. Saunders. 1981.)

passes through the membrane CS until the inner surface of the membrane is reached. At this point a reaction occurs (a reaction which is made possible by enzymes) which breaks up the CS into the carrier C and the substance S, consuming energy (from adenosine triphosphate (ATP), which we will discuss later) in the process. The substance S is released to the inside of the cell and the carrier repeats the process or it may take back another type of substance to the outside of the cell (e.g. K^+ in and Na^+ out). It should be noted that the carrier C is specific, and will transport only a particular type of substance(s), so that different carriers transport different types of substances. The sodium-potassium pump is an example of a carrier that will transport only these two ions. Furthermore, the enzyme involved is specific to each reaction in active transport.

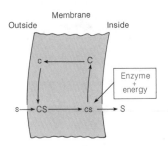

Figure 6.14. Basic mechanism of active transport. (From Guyton: *Textbook of Medical Physiology.* 6th Ed. Philadelphia. W.B. Saunders. 1981.)

This theory embraces the idea that some carriers may be double carriers, i.e. transport more than one ion at a time. However, in any given situation, active transport may be limited by:

- insufficient carrier(s);
- insufficient energy;
- insufficient enzymes.

Although these mechanisms and the theories concerning the way in which they operate may seem relatively straightforward, it should be appreciated that some transport mechanisms are more complex than those described so far. Exactly how the carrier process functions is still debated and several theories exist. Also some mechanisms, like sodium co-transport, are more complex again – it is neither pure diffusion nor active transport. In this case sodium is transported together with glucose or else amino acids in the intestine and the kidneys.

It should also be noted that any transport of a positively charged ion such as sodium may lead to an electrical gradient being created. This may, in turn, cause a movement of negatively charged ions such as the chloride ion, which could then cause a change in osmotic pressure.

Endocytosis

Endocytosis is a general term used to describe processes in which a cell ingests materials as a method of moving them to the interior of the cell.

Phagocytosis

This refers to the ingestion of large particles into the cell by the formation of vesicles (small sacs). The particles involved may be

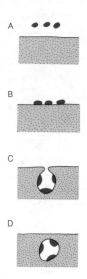

Figure 6.15. Mechanism of pinocytosis. (From Guyton: *Textbook of Medical Physiology*. 6th Ed. Philadelphia. W.B. Saunders. 1981.)

other cells, damaged micro-organisms, cellular debris or foreign material. One example of this is the ingestion of bacteria by white blood cells. This process is of great importance to the immune or defence system of the body since it is capable of destroying bacteria. Not all cells have this phagocytotic capability. Those that do (white blood cells) ingest foreign substances by flowing around them in amoeboid fashion and engulfing them. That part of the cell membrane around the foreign matter is pinched off, forming a sac. Inside the cell the contents of the vesicle are destroyed.

Pinocytosis

This is a very similar process to phagocytosis, the essential difference being one of scale. Minute quantities of fluids and other substances adhere to the cell membrane which invaginates, surrounding these materials and forming tiny vesicles which can be detected only with an electron microscope. The vesicles are pinched off and migrate to the interior of the cell (see Fig. 6.15). The particular importance of pinocytosis is that it is the only mechanism by which very large molecules such as protein, can be transported into a cell.

Exocytosis

This is a method by which substances such as cell secretions and products may leave a cell to enter the extracellular fluids (Fig. 6.16). Many substances produced within a cell are sealed within membrane bound vesicles. These vesicles migrate to the cell membrane where they fuse with the membrane and the contents are released into the interstitial fluids. This process is another energy-consuming process.

Thus we see that active transport, endocytosis and exocytosis are active or physiological energy-requiring processes, compared to diffusion, facilitated diffusion, osmosis and filtration, which are passive or physical processes not requiring energy. It is important to realise that a substance may move by different mechanisms at different times depending on the circumstances. For example Na^+ ions frequently move by active transport, but may move by diffusion if the membranes become permeable to them.

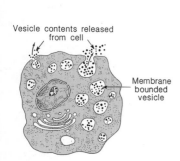

Figure 6.16. The process of exocytosis. A membrane-bounded vesicle fuses with the plasma membrane, and the contents of the vesicle are released from the cell.

Example of Transport Mechanisms

We will now look at one important example of transport mechanisms in the body to illustrate some of the points discussed above. Let us consider the transport of fluids from the blood capillaries into the interstitial fluid and thence into the cells, thus:

blood   ⟶   interstitial   ⟶   body
capillaries   (1)   fluid   (2)   cells

Step 1 apparently occurs by a passive diffusion mechanism. The plasma, with the exception of the very large protein molecules, is able to move through the capillary walls into the tissue spaces.

                   tissue
plasma   ⟶   plasma in tissue spaces
            walls   (except very large proteins)

Now:

(a) Normal blood pressure (as well as hydrostatic pressure – the pressure of the blood at rest, caused by the force of gravity acting on the blood) is exerted on the selectively permeable capillary walls and this tends to force plasma out by filtration.

(b) Opposing this, however, is the fact that the protein molecules in the capillaries give rise to an osmotic pressure with respect to water – the water concentration is higher outside the capillary than inside.

(c) Furthermore, the concentration of small molecules, glucose, electrolytes and water inside the capillary at the arterial end is greater than that outside, so that these tend to diffuse out of the capillary also (see Fig. 6.17).

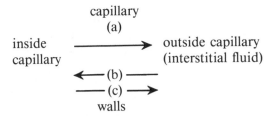

This gives rise to an osmotic pressure difference of about 22 mmHg (3.0 kPa). This needs to be compared to the blood pressure in capillaries, which is variable, but in which there is a consistent drop in pressure between the arteriolar (joined to arteries) end and the venular (joined to veins) end – from about 35 mmHg (4.7 kPa) to about 15 mmHg (2.0 kPa).

As can be seen in Fig 6.17, the net pressure at the arteriolar end is (35–22) mmHg or 13 mmHg (1.7 kPa) *outwards*. Similarly, the net pressure at the venular end is (22–15) mmHg or 7 mmHg (10 kPa) *inwards*. Since blood pressures still tend to be quoted in the old units, both sets of units have been given.

Note: Figure 6.17 is a simplified diagram. The reader is invited to pursue this matter further in texts such as Guyton's

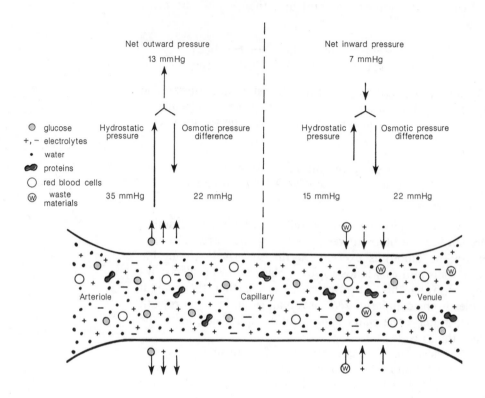

Figure 6.17. Molecular transfer in the capillary system. (From Nave & Nave: *Physics for the Health Sciences*. 3rd Ed. Philadelphia. W.B. Saunders. 1985.)

Medical Physiology. However, **Starling's Equilibrium for capillary exchange** still becomes apparent – that the movement of materials in and out of the capillaries at the two ends is in near equilibrium, with a slightly higher outward pressure. The slight outward movement of fluid which results from this is balanced by an inward input by the lymphatic system.

Many of the large molecules which stay in the capillaries are blood proteins so that loss of these would upset the balance of water and solute movement described. In fact, this lowers the osmotic pressure with the result that:

1. The difference between the osmotic and the hydrostatic pressures *increases* at the *arteriolar* end, so that the net outward pressure increases, and more fluid leaves the capillaries and passes into the tissues.

2. The difference between the osmotic and the hydrostatic pressures *decreases* at the *venular* end, so that the net inward pressure decreases, and less fluid leaves the tissues and passes into the capillaries

3. Both of these results lead to an *increase in tissue fluid* levels, i.e. to oedema.

FACTORS WHICH INFLUENCE FLUID MOVEMENT

1. **Plasma proteins** – as described above, the loss of these from the blood, through injury or surgery for example, will lead to an increase of tissue fluid levels.

2. **The concentration of electrolytes** which, of course, exist as ions such as Na^+, K^+, Cl^- and HCO_3^- and other constituents such as acetoacetic acid resulting from the breakdown of fats in people suffering from *diabetes mellitus*.

3. **Hormones** – These control the concentration of electrolytes and other blood constituents such as glucose. In Addison's disease, for example, lack of ADH (antidiuretic hormone) leads to a failure of the kidneys to re-absorb sodium and chloride ions. People suffering from Cushing's disease (an increased secretion of cortisol) have elevated blood levels of glucose.

4. **Changes in capillary pressure** which lead to changes in water volume.

As an example, if the kidneys are malfunctioning due to renal disease, proteins can be lost from the blood.

Returning now to our two-stage process, viz.,

$$\text{blood capillaries} \xrightarrow{(1)} \text{interstitial fluid} \xrightarrow{(2)} \text{body cells}$$

we are now in a position to discuss the second step.

Step 2 involves more than diffusion, because diffusion can not explain the transfer of fluid from the interstitial fluid to the body cells. Various cells of the body have different needs and maintain different concentration gradients with respect to the plasma. The interchange of substances between the interstitial fluid and the body cells is meticulously regulated by the cell membrane, as discussed above in relation to blood cells. Similarly, all of the discussion above regarding the movement of ions in and out of cells, the maintenance of an electrical potential inside and outside a cell membrane and the presence of pumps in cells, applies just as well to the different body cells as it does to the red blood cells, so there is no need to repeat that discussion here.

Dialysis

In our discussion of osmosis we have spoken of the transport of only one material – the solvent – across a membrane. However membranes exist in the body which are permeable to a number of different molecules. For example, some membranes are permeable to water, salts, glucose, urea and other organic molecules (molecules of compounds of carbon). Larger molecules

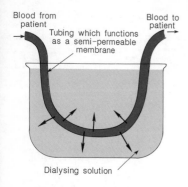

Blood from patient

Blood to patient

Tubing which functions as a semi-permeable membrane

Dialysing solution

Figure 6.18. The principle of dialysis.

such as haemoglobin, albumin, globulin and other protein molecules are normally not able to pass through the membrane. The process of liquids, small molecules and ions passing through a membrane is called **dialysis** (Fig. 6.18).

Haemodialysis and Peritoneal Dialysis

Many of the concepts and principles discussed in this chapter are utilised in the dramatic medical treatments known as hae-modialysis and peritoneal dialysis. The term dramatic is used because they can have very rapid effects and because they are life-saving measures in most patients. It is therefore appropriate that we have a brief look at these measures which are able to replace some of the roles of the kidneys.

When partial or total kidney dysfunction occurs, their major roles of waste eliminators, acid-base regulators (see Chapter 8) and fluid and electrolyte regulators may need to be assisted or be taken over completely on either a temporary or permanent basis. If such measures are not taken, death may occur because these roles are not being fulfilled.

Haemodialysis and peritoneal dialysis are two methods of assisting or replacing normal kidney function.

Haemodialysis
This is a process by which blood is passed over one side of a semipermeable, artificial membrane, and a suitable fluid is passed over the other side of the membrane in the opposite direction. The membrane is porous enough to allow all constit-uents of plasma, except the colloidal plasma proteins, to diffuse freely in both directions.

The basic objective of this technique is to rid the blood of *unwanted or excess substances*, a function which the kidneys are not performing or, at least, not performing satisfactorily. The unwanted substances are waste products such as urea and creatinine; excessive or abnormal quantities of essential sub-stances (electrolytes, acids, bases, glucose, water etc.) and toxic substances, e.g. drugs (such as an overdose of barbiturates). Another objective may be to increase the concentration of certain substances, such as electrolytes.

The dialysing solution will be designed to meet some or all of the objectives which have been outlined. For example, the osmolarity (concentrations of various substances) of the dialysing solution will facilitate diffusion of liquid (water) out of the vascular compartment when the water concentration there is too high by establishing a concentration gradient in the direction of the dialysing solution. Water will then diffuse into the dialysing solu-tion and be removed from the vascular compartment (the blood).

The diffusion of water in the opposite direction (i.e. into the blood) can be arranged if the water content of the blood is too low, by changing the osmolarity of the dialysing solution so that a concentration gradient exists in the direction of the blood. If the water content of the blood is as it should be, an equilibrium concentration can be established so that no water diffuses in either direction.

The solute concentration of the dialysing solution will also be designed to re-establish normal concentrations of solutes in the plasma. No urea or creatinine will be present in the solution so that almost all of the waste products will diffuse outwards from the blood. Electrolyte concentrations will be almost identical to normal plasma levels, so that only excess concentrations will diffuse out, leaving almost normal plasma levels in the blood.

The continuous but *opposing flow* of the dialysing solution ensures that the blood is continually running over fresh fluid on the other side of the membrane, resulting in a *continuous* diffusion of substances across the membrane. The substances which have diffused out of the blood are thus being constantly and immediately carried away in the dialysing solution.

In addition, pressure can be utilised, by controlling the flow of the dialysing solution in such a way that a pressure gradient is established across the membrane in the direction of the dialysing solution. This promotes *filtration*.

This is the major method of removing relatively large quantities of fluid from the vascular compartment in a short time.

Blood is diverted from the patient (by an arteriovenous shunt for example), by insertion of needles and with the aid of a pump, and passed through the artificial kidney and back to the patient. A number of different kinds and designs of dialyser exist, from the very large types like the Kiil (Fig. 6.19) to the more compact units which clean the dialysing solution and re-use it. The needs of the individual patient, the medical situation and the preferences of the medical staff usually dictate the particular type of artificial kidney chosen for the patient. Figure 6.20 (a) shows one type.

However, all types work on the same basic principle – the principle of diffusion as discussed; all have the same requirements – a membrane, access to the patient's blood and a dialysing fluid. Research is currently being conducted towards the development of an artificial kidney which can be carried on, or even in, the body of a patient.

Peritoneal Dialysis
Here diffusion and osmosis are the major players in the act. This type of treatment is appropriate for the same reasons as have been discussed for haemodialysis. However, there are a few major differences between this method and haemodialysis. The

Figure 6.19. Diagram of the artificial kidney. (From Guyton: *Textbook of Medical Physiology.* 6th Ed. Philadelphia. W.B. Saunders. 1981.)

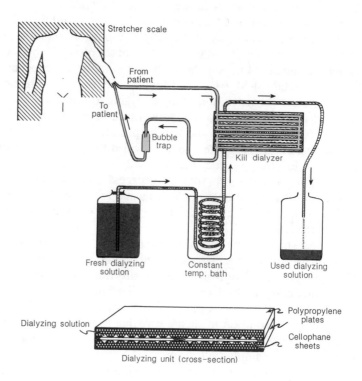

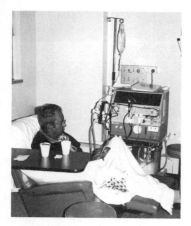

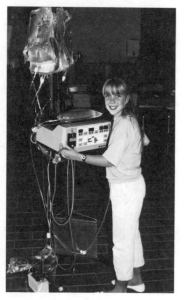

Figure 6.20 (a) top. Haemodialysis in comfort at home.
(b). Peritoneal dialysis with some mobility.(Courtesy of Gambro Pty Ltd.)

membranes used in this case are not artificial, but are those surrounding the abdominal cavity – the peritoneal membranes. In this technique, a dialysing solution, having similar characteristics as that employed in haemodialysis, is run into the abdominal cavity, left for a short, controlled, period of time and drained out. This is repeated, using new fluid each time, over a 24 or 36 hour period, for example. (See Figure 3.1).

During the time that the solution is contained in the abdominal cavity, diffusion and osmosis will occur across the membranes, as determined by plasma and dialysing solution concentrations.

This type of dialysis is slower and is not as effective as haemodialysis in some situations. An example is shown in Figure 6.20 (b).

A more detailed study of these treatments would reveal that they both present very real hazards to the patient which are not present if his own kidneys are operating satifactorily. These hazards include infection, damage to blood cells, haemorrhage, excessive removal of some substances (such as water) leading to shock and other problems. Against these dangers, however, is the very life of the patient. Indeed, in cases of renal failure, there is no doubt that this application of the concepts and principles of solute and solvent movement through membranes is the most effective form of artificial treatment available – not counting kidney transplants – to replace kidney function and thus sustain the life of the patient.

DEHYDRATION

If water losses from the body are severe (as can occur in hot conditions or as a result of fever, continued vomiting and/or diarrhoea) and this water is not replaced, **dehydration** can occur. In such a case, extracellular fluid is lost and is then constantly being replaced by water from within the cell, which interferes with the proper functioning of that cell. This condition can rapidly prove fatal if not corrected.

Because of the seriousness of this condition and the fact that it is a frequent cause of death, particularly in young children, we will consider it in more detail.

Hypertonic Dehydration

In this case body water is lost faster than electrolytes are, causing body fluid volume to be reduced. The effect of this is that body fluids become hypertonic to their normal state – the concentration of salts is higher than it should be because the water content is lower. This results from the causes listed above, particularly from chronic diarrhoea in infants.

It is most important that this type of loss be corrected by an intake of water. Such home remedies as boiled skim milk are dangerous because they only serve to make the condition worse. In the case of skim milk, its very high sodium content would tend to cause even further water loss into the gut.

The ultimate effects of this water loss include very viscous (thick) blood, a fall in blood pressure, sluggish circulation and eventual heart failure. Prior to this, kidney malfunction occurs resulting in excessive urea production and blood pH alteration; and urine flow (which has already decreased because of increased ADH production), decreases further and may stop. Respiratory secretions also become viscous, giving rise to breathing difficulties, and the skin may become doughy in texture, particularly in children, because of water loss in tissues.

Finally, shrinkage in the brain and the blood vessels in the brain can eventually produce brain haemorrhage, with all that this implies.

Isotonic Dehydration

This is the most common form of depletion of fluids; it involves *fluid loss without any real change of electrolyte* concentration, since electrolytes are lost as the fluid is lost. Isotonic dehydration can result from haemorrhage, fluid loss from severe or extensive burns, severe vomiting and/or diarrhoea etc. Homeostatic mechanisms tend to rapidly compensate for this loss by restoring blood pressure and transferring fluid (containing electrolytes) from tissues to the blood to offset depletion of blood volume. However, if volume loss continues these mechanisms can no longer cope, the blood pressure drops and death eventually follows.

Hypotonic Dehydration

In this case both body fluid volume and electrolyte concentration are depleted. It commonly occurs following hypertonic or isotonic dehydration in which fluid volume is replaced without any replacement of lost electrolytes. The water intake means that the depletion of volume may not be very great, but the depletion in electrolytes in the body fluids is very significant.

Persistent vomiting and inability to drink (or the unwilling-ness of very young children to drink), will often result in the depletion of such ions as chloride and hydrogen as the gastric juice is regurgitated.

The loss of hydrogen ions results in **alkalosis** (a condition in which the blood is more alkaline than it should be; as discussed later). Hypotonic dehydration leads to muscular disorders and weakness, cardiac disturbances and seizures.

The overwhelming importance of an understanding of body fluids now should be apparent to the reader. It will also be apparent that the welfare and indeed the very life of the patient will very much depend on this understanding.

REVIEW

1. Distinguish between:
   (a) an homogeneous and a heterogeneous mixture
   (b) a solution and a suspension
   (c) an emulsion and a gel.
2. What is the difference between a mole and an osmole?
3. What is the essential difference between a semipermeable membrane and a selectively permeable membrane?
4. What are the three principal factors which determine the rate at which electrolytes diffuse in the body?
5. Describe the transport of liquids and solids from the capillary into the cell.
6. Explain the method by which cells can ingest bacteria during an immune response.
7. Describe the effect on a red blood cell of a hypertonic sodium chloride solution and a hypotonic sodium chloride solution.
8. A patient suffering from a disease lost a large volume of water from the vascular compartment.
   (a) What effect would this have on the vascular compartment?
   (b) What type of dehydration is this?
   (c) How would the body attempt to restore homeostasis?

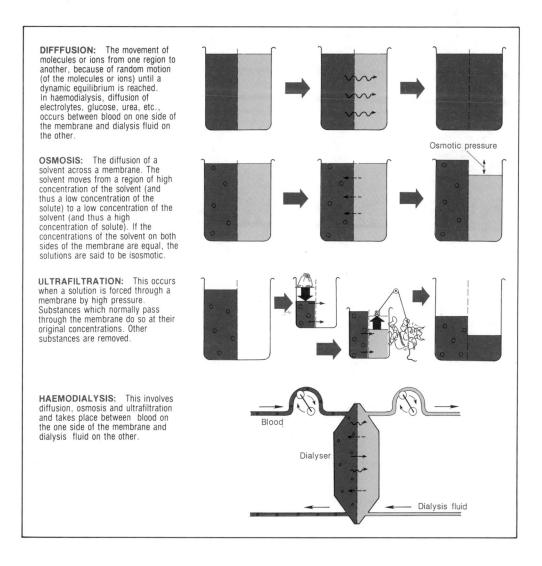

DIFFFUSION: The movement of molecules or ions from one region to another, because of random motion (of the molecules or ions) until a dynamic equilibrium is reached. In haemodialysis, diffusion of electrolytes, glucose, urea, etc., occurs between blood on one side of the membrane and dialysis fluid on the other.

OSMOSIS: The diffusion of a solvent across a membrane. The solvent moves from a region of high concentration of the solvent (and thus a low concentration of the solute) to a low concentration of the solvent (and thus a high concentration of solute). If the concentrations of the solvent on both sides of the membrane are equal, the solutions are said to be isosmotic.

ULTRAFILTRATION: This occurs when a solution is forced through a membrane by high pressure. Substances which normally pass through the membrane do so at their original concentrations. Other substances are removed.

HAEMODIALYSIS: This involves diffusion, osmosis and ultrafiltration and takes place between blood on the one side of the membrane and dialysis fluid on the other.

Osmotic pressure

Blood

Dialyser

Dialysis fluid

A summary of dialysis and associated terms. (*Courtesy of Gambro Pty Ltd.*)

7

Fluids – liquids and gases

OBJECTIVES

After studying this chapter the student should be able to:

1. Apply a knowledge of the gas laws to describe the process of breathing.
2. Describe the role of a surfactant in the breathing process.
3. State Dalton's law and Henry's law. Use these laws to explain the movement of oxygen and carbon dioxide into and out of the blood at the lungs and tissues.
4. List the properties of oxygen that make it most suitable for use in the body.
5. Identify the safety measures that must be observed whenever oxygen is being used.
6. Describe the measures that must be taken to prevent oxygen toxicity.
7. State Pascal's principle and describe its importance in terms of cardiac output and venous return.
8. Describe the pressure changes involved in the circulation of the blood.
9. List and describe the factors that affect the flow of blood through blood vessels.

INTRODUCTION

We would now like to present a series of nursing problems. If you know the answers and can present a basis for those answers, you already have a knowledge of some of the principles of dynamics and pressure in liquids. If not, after having read through the problems, join us in our journey through these important principles and properties so that you will then be able to apply them to nursing practice. Then when you have finished reading the chapter, why not come back and try answering these questions to see how you fare?

Questions

1. We have an elderly patient who has had complete bed rest for a time and who is showing signs of skin problems, such as redness and tenderness, particularly over bony prominences, in spite of receiving good basic skin care. Would placing the patient on a water bed or mattress be likely to make any difference? Why?

2. If a nurse is irrigating a patient's eye with a prescribed, sterile liquid, is there any particular danger associated with running the liquid over the cornea (the outer layer) of the eyeball?

3. If a patient is suspected of having a growth (tumour) in the brain, why could it be expected that a lumbar puncture (the insertion of a special needle into the lower back region of the spinal canal) might be one of the diagnostic procedures for which you would prepare?

4. Imagine a situation where a nurse is administering an enema to a patient (i.e. inserting a solution into the lower bowel area through the anus) to assist evacuation and cleansing. The solution does not seem to be flowing satisfactorily from the suspended container through the tube to the bowel. After the nurse has checked the equipment and the patient, would it make any difference to the patient if she just kept raising the level of the container to increase the flow? Is there any better way of increasing the flow?

5. A patient has been told that she should keep moving or flexing her legs and feet when she returns to work as a cashier in a supermarket. Why?

6. Why should an intravenous fluid bottle or container be kept above the level of the patient's body?

7. In another case, a patient is being transported by trolley. It is noted that an open urinary drainage system is lying on top of the bed. Is there anything wrong with this situation?

PRESSURE IN FLUIDS

Most people probably have a general idea of the meaning of pressure, but falter when asked to explain what it means. It is appropriate, then, to begin with a simple definition. Pressure may be defined as **force per unit area**. Thus:

$$\text{pressure (Pa)} = \frac{\text{force (newtons)}}{\text{area (m}^2\text{)}}$$

Since this concept is often not well understood, let us consider some examples that may help to make it clearer. Stiletto heels are quite popular for women's shoes, although they are less than popular with the owners of polished wooden floors because of the marks that they leave. Why should this be the case? The wearers of the shoes do not suddenly put on weight, of course; they are exerting the same downward force whether they are wearing stiletto-heeled shoes or sneakers. However, that same force was being exerted over a very small area in the case of the stiletto heels. Since a constant force is being divided by a very small number (the small area), this gives rise to a much larger pressure. This larger pressure then causes indentations in floors. As a comparison, the same force is distributed over a much larger area in the case of the sneakers, so that the pressure exerted on the floor is much less.

To further illustrate this point, let us consider a woman of mass 70 kg. The 'downward' force that she exerts is given by her weight:

Weight (w) = mg (where m = mass and g = the acceleration due
to gravity)
= 70 × 9.8

Therefore

$$\text{weight} = 686 \text{ newtons.}$$

If she is wearing conventional heels, they could have a total area on both shoes of 40 square centimetres. We are using this unit rather than the SI units (square metres) for convenience.

$$\text{pressure} = \frac{\text{force}}{\text{area}} \qquad = \frac{686}{40}$$
$$= \text{approximately 17 newtons/cm}^2$$

If we now take the same woman in a pair of stiletto heels, the area might be 0.6 cm^2.

$$\text{pressure} = \frac{\text{force}}{\text{area}} \qquad = \frac{686}{0.6}$$
$$= \text{approximately 1140 newtons/cm}^2$$

This is comparable to the pressure which would be exerted by the mass of about 10 elephants acting on one elephant's foot (provided that the elephant was not wearing stiletto heels!).

The second illustration of this concept is that of holding a weight by one's finger. If the weight is suspended by a wide piece of tape it is much more comfortable over one's finger than if it is suspended by a piece of thin wire. In both cases the force is the same, but the thin wire is acting over a much smaller area, once again giving rise to a much greater pressure than is the case with the tape, where the area of contact with the finger is much larger.

The concept of pressure applies equally well to solids, liquids and gases, since the force involved may be applied equally well by any one of these. In nursing, some examples of pressure exerted on or by solids do arise, for example:

1. When a patient is lying in bed on a conventional mattress, the weight of the patient tends to be concentrated at just a few points of contact with the mattress – the sacral area and the heels, for example. It should be noted that all these contact points lie over sharp and/or prominent bones and the tissues involved are not adapted to *weight-bearing* as are the soles of the feet.

Since the heels are only small in area, the pressure on them is very considerable and it is no wonder that skin problems occur with patients who are confined to bed for prolonged periods. Skin breakdown may occur because of compression of skin tissue, small blood vessels and even nerves in some patients, all of which can cause numerous complications for the patient. In addition to *compression*, a shearing force or drag occurs when the body is inadequately supported so that skin tissue is dragged or slides over bed linen (see Fig. 7.1).

2. The jagged end of a broken bone has a very tiny cross-sectional area on any protruding portions, so that any force exerted on tissue by that protruding portion is manifested as a very high pressure.

3. It should be remembered that our bodies are designed to function while a *constant pressure* of just over 100 kPa (kilopascals, where the pascal [Pa] is the SI unit of pressure) is exerted by the atmosphere on every external surface of the body. If the body is suddenly placed in a situation where the pressure is lower than this – a pilot of a jet aircraft who ejects at a high altitude, for example – the effect on the body can be traumatic and even fatal. Many of the fine blood vessels in the ears and nose tend to bleed profusely, because the lower atmospheric pressure at high altitudes cannot prevent these fine blood vessels from bursting.

However, since our chief concern in this section is with liquids, we will now look at these in more detail.

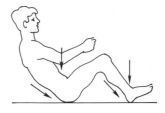

Figure 7.1. The shearing force exerts a downward and forward pressure.

Pressure in Static Liquids

Pressure is exerted *equally in all direction* in an enclosed or static liquid. Since there is no fluid movement, the liquid is in a state of balance. The forces on any one molecule in the body of the liquid would be acting in pairs (up/down, side to side) such that the net force is zero. The molecule would be in equilibrium. The concept that pressure acts in all directions makes the transmission of pressure by fluids possible in static liquids even through tubing such as intravenous tubing.

Pascal's Principle

This states that **any change in pressure in an enclosed fluid is transmitted equally and undiminished to every part of the fluid.** This principle is utilised in the hydraulic press, where an effort exerted on a small cylinder creates a change in pressure which is then transmitted to a large cylinder, enabling the operator to exert a stronger force (Fig. 7.2).

The hydraulic lifts used to move patients from or into beds, or into swimming pools for therapy, particularly if the patient is heavy or disabled, utilise this principle, as shown in Fig. 7.3. Operating tables are raised and lowered using the same principle.

Another interesting example is that of *water or air mattresses*. These have particular applications for patients who are susceptible to the development of pressure sores – those who are unconscious, paralysed or confined to bed. Whereas the body tends to be supported on a limited area in a conventional bed, the even distribution of pressure to all parts of the body by an air or water bed (in accordance with Pascal's principle) helps to make the patient very much more comfortable. Furthermore, the reduction in the possibility of skin damage from pressure is most important. However, for maximum benefit the patient must be *fully supported over the entire body area*, be in direct contact with

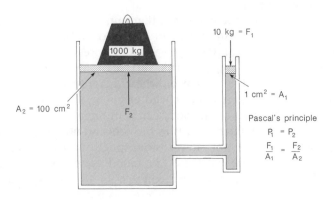

Figure 7.2. The operation of a hydraulic press. A small effort force on the small piston overcomes a large resistance force on the large piston. (From Nave & Nave: *Physics for the Health Sciences*. 3rd Ed. Philadelphia. W.B. Saunders 1985.)

10 kg = F_1

1 cm^2 = A_1

A_2 = 100 cm^2

F_2

Pascal's principle

$P_1 = P_2$

$\dfrac{F_1}{A_1} = \dfrac{F_2}{A_2}$

the mattress and the mattress must contain sufficient fluid to ensure that the patient's body does not touch the mattress base. The use of this device does not eliminate the need for the usual nursing care given to all patients confined to bed – turning, position changing, pressure area care – as it is an aid to care, not a replacement for it.

The cerebrospinal fluid (CSF) of the brain and spinal cord may be regarded as a *closed system*, and thus Pascal's principle will apply. This means that any increase in pressure at any location within the system will cause an increase in pressure throughout the whole system. Thus any abnormal growth or tumour that intrudes into space normally occupied by CSF will give rise to an increased pressure in all parts of the fluid. This increase in pressure may be measured at any convenient location, such as between the third and fourth lumbar vertebrae, by means of a spinal tap.

An instrument called a manometer is used to measure this pressure, and the liquid employed in this case is water. In the **Queckenstedt test** for detecting obstruction of the CSF flow, pressure in the cranium (those bones of the skull which together with the CSF form a protective cavity for the brain) is increased by squeezing the jugular veins. If no obstruction to the passage of CSF exists, the application of Pascal's principle indicates that this increase in pressure will be transmitted to all parts of the fluid and thus the water level in the manometer (being used in the spinal tap) will rise. If, however, an obstruction exists, the water level in the manometer will be unaffected because the pressure cannot now be transmitted to other parts of the fluid.

One other example of Pascal's principle is that of **central**

Figure 7.3. Example of a hydraulic lift. (From Nave & Nave: *Physics for the Health Sciences*. 3rd Ed. Philadelphia. W.B. Saunders. 1985.)

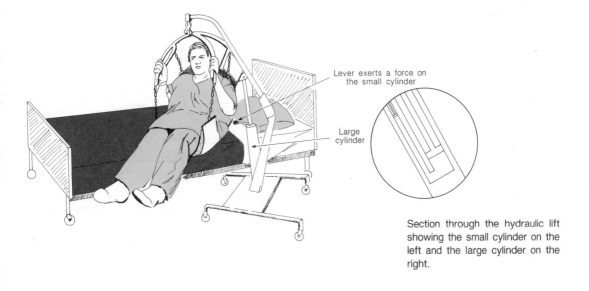

Lever exerts a force on the small cylinder

Large cylinder

Section through the hydraulic lift showing the small cylinder on the left and the large cylinder on the right.

venous pressure (CVP), which is the pressure of the blood in the right atrium. As in the case above, the pressure is measured with a manometer, although of a different type (see Fig. 7.4).

In another application, a fetus may suffer a deformity if the mother increases the pressure on the amniotic fluid by frequently or continually wearing tight clothing. Any increase in pressure in any part of the fluid will be transmitted throughout the fluid and this may cause damage to the fetus. The advantage of this arrangement, however, is that the effect of any blow is distributed uniformly throughout the fluid, and thus the fetus is protected.

Similarly, any abnormal increase in enclosed fluid pressures in the body may cause damage or acute discomfort. Examples include the pericardial and pleural cavities, and the eye. In the case of the eye, damage to the optic nerve may result. For example, if the eye receives a severe blow or if proper care is not exercised during eye irrigations, the high pressure applied to the cornea can be transmitted to the interior of the eye – to the retina or the optic nerve. **Glaucoma** involves a build-up of pressure in the eyeball as a result of increased fluid production which, if not treated, can damage the retina and then the optic nerve, leading to blindness. Under normal circumstances, the fluid in the eye does protect the retina.

One other example of the build-up of pressure is that of the bladder. As the reader well knows, this can be distressingly uncomfortable until relieved by micturition (passing urine). This is stimulated by the general pressure exerted by the enclosed fluid on nerve receptors in the walls of the bladder.

Pascal's principle and other background understanding will

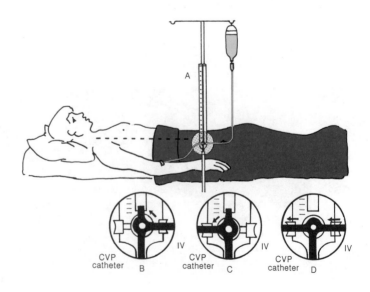

Figure 7.4. Procedure for measuring CVP with a manometer. A. Manometer and IV tubing in place. B. Turn the stopcock so that the manometer fills with fluid above the level of the expected pressure. C. Turn the stopcock so that the IV is off and the fluid in the manometer flows to the patient. Obtain a reading after the fluid level stabilises. D. Turn the stopcock to resume the IV flow to the patient.

also be applied to the flow of blood in the human body. However, there are a few points that need to be covered to complete this background knowledge.

Liquids in Enclosed Containers
One of the properties of a liquid is that it will adopt the shape of the container in which it is placed. It follows, then, that the shape of the container is not important and does not affect the properties of the liquid inside. This same applies to the size of the container.

Pressure at any point below the surface of a liquid in an enclosed container depends upon two factors:

1. The **height** of the liquid column. In the example of the metal can, we see that the lower the hole is (or the higher the liquid column is), the greater will be the pressure. This means that the *pressure is proportional to the height of the liquid column*, sometimes called the 'head'.

2. The **density** of the liquid. Mercury, for example, has a very high density which means that the weight of the liquid above each of the holes will be *greater*. Since the density of mercury is 13.6 times as great as the density of water, a column of mercury will weigh 13.6 times as much as a column of water of the same height and thus give rise to a pressure 13.6 times as great as that caused by water. Once again, we say that the pressure exerted by the liquid is proportional to the density.

Combining these two conclusions we then have: **The pressure exerted by a column of a liquid is proportional to the height of the column and the density of the liquid.**

These facts should be borne in mind by the practising nurse when administering solutions such as intravenous infusions and transfusions, etc.

Pressure in Flowing Liquids

It has been stated that pressure in static liquids is transmitted equally in all directions and is dependent on the height and density of the column of liquid, at any point below its surface. These concepts underlie the use of intravenous infusions (Fig. 7.5) and medical treatments such as some types of enemas. In the static situation (intravenous infusion not flowing) the pressure at the point of input to the patient will be *proportional* to the *height of the open surface of the solution* and *the density of the solution*, e.g. five per cent glucose or whole blood. However, once the

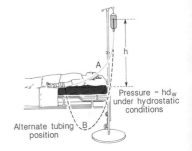

Figure 7.5. Intravenous apparatus as an example of the transmission of pressure. Under hydrostatic (no flow) conditions, the pressure at the patient's arm would be the same in configuration *A* and *B*. (From Nave & Nave: *Physics for the Health Sciences*. 3rd Ed. Philadelphia. W.B. Saunders. 1985.)

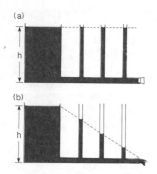

Figure 7.6. (a) The pressure is the same at all points along the horizontal tube when there is no flow. (b) A uniform pressure drop occurs when there is smooth flow through a uniform tube. (From Nave & Nave: *Physics for the Health Sciences*. 3rd Ed. Philadelphia. W.B. Saunders. 1985.)

infusion starts to flow into the patient, the situation changes, and other factors become involved that affect the pressure (Fig. 7.6). In fact, there will be a *drop in pressure* between the beginning of the tube and the exit point. This is not to say that relatively large pressures cannot be created at the exit point of tubes of flowing fluids, but rather that the additional factors may have to be overcome.

This pressure gradient in flowing liquids in a tube is caused by *fluid friction*, leading to resistance to the flow of the liquid and thus altering the *volume flow rate*. Friction may result from several factors:

- the walls of the tubing;
- the diameter of the tube
- the consistency of the liquid (viscosity)
- the type of flow pattern (smooth, rough).

Each of these and others will be discussed later in detail in relation to blood flow, since blood is the flowing liquid of greatest importance in the body. However, it should be pointed out that the law governing the flow of an ideal fluid does not completely apply to blood flow. The law, **Poiseuille's law**, may be simplified to the following statement: **the volume flow rate will be equal to the pressure drop divided by the resistance**, under laminar flow, or smooth conditions where wall friction is not significant. Pure liquids such as water obey this law, but the presence of blood cells, colloids, etc., make blood too complex a liquid. For example, water viscosity does not depend on pressure, so that if pressure changes it does not alter the viscosity. The same cannot be said for blood, as changes in viscosity seem to occur under some conditions in relation to pressure changes. However, Poiseuille's law has some general application, as will be seen.

Application of Pressure Concepts

In intravenous infusions, it is found that an increase in the height of the liquid container will cause an increase in pressure at the point of entry of the needle. Since the pressure increases, this may be damaging and/or painful for the patient, particularly if the needle slips into the tissues, so that care is required.

At this point, it may well be appropriate to ask why pressure is needed at all. Remember that a certain pressure does exist in the veins, so that the applied pressure is needed to push the fluid into the vein against this. If the nurse momentarily lowers the pressure at the entry point, by laying the flask on the bed or lowering it below the level of the patient, a backflow of blood will occur, because the height of the solution level is lower and so is the pressure.

At the beginning of this chapter, we gave the example of the administration of an enema. In this case as before, raising the height of the container will increase the height of the fluid column in relation to the entry point of the fluid, and thus cause an increase in pressure and an increase in volume flow rate. However, this increase in pressure can cause discomfort or cramping to the patient, and might damage bowel tissue in some circumstances. A much more satisfactory method of increasing the volume flow rate is to use tubing with a larger bore. This will serve to increase the volume flow rate without increasing the pressure.

Other factors may be significant, of course. In the above example, the wider bore tubing will only do its job if the opening or orifice at the end of the tubing is as large (or almost as large) as the bore of the tubing.

BLOOD FLOW IN THE BODY

This very important section will be treated under a number of sub-headings, all of which are significant in explaining our present knowledge of the operation of the circulatory system.

Blood flow through blood vessels is determined by two overall factors:

1. Pressure difference between the two ends of the vessel – this is the force that pushes the blood through the vessel.
2. Resistance.

Pascal's principle has almost universal application in the circulatory system. Whenever blood is considered, whether it be in a chamber of the heart or a tiny capillary, the principle holds true. For example, the large increase in the pressure of the blood in the left ventricle in the early stages of ventricular systole (the contraction or pumping phase) is transmitted throughout the chamber and is then responsible for opening the aortic valve when the pressure in the left ventricle exceeds that in the aorta.

It should be noted, however, that while Pascal's principle applies equally well to a fine capillary, the nature and characteristics of capillaries change from the arterial end to the venous end and, as we have already seen in Chapter 6, this results in a considerable change in pressure from one end of the capillary to another.

Blood Pressure, Blood Flow and Resistance

Any fluid will flow down a **pressure gradient**. That is, the fluid will flow from a point of higher pressure to a point of lower

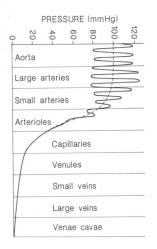

Figure 7.7. Blood pressures in the different portions of the circulatory system. (From Guyton: *Textbook of Medical Physiology*, 6th Ed. Philadelphia. W.B. Saunders. 1981.)

pressure. Note that it is a *difference* in pressure that is significant, not the actual values of the pressure.

For example, if the pressure at one end of a tube is 100 mm mercury (Hg) and the pressure at the other is 0, the pressure difference is 100 mmHg; and if the pressure at one end of another tube is 1100 mmHg and the pressure at the other end is 1000 mmHg, the pressure difference is also 100 mmHg. Thus the pressure available to drive the fluid along the tube is exactly the same in both cases.

In the circulatory system, a large pressure gradient exists between the beginning of the system – the aorta – and the end outside the right atrium of the heart (Figs 7.7 and 7.8). Pressure in the aorta is highest, averaging 100 mmHg, since blood is pumped directly into it. Blood pressure falls progressively as it passes through the systemic circulation, dropping to approximately 0 mmHg at the right atrium. The decrease in pressure is directly proportional to vascular resistance. This does not necessarily mean, however, that fluid flow will be the same in all cases – for different fluids or for different tubes. This leads us to the concept of resistance. **Resistance** to the flow of fluid through a tube is the *tendency to oppose that flow*.

Resistance depends upon:

1. The **viscosity** of the liquid. Viscosity is a measure of the resistance of a liquid to flow. Thus, treacle is more viscous than water because it does not flow as readily as water. Blood is similarly more viscous than water. Viscosity arises from the mutual cohesive forces of the molecules in the liquid. The stronger the cohesive forces, the greater is the resistance to flow. Factors that break or disrupt these forces or strengthen them will affect viscosity.

This effect is illustrated in Fig. 7.9.

In each case the rate of flow is the same (100 mL/min), and all other conditions are equal, except that the pressure necessary to generate that flow is different for water, plasma and normal blood as indicated by the height of the fluid in the tubes. Thus we could make up a 'pecking order' for viscosities:

normal blood > plasma > water

As far as blood is concerned, the most significant factor controlling blood viscosity is the concentration of red blood cells. If, for example, the red blood cell concentration is one-half normal, the viscosity falls from 3.5 times that of water (as above) to only twice that of water. Alternatively, if the red blood cell concentration doubles, the viscosity can be as high as 20 times normal.

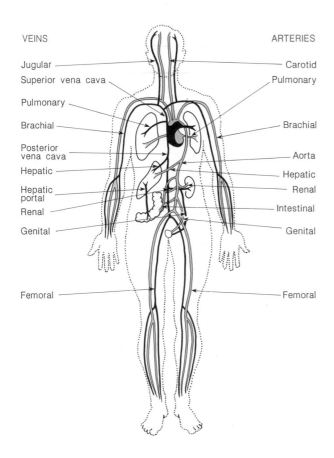

VEINS   ARTERIES

Jugular ——————   —————— Carotid
Superior vena cava ——   Pulmonary

Pulmonary ——

Brachial ——   —————— Brachial

Posterior
vena cava ——   —————— Aorta
Hepatic ——   —————— Hepatic

Hepatic
portal ——   —————— Renal
Renal ——   —————— Intestinal

Genital ——   —————— Genital

Femoral ——————   —————— Femoral

Figure 7.8. The blood transport system –
the heart and the main blood vessels in
humans. (From Cree & Webb: *Biology Outlines.* Sydney. Pergamon Press. 1984.)

It is important when administering intravenous infusions to
maintain blood viscosity within normal levels. This applies
particularly when blood volume is being replaced, so that care
must be taken that viscosity is not lowered by less viscous
liquids.

Other factors that affect the viscosity of the blood include:

(a) *Temperature.* An increase in temperature lowers the
viscosity by reducing and weakening cohesive forces (increases
kinetic energy of molecules). For example, increased muscular
activity during prolonged exercise will cause an increase in local
tissue temperature, thus lowering the viscosity of the blood. This
lower viscosity will allow the blood to flow more readily and
increase the rate of delivery of oxygen and nutrients to the
tissues, and in the process relieve the workload on the heart.
Lowering the temperature has the opposite effect.

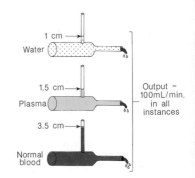

1 cm →
Water

1.5 cm →   Output =
Plasma   100mL/min.
                                  in all
3.5 cm →   instances

Normal
blood

Figure 7.9. Effect of viscosity on flow.
(From Guyton: *Physiology of the Human
Body.* 5th Ed. Philadelphia. W.B. Saunders.
1979.)

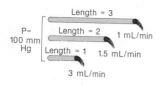

Figure 7.10. Effect of vessel length on flow. (From Guyton: *Physiology of the Human Body*. 5th Ed. Philadelphia. W.B. Saunders. 1979.)

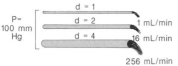

Figure 7.11. Effect of vessel diameter on flow. (From Guyton: *Physiology of the Human Body*. 5th Ed. Philadelphia. W.B. Saunders. 1979.)

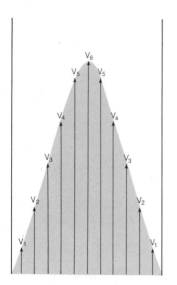

Figure 7.12. Streamlined flow of liquid in a tube. The velocity of the streamliness is greatest in the centre (V_6) of the tube, lowest adjacent to the sides (V_1), and with a gradual decrease between $V_6 \rightarrow V_1$.

(b) *Dehydration.* If the water content of the blood is decreased, the viscosity of the blood will increase (molecules are brought closer together and cohesive forces strengthened).

(c) *Diseases or disorders* such as asphyxia, loss of blood proteins and alteration to the water volume in the circulatory system. Exposure and shock cause lower body temperature, which increases the viscosity of the blood and increases the workload on the heart.

(d) *The use of additives.* Intravenous solutions may alter the viscosity of the blood or be deliberately added to maintain that viscosity, e.g. in a patient who is dehydrating.

2. **The length of the tube.** Since friction causes a resistance to rate of flow, it follows that the longer the tube through which the fluid has to flow, the greater will be the resistance – *the longer the tube, the greater the resistance.* This is illustrated in Fig. 7.10.

3. **The diameter of the tube.** When fluid is flowing through a tube, friction causes the outermost 'layer' of fluid to be retarded more than the next layer, which in turn is retarded more than the next layer and so forth. This means that the blood in the centre, for example, flows very much faster than the blood forming the outermost layer. This has the further consequence that the blood flow through a blood vessel *increases very rapidly as the diameter of that vessel increases.* In fact, the blood flow (as millilitres per minute or similar unit) increases as *the fourth power* of the diameter of the vessel.

In Fig. 7.11, we have three vessels of the same length and all other conditions identical, but with diameters of one, two and four units. The very large difference in flow rates is readily apparent. This has considerable physiological significance, since the diameter of most blood vessels in the body can change fourfold, meaning that their capacity to carry blood increases by a factor as high as 256! However, normal blood vessel size does change dramatically from the large aorta through to the small capillaries, increasing yet again as blood flows into the venous system.

Thus these three factors: viscosity, and the length and the diameter of the tube, determine the resistance offered to the flow of blood in blood vessels. We are now in a position to state the relationship that applies in these circumstances:

$$\text{blood pressure} = \text{blood flow} \times \text{resistance}$$

Type of Flow

If we were able to take a cross-section of a tube while a liquid was flowing through it, two types of flow could be observed:

1. **Laminar** or **streamlined flow.** The characteristics of this type of flow are listed in Table 7.1. The liquid closest to the inner surface of the tube will experience the greatest amount of friction and thus travel slowly (as indicated by the arrows V_1 in Fig. 7.12). The liquid that is next closest to the inner surface of the tube will experience a little less friction and will thus travel a little less slowly, as indicated by the arrows V_2, and so forth. The liquid in the centre will travel fastest, as indicated by the arrow V_6.

It must then be remembered that, in a tube, each set of arrows represents a cylinder of liquid moving through the tube. In Fig. 7.13 the cylinder inside the tube might be the one which we have represented by the arrows V_4, for example.

2. **Turbulent flow.** This is represented in Fig. 7.14.

In Table 7.1 the characteristics of turbulent flow are compared with streamline flow.

If streamline blood flow encounters a bifurcation, that is a division of blood vessels (e.g. the aorta), some turbulence may occur. Such localities are more prone to develop problems and obstructions.

A common cause of turbulent flow in a blood vessel is arteriosclerosis of the following types:

• Atherosclerosis, in which fatty plaques form in the inner layer of the arteries, called the *intima*.
• Medial calcific sclerosis, involving the middle or medial layer, in which calcium compounds are deposited and some tissue destruction occurs.

In these cases, the plaques intrude into the arteries and

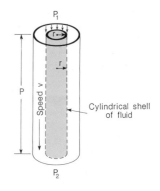

Figure 7.13. A cylindrical shell of the flui flowing through a tube. (From Greenberg: *Physics for Biology & Pre-Med. Students.* New York. Holt, Rinehart & Winston. 1975.

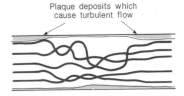

Figure 7.14. Turbulent flow.

TABLE 7.1

Laminar/Streamline Flow	Turbulent Flow
1. This is an organised, regular flow, with the particles at the centre flowing fastest and those just inside the inner surface of the tube flowing very slowly.	1. In this case, the flow is disorganised and follows no real pattern. Some particles may move across the tube or backwards up the tube.
2. The flow consists of 'cylinders' of molecules moving inside each other.	2. There are more collisions, a great deal of kinetic energy lost and the flow is inefficient.
3. It is a smooth, uniform flow which occurs naturally in most blood vessels.	3. This type of flow occurs in blood vessels only when some obstruction to normal flow exists.

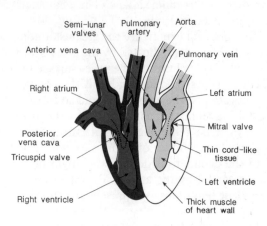

Figure 7.15. Blood flow through the heart
(From Cree & Webb: *Biology Outlines.*
Sydney. Pergamon Press. 1984.)

interfere with the normal streamline flow. The same effect will
occur in any situation where the inner lining of the blood vessel
is not smooth.

Cardiac Output

No discussion of blood flow can be complete without considering
the output of blood from the heart (Fig. 7.15). Cardiac output is
then defined as **the quantity of blood pumped by the left ventricle
into the aorta each minute.** It is usually quoted in litres per
minute. This is most significant in the body since it directly
determines the rate at which oxygen and nutrients are delivered to
the tissues of the body.

cardiac output (L/min) = heart rate (beats/min) × stroke volume
(L/beat)

As an example, if we take a heart rate of 72 beats per minute
and a 'typical' 70 millilitres (0.070 L) as the stroke volume, we
have:

cardiac output = 72 beats/min × 0.070 L/beat
= 5.0 L/min

This is a typical value for an adult at rest, but during exercise
cardiac output may rise to as much as 25 L/min.

Venous Return and the Starling Law of the Heart

An examination of Fig. 7.7 shows that venous blood pressure is
very low and thus the pressure of the blood filling the right

atrium is also very low. This atrial filling is then a passive process.

However, it is a most important process, since *the major factor determining cardiac output is venous return,* under normal circumstances. Let us examine the reason for this.

The Starling (or Frank-Starling) law of the heart states that **within the physiological limit, the heart will pump whatever volume of blood enters the right atrium.** In addition, it will do so without significant build-up of back pressure in the right atrium. This is another way of saying that the heart is an automatically controlled pump that simply pumps out all the blood that comes in. It is capable of pumping far more blood than the five litres or so that normally returns to it from the veins each minute.

Thus, the heart is prepared to work as hard as it is asked – no more, no less! This confirms our statement above, since it is venous return that determines how hard the heart needs to work, under normal circumstances. The output of the heart under the control of venous return can rise to a maximum of about 15 litres per minute. It should be noted, however, that neural or hormonal stimulation can virtually double this output (up to 35 litres per minute in well-trained athletes engaged in heavy exercise). This can happen very quickly within a few seconds of beginning the exercise and before most of the increase in venous return occurs – by increasing both the heart rate and the force of contraction.

This *active increase* in cardiac output should be contrasted with that *passive increase* dictated by the Starling law. In the latter case, the increase in venous return causes the muscles of the ventricular wall to stretch, so that the ventricle is enlarged to accommodate the increased volume of blood. As with most muscles, the more they are stretched, the greater is the energy of contraction. This then results in greater cardiac output.

Gravity and Venous Return

When blood has passed through capillary beds the blood pressure is very low. However, the person who is standing, walking, running, etc., still has to have a return flow of blood to the heart, even if this return is acting against the force of gravity. This is achieved in two ways:

1. The veins are equipped with valves, which prevent the blood from flowing backwards (Fig. 7.16).
2. *Extra mechanisms* operate to assist venous return, as listed on the following page.

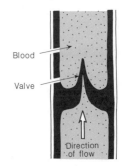

Blood

Valve

Direction of flow

Figure 7.16. Section along a large vein. (From Cree & Webb: *Biology Outlines.* Sydney. Pergamon Press. 1984.)

(a) Veins often pass between skeletal muscles and bone or other tissue, enabling the movement of the muscles to tend to squeeze veins and pump blood towards the heart. Our normal activity – whether walking, running or sitting at a desk and moving feet and legs from time to time – assists venous return in this way.

People who are sitting in cramped aeroplane seats for long periods of time, standing on parade, or standing to attention for some other reason need to wriggle their toes as much as possible to assist venous return. It is surprising just how much this activity does assist venous return and prevents people from fainting. Note that fainting is the body's very natural way of dealing with diminished venous return, since fainting causes a supine position to be adopted and venous return to improve. The fact that the body does not now have to cope with gravity makes the task much easier! Elevation of the limbs will obviously be advantageous for the same reason.

(b) Veins that pass around the thoracic area are assisted in their task by the normal breathing action, which aids venous return in a similar way to the muscle 'pump' described above. This effect is sometimes referred to as the 'respiratory pump' or the 'abdominal-thoracic' pump.

(c) The walls of the veins are richly equipped with nerves, which cause the smooth muscle of the veins to constrict, and this in turn gives rise to an increase in pressure within the veins and forces the blood towards the heart.

GASES

We will now examine that other group of fluids in the body – gases. We are all aware of being surrounded by air, which is a mixture of gases, and we know that it is essential to our existence. If we stop breathing air (or rather the oxygen it contains), it becomes immediately apparent how important air is!

It is, of course, all too easy to simply go on breathing without thinking of what is involved. However we do become more aware of our breathing processes when we exercise, work hard, go diving, engage in work or activity at high altitudes such as skiing, mountaineering or sky-diving, or try to breathe freely in polluted cities. We may also consider the significance of a laboratory report that says a patient's arterial partial pressure of oxygen is 50 mmHg, and wonder if that is a problem. In furthering your knowledge of gases and their behaviour you should come to a greater understanding of some of the complexities of breathing and some of the factors affecting gases in the body.

The Atmosphere and the Pressure It Exerts

Air is a mixture of gases of which oxygen is the most important. It will be recalled by the reader that a gas (in terms of the kinetic theory):

1. takes the shape of the container in which it is found and fills that container;
2. consists of molecules that move around at high velocities and bump into each other and into the walls of the container.

Table 7.2. lists the composition of dry air (air from which the moisture has been removed). The term 'partial pressure' (which is defined later in this chapter) refers to the contribution that each gas makes to the total pressure exerted by the atmosphere, called atmospheric pressure.

The very small component (0.01 per cent) not mentioned consists of the rare gases neon (18 ppm), helium (5 ppm), krypton and xenon (1 ppm each). A 'ppm' is a part per million.

Atmospheric pressure arises by virtue of the weight of the air above any point on the earth's surface. It is for this reason that atmospheric pressure decreases as altitude increases and effectively disappears at an altitude of about 150 km, although the atmosphere has become so sparse that it is difficult to say precisely at which altitude it 'disappears'.

Atmospheric pressure is not constant even at a particular altitude, but varies according to atmospheric conditions, as the weather experts are quick to tell us. In most cases, water vapour makes a contribution to the total atmospheric pressure, and this contribution is variable. In desert conditions its contribution is minimal, but it can be quite high in tropical or semi-tropical conditions, or elsewhere at various times.

Other gases may sometimes make a contribution to atmospheric pressure in particular environments. Cave explorers have to be very conscious of the build-up of carbon dioxide which, being heavier than air, tends to settle in the lower levels of caves. Miners can have similar problems, with the additional complica-

TABLE 7.2

Component	Percentage	Partial Pressure	
		mmHg	kPa
Nitrogen(N_2)	78.08	593.4	79.10
Oxygen (O_2)	20.95	159.2	21.21
Argon (A)	0.93	7.1	0.95
Carbon dioxide (CO_2)	0.03	0.2	0.03
Total	99.99	759.9	101.3

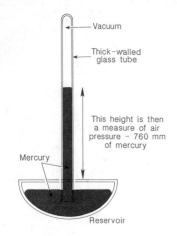

Vacuum

Thick-walled glass tube

This height is then a measure of air pressure - 760 mm of mercury

Mercury

Reservoir

Figure 7.17. A simple barometer.

tion of gases that are flammable or explosive, such as methane (natural gas).

Flyers, climbers and such are not normally troubled by changes in the composition of the air, but by the decrease in air pressure that occurs at high altitudes. Parties attempting to climb very high mountains such as Mt Everest often have to resort to breathing from bottled oxygen supplies. Many athletes had great difficulty during the Olympic Games at Mexico City because of the very high altitude there. Also, the lower pressure outside the body allows gas to expand inside the body, which may cause problems as we shall see later in this chapter.

Air pressure is normally measured using a thick-walled glass tube which has been inverted over a container of mercury, as shown in Fig. 7.17. The Fortin barometer has refined the technique considerably, but the principle is the same. The original barometer used water, but required a tube over ten metres long! The fact that the density of mercury is 13.6 times greater than that of water means that, if mercury is used instead of water, the length of tube required is less than a metre. The older units for air pressure were derived from this, as indicated in the diagram, but in meteorological work they have been replaced by hectopascals. In all other work, the kilopascal is the unit used. Thus, the normal atmospheric pressure at sea level

= 760 mmHg (old units),
= 1013 hectopascals (meteorological),
= 101.3 kPa(SI units)

The Concepts of Negative and Positive Pressure

In discussing pressures in the lungs and thoracic cavity, the terms 'negative pressure' and 'positive pressure' are frequently used in clinical practice. This is done as a matter of convenience and means that all the pressures involved are compared to normal atmospheric pressure. It follows that:

1. Any pressure above normal atmospheric pressure (760 mmHg) is regarded as a *positive pressure* (+); e.g. a pressure of +4 mmHg is the same as (760 + 4) mmHg or 764 mmHg (102 kPa).

2. Any pressure below normal atmospheric pressure is called a *negative pressure* (−); e.g. a pressure of −2 mmHg is equivalent to (760−2) mmHg or 758 mmHg (101 kPa).

While the pressure differences quoted in the examples do not seem to be dramatically different from normal atmospheric pressure, these pressure differences are more than sufficient to form a pressure gradient to enable the gases involved in inhalation and exhalation to move in the desired direction. In fact, the pressure differences in normal breathing are only + 1 mmHg (.1333 kPa) and −1 mmHg (−.1333 kPa). However, during maximum expiratory effort, the pressure in the lungs can be increased to over + 100 mmHg (13.33 kPa) in a strong and healthy male. During a maximum inspiratory effort, it can be reduced to as low as −80 mmHg (−10.7 kPa).

It is also important to note that reference has been made to normal atmospheric pressure for convenience. However, the pressure differences occurring at any time are differences that exist in relation to the atmospheric conditions prevailing at that time and for the person concerned.

Some other terms should be mentioned:

Vacuum: this means the total absence of any substance. However, a vacuum is never generated in a patient. What *does* happen is that a 'negative pressure', as defined above, is created.

Sub-atmospheric pressure: this term is used to indicate any pressure that is below the atmospheric pressure at a certain place and time.

Suction: in practice, this amounts to a decrease in pressure compared to atmospheric pressure. Any liquid between a suction device and the atmosphere will be forced into the device. For example, during surgery, blood is removed from open cavities this way.

Clinical Applications of Atmospheric Pressure

Pressure (whether atmospheric or otherwise) can shift fluids from high pressure areas to low pressure areas. Advantage is taken of this phenomenon to fill syringes, etc., or to remove fluids from patients. Examples include:

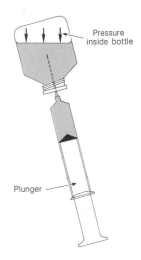

1. The filling of medicine droppers, hypodermic syringes (Fig. 7.18) and asepto syringes (used for irrigating cavities or spaces such as the bladder). The squeezing of the bulb on the medicine dropper evacuates some of the air from the dropper and bulb. When the bulb is released with the lower end of the dropper under a liquid, the rubber bulb tends to regain its shape. This creates a lower pressure inside than the atmospheric pressure outside, causing the atmospheric pressure to force some of the liquid up into the dropper.

In the case of the syringes, when the plunger is withdrawn while the needle end is immersed in a liquid, the pressure inside the syringe is decreased with respect to atmospheric pressure, and atmospheric pressure then forces the liquid up through the needle and into the body of the syringe.

Figure 7.18. Filling a hypodermic syringe.

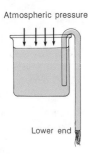

Atmospheric pressure

Lower end

Figure 7.19. Siphon. The end from which the liquid flows must always be lower than the end in the liquid for the siphon to function.

2. The same principle applies to a drinking straw or tube, the decrease in pressure within the straw being caused by an inhalation of air into the lungs. It should be emphasised that the work of drawing the liquid into the straw and thus into the mouth is effected by maintaining a lower pressure inside the straw than the atmospheric pressure outside.

3. Barometers, as previously explained.

4. The siphon operates in a similar way (Fig. 7.19). The siphon is started by decreasing the pressure inside the tube, by removing air from it – sometimes by 'sucking' the air out. It may also be started by filling the tube with liquid, then placing one end under the surface of the liquid and allowing the liquid to flow from the other end. The flow of liquid from the lower end causes a lowering of pressure inside the tube, and atmospheric pressure then forces the liquid into the tube.

The siphon is used for gastric lavage – a procedure by which a patient's stomach is irrigated to remove and drain substances such as poisons and stomach contents following a drug overdose.

5. Suction devices have already been mentioned and include:

(a) Suction machines or pumps

These are mechanically able to create negative pressure in receptacles and tubes attached to them.

Drainage bottles (which collect fluids from a cavity in a patient via tubing) are frequently attached to suction pumps to promote or increase the removal of fluids. Regions of the body which are drained in this way (particularly following surgery), include the chest cavity and the stomach. The removal of secretions from the upper and lower respiratory tract is highly dependent on the use of suction devices.

With any suction device, a pressure control valve and gauge must always be used to regulate the amount of 'negative pressure' being created, since the membranes of the body would be susceptible to damage if the suction was too strong.

In addition to the use of these small machines, 'wall suction' is available in many institutions. Wall suction involves the setting-up of a general or common suction system throughout institutions or specific areas. The central machine has inlets available in various treatment areas. These inlets are located on a wall area near the patient or treatment beds.

A pressure control valve, gauge and receptacle is plugged into the suction inlet and can then be used with tubing for the various treatments mentioned above. This system reduces the need for many machines to be kept and maintained by the institution, removes obstacles from the floor in treatment areas and reduces electrical hazards.

(b) Portable wound suction receptacles. These function in a very similar way to the bulb of a medicine dropper – the compression of the receptacle itself expels air and the elasticity of the receptacle causes it to tend to regain its shape, thus decreasing the pressure inside and allowing atmospheric pressure to force liquid into the drain tube. An example of this type of device is a haemovac.

6. Positive pressure ventilators or respirators. Gas mixtures are delivered intermittently into a patient's airway by producing a positive pressure; they are also used to humidify the respiratory tract and to deliver medications in the form of aerosols.

7. Vascular boots are closed devices that fit over the lower leg like a boot and can be filled with air. Air is pumped in and out in such a way as to provide alternate constriction and release of the blood vessels in the lower leg. During constriction, blood is forced past the one-way valves in the veins back towards the heart. During release, the veins can fill again with the valves in the veins closed. Vascular boots may be used on patients with circulatory problems.

8. Artificial respiration, cardiopulmonary resuscitation and rocker bed techniques all make use of differences in pressure to achieve their goals.

Consequences of Pressure Variations on the Body

1. If one or both of the eustachian tubes are blocked as a result of a cold, the pressure on each side of the tympanic membranes in the ear is not able to equalise in the normal way, when air pressure on the outside is balanced by air pressure transmitted through the mouth and up the eustachian tubes to the inside. A blockage in the tubes prevents this from happening. This means that flying or even travelling in hilly country in a car can be not only painful but dangerous for the ears. Even today, members of flight crews who have colds but still fly often end up with ruptured eardrums. It may come as no surprise then, to learn that aircrews on our major airlines are not allowed to fly if the airline is aware that they have a cold, or even a trace of a cold.

2. A similar effect is observed if sinuses are blocked. The main problem here is that haemorrhaging into the sinuses can occur.

3. Gas in the gastrointestinal tract (GIT) can also be a problem. Qantas aircraft, for example, are pressurised to the equivalent of about 2000 metres altitude. Under normal conditions, a gas expansion of about 20 per cent occurs, but passengers and crew are not usually aware of this problem, since any excess gas tends to be eliminated through the mouth or anus. However, should explosive decompression occur – if the plane's skin is suddenly ruptured and the air in the plane rushes out explosively – the gas in the GIT will suddenly expand to about four times its

volume, causing considerable discomfort. Furthermore, the possibility of blood vessel rupture in the GIT and of transmission of this increased pressure to other sensitive parts of the circulation system is very real.

THE BREATHING PROCESS AND THE GAS LAWS

Before attempting to understand breathing, we must look at the laws which describe the behaviour of gases.

Boyle's Law

This is stated as follows: *the volume of a given mass of gas is inversely proportional to the pressure to which it is subjected, provided that the temperature remains constant.*

In mathematical terms:

$$V \, \alpha \, \frac{1}{P} \text{ (for constant T)}$$

or PV = constant (for constant T)
where V = volume,
P = pressure
and T = temperature

This means that, provided the temperature remains constant, an increase in the pressure of an enclosed mass of gas will result in a decrease in volume. Under the same conditions, a decrease in pressure will cause an increase in volume.

Fig. 7.20 will perhaps clarify this law. If we look at Fig. 7.20(a), we see a representation of an enclosed mass of gas occupying a volume that we have called 2V when subjected to a pressure, 2P. In Fig. 7.20(b), the double pressure of 4P is applied to the gas and the volume decreases proportionately to V. In Fig.7.20(c), the halved pressure of P is applied and the volume increases proportionately to 4V.

In Fig. 7.21, we consider a system in which a mass of gas is enclosed in a container with a piston (or plunger) which can be set to accommodate various volumes as indicated. A pressure gauge provides a means by which the effect of these volume changes on the pressure of the enclosed gas can be measured.

It is appropriate to remind the reader that we are now making reference to a mass of gas inside the container and we are considering the effect of changing the volume that this mass of gas occupies. In terms of the kinetic theory, if the gas is

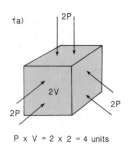

(a)

P x V = 2 x 2 = 4 units

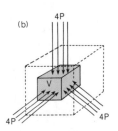

(b)

P x V = 4 x 1 = 4 units

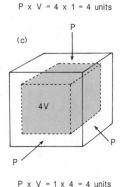

(c)

P x V = 1 x 4 = 4 units

Figure 7.20. In each case we have an enclosed mass of gas at *constant temperature*. It may be observed that, in each case the relationship between the pressure and volume of the gas is: P × V = constant (for constant temperature).

occupying a smaller volume, collisions with the walls of the container will be more frequent and thus the pressure will be greater. If the gas is occupying a larger volume, collisions with the walls of the container will be less frequent and the pressure exerted will be less.

As indicated, three different volumes are considered, and the pressures read from the gauge in each case.

In both sets of diagrams the relationship known as Boyle's law is illustrated – that for constant temperature, the product of the pressure and volume (PV) of an enclosed mass of gas is constant.

It should be noted that under normal conditions of temperature and pressure (the conditions with which we are concerned in the human body) this law holds true for gases such as air.

The functioning of syringes (and previously discussed droppers) combines both Boyle's law and atmospheric pressure. When the plunger is withdrawn while the needle end is immersed in a liquid, the volume of air below the plunger increases while the pressure decreases. Atmospheric pressure will then force liquid up through the needle into the body of the syringe to equalise the pressure.

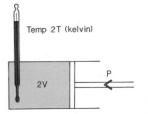

Figure 7.21. The relationship between pressure and volume of an enclosed mass of gas at constant temperature (PV = constant).

Charles' Law

Charles' law states: *The volume of a given mass of gas is directly proportional to its absolute temperature (provided the pressure remains constant)* (Fig. 7.22)

This means that if the temperature (K) doubles, the volume doubles; and if the temperature (K) is halved, the volume is halved. Also, if the volume is doubled, the temperature (K) is doubled; and if the volume is halved, the temperature (K) is halved, provided in all the above cases that the pressure remains constant.

In mathematical terms:

$$\frac{V_1}{T_1} = \frac{V_2}{T_2}$$

Once again, in terms of the kinetic theory, we have an enclosed mass of gas, occupying a particular volume at a particular temperature. If we now heat up the gas and so increase the temperature, the molecules of gas will have more energy: they will travel faster and each collision with the walls of the container will be more energetic. Furthermore, because they are travelling faster, they will collide with the walls of the container more often. Since one of the walls of the container is the piston, it will

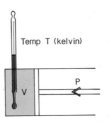

Figure 7.22. The relationship between the temperature (kelvin) and the volume of an enclosed mass of gas at constant pressure: V/T = constant.

tend to cause an increase in the pressure acting on it. However, we have been told that the pressure pushing on the piston from the outside is constant, so that the piston will move out to equalise the pressure (inside and outside) once more, thus increasing the volume.

If we cool the gas, collisions with the piston will have less energy and will be less frequent, the pressure on the gas will decrease and the constant pressure acting on the piston will cause it to move in, thus decreasing the volume.

The General Gas Law

In the normal breathing process, as we shall soon see, we are particularly interested in pressure volume relationships and thus in the implications of Boyle's law. However, Boyle's law assumes constant temperature, which is not really the case in breathing. It would, of course, be true if the atmospheric temperature and the core body temperature were exactly the same, e.g. 37°C. This is usually not the case: if an individual breathes air at 0°C, there is a difference in temperature between the air being breathed and core body temperature of some 37 Celsius degrees.

This in turn suggests the application of Charles' law (although the extent to which incoming air is heated by the body may not be easy to determine). However, Charles' law assumes constant pressure, which is once again not the case.

It is possible to overcome these difficulties by using the *general gas equation*, which considers all three variables (P,V and T) at once.

$$\frac{P_1 V_1}{T_1} = \frac{P_2 V_2}{T_2}$$

where:

P_1 = initial pressure $\qquad$ P_2 = final pressure
V_1 = initial volume $\qquad$ V_2 = final volume
T_1 = initial temperature $\qquad$ T_2 = final temperature

This means that if we have a mass of gas held under a given set of conditions (the initial conditions above), and these conditions are altered to what we have called the final conditions, then by measuring, say, V and T, we can calculate P; given P and T, we can calculate V and so forth.

It should be noted here that some books refer to the need to keep pressure packs and gas cylinders out of the sun and away from direct heat. This is a perfectly valid safety consideration, but is not an application of Charles' law as is often suggested. If we think about this, we realise that the volume is constant in such packs and cylinders and that the variables involved are pressure and temperature. It follows that this example is an application of the general gas law under constant volume conditions. Therefore:

$$\frac{P_1}{T_1} = \frac{P_2}{T_2}$$

This simply means that if the temperature is increased, the pressure is increased proportionally. Pressure packs, gas cylinders and the like should not therefore be exposed to high temperatures, which increase the risk of explosion.

The Process of Breathing

For simplicity, it will be assumed that the atmospheric temperature and the core temperature of our patient are identical, so that we are able to apply Boyle's law to our discussion. However, the reader should bear in mind that temperature difference is significant at times, and that a precise assessment of what is happening during breathing under these conditions is possible only by using the general gas equation.

We will start by looking at the breathing process in basic terms.

During **inspiration:**

- the sternum or breastbone moves outwards and upwards;
- the ribs move upwards and outwards;
- the diaphragm moves downwards.

These movements serve to increase approximately twofold the volume of the thoracic cavity (that is the volume of space contained within the rib cage and diaphragm). By Boyle's law, this means that the pressure in the thoracic cavity is decreased below atmospheric pressure. Since the lungs are in direct contact with the atmosphere through bronchial tubes and the trachea, atmospheric pressure forces air into the lungs down the pressure gradient, i.e. the pressure outside the lungs is higher than the pressure inside the lungs and air is forced *into* the lungs.

During **expiration:**

- the sternum moves downwards and inwards;
- the ribs move downwards and inwards;
- the diaphragm moves upwards.

These movements serve to decrease the volume of the thoracic cavity, which, by Boyle's law, means that the pressure in the thoracic cavity is increased above atmospheric pressure.

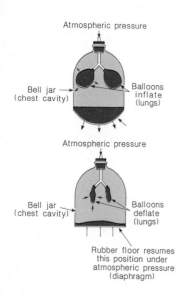

Figure 7.23. The chest during exaggerated breathing: inspiration, and expiration. The schematic diagrams illustrate the mechanics of breathing. (From Otto *et al. Modern Biology.* New York. Holt, Rinehart & Winston. 1981.)

Once again, the direct contact of the lungs with the atmosphere means that the gases in the lungs can be expelled into the atmosphere down a pressure gradient. In this case, the pressure inside the lungs is higher than atmospheric pressure and the gases in the lungs are forced outwards.

These processes are illustrated in Fig. 7.23, where the balloons in the bell jar represent the lungs, the rubber membrane represents the diaphragm and the bucket handle represents the action of the ribs and the sternum.

It should be noted at this stage that inhalation is an *active process*, in which muscles contract to effect the changes described, whereas exhalation (during normal breathing) is a *passive process* involving muscle relaxation aided by the elasticity or elastic recoil of the lungs and chest structure, and by surface tension, as described below. During exercise, exhalation can be a partly active process. The most important of the factors involved in breathing is the use of the diaphragm, although it moves only about one centimetre in normal breathing. However, during heavy exercise, it may move as much as ten centimetres.

All of the above presupposes that it is possible for air to freely move in and out of the airway, which of course is normally possible. However, if the airway becomes blocked, the effects can be serious and an immediate response is indicated, e.g. Heimlich manoeuvre.

In a disorder known as sleep apnoea ('apnoea' is a Greek word meaning 'without breath'), soft tissues in the back of the throat, viz. the uvula, soft palate, pharynx and the back of the tongue, collapse into the airway during sleep and completely block it. This occurs particularly during the deep or dreaming stage of sleep known as REM (rapid eye movement) sleep. This results in fragmented sleep, low blood oxygen levels (sometimes disastrously so), general daytime sleepiness, impaired intellectual function et cetera, and may lead to heart attack, hypertension and stroke.

The treatment of choice worldwide for this disorder is nasal CPAP (**C**ontinuous **P**ositive **A**irway **P**ressure) which was developed at Sydney University by Professor Colin Sullivan. It consists of a pump which delivers air at a constant pressure (predetermined for each patient) through tubing to a nasal mask and thence to the soft tissues around the airway. The pressure keeps the soft tissues away from the airway and the person breathes normally, i.e. it acts as a pneumatic splint.

Pressures Involved in Breathing

Intra-alveolar pressure
We have already mentioned pressure differences between the atmosphere and the lungs. The pressure in the lungs is transmitted all the way down to the alveoli (remember Pascal's principle?), so that all that we have said about pressures inside the lungs also refers to intra-alveolar pressures (Fig. 7.24).

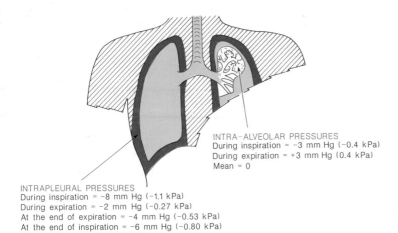

INTRA-ALVEOLAR PRESSURES
During inspiration = -3 mm Hg (-0.4 kPa)
During expiration = +3 mm Hg (0.4 kPa)
Mean = 0

INTRAPLEURAL PRESSURES
During inspiration = -8 mm Hg (-1.1 kPa)
During expiration = -2 mm Hg (-0.27 kPa)
At the end of expiration = -4 mm Hg (-0.53 kPa)
At the end of inspiration = -6 mm Hg (-0.80 kPa)
Mean = -5 mm Hg (-0.67 kPa)

Figure 7.24. Intra-alveolar and intrapleural (intrathoracic) pressures during normal breathing. (From Guyton: *Physiology of the Human Body*. 5th Ed. Philadelphia. Saunders College Publishing. 1979.)

Intrapleural pressure

The elastic tendencies of the lungs that cause them to move constantly towards a state of collapse can be measured by the amount of *'negative pressure' in the intrapleural spaces* (between the lungs and the pleural sac surrounding them) that prevents their collapse. This is called intrapleural pressure and is normally about -4 mmHg (-0.53 kPa). This means that a pressure of -4 mmHg is needed in the intrapleural space to prevent lung collapse when the alveoli are at atmospheric pressure. Immediately after expiration, the pressure in the cavity between the pleural sac and the lungs must still be *lower* than atmospheric pressure, so that atmospheric pressure will force the walls of the lungs out against the pleural sac.

This is the normal case when the lungs are of normal size, but during a large inspiratory effort, the intrapleural pressure needed to expand the lungs may be as high as -18 mmHg (-2.4 kPa).

If we watch a patient breathing, the rise and fall of the chest can be observed. The same effect can be observed in pleural drains and, from what we have said above, this is not unexpected – since the pressure in the pleural cavity is changing. This highlights the need for the nurse to ensure that a pleural drain is not open to the atmosphere at any time. The consequences of this would be the same as opening the chest to the atmosphere, as occurs with a stab wound – air would rush in, the negative pressure would no longer exist and the elastic nature of the lung would cause it to contract and collapse. This is why the drainage tube must be well anchored into position in the patient (sutures) and supported against pulling (taped to skin). The distal end of connecting tubing must also be submerged below the surface of sterile liquid at all times. This latter protection acts as a water seal to prevent air entry. The density and weight of water is so much greater than air that it is not forced up into the chest by the atmosphere, although it rises slightly in the tube (see Fig. 7.25).

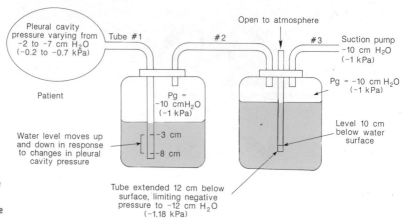

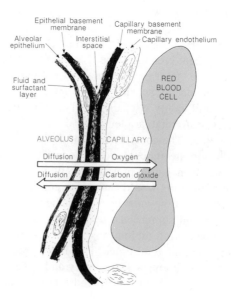

Figure 7.25. Underwater sealed drainage arrangement involving a regulator bottle on the right, which limits the negative pressure created by the pump. (From Nave & Nave: *Physics for the Health Sciences*. 3rd Ed. Philadelphia. W.B. Saunders. 1985.)

Intrapleural pressure is caused by two factors:

1. The *elastic fibres* that are present in the structure of the lungs, and which, under normal circumstances, account for about one-third of the recoil tendency of the lungs.

2. The *surface tension* of the fluid lining the alveoli (Fig. 7.26), which exerts continuous forces that tend to cause the alveoli to collapse and, in turn, tend to cause the whole lung to collapse. Surface tension is caused by forces of attraction between molecules of a liquid. It is these forces that give rise to the 'skin' on water that we try to overcome with soap when washing ourselves, our clothes or our car.

Figure 7.26. Fine structure of the respiratory membrane and relationship to red blood cells.

These forces account for the other two-thirds of the recoil tendency of the lungs in normal conditions. However, these forces are rather powerful and, just as we require soap to lower the surface tension of water to enable it to wash properly, our lungs use a similar type of compound called a **surfactant** to lower the surface tension. The term surfactant means 'surface active agent' and covers soaps (including detergents) and the phospholipid (dipalmitoyl lecithin) that is the chief constituent of the substance utilised by the lungs for this purpose.

In the absence of a surfactant, lung expansion is so difficult that intrapleural pressures of the order −20 to −30 mmHg (−2.67 to −4.0 kPa) are required to overcome the tendency of the alveoli, and thus of the lungs, to collapse. Some newborn babies (particularly premature ones) have an insufficient supply of surfactant, which makes breathing extremely difficult for them. In the absence of immediate and very careful treatment, this condition – hyaline membrane disease or respiratory distress syndrome – is usually fatal.

The essential function of the surfactant is to form a mono-molecular layer – a layer just one molecule thick – at the interface between the air in the alveoli and the fluid lining the surface of the alveoli. In this way, the formation of a water-air interface is prevented. Such an interface has a surface tension two to 14 times as great as the surfactant-air interface. Thus the surface tension is reduced and the individual can breathe much more easily.

Surfactant also assists in keeping all of the alveoli in any one region of the lungs from becoming much larger or smaller than their fellows – something which would tend to occur without the presence of the surfactant. However, the *interdependence* of the alveoli – the fact that the alveoli walls are joined together – also helps to keep their size uniform.

Yet another vital role of the surfactant is to prevent the filtration of fluid from the alveolar wall capillaries into the alveoli. If an insufficient supply of surfactant is present, extensive movement of fluid results in the alveoli becoming fluid-filled and severe pulmonary oedema occurs. This is one of the key factors in the breathing difficulties experienced by babies that suffer from respiratory distress syndrome.

Finally, we have a series of diagrams to show these processes (see Fig. 7.27). It is most important for the reader to remember that we are discussing three cavities:

1.   The **alveolar space**, in which the actual exchange of gases takes place.

2.   The **intrapleural cavity** (or space between the lungs and the pleural sac) in which a negative pressure is maintained to prevent lung collapse.

3.   The **thoracic cavity**, which controls the breathing process.

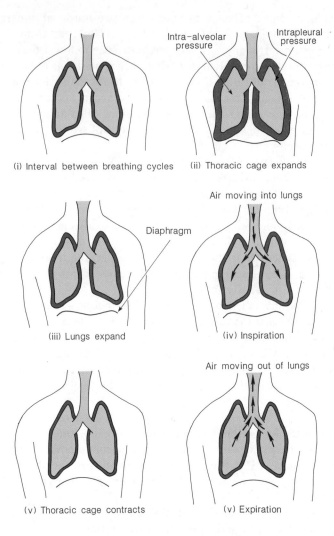

Figure 7.27. The breathing process.
(i) The lungs and the thoracic cage in the short interval between breathing cycles: pressure in lungs (intra-alveolar pressure) = atmospheric pressure.
(ii) Thoracic cage expands (diaphragm contracts and ribs and sternum move upwards and outwards): intrapleural pressure < pressure in lungs (intra-alveolar pressure).
(iii) The pressure difference causes the lungs to expand until: intrapleural pressure = pressure in lungs (intra-alveolar pressure) *but now:* pressure in lungs < atmospheric pressure, i.e. negative lung pressure exists.
(iv) Atmospheric pressure drives air in (air is moving down a pressure gradient) to the lungs until intrapleural pressure = pressure in lungs (intra-alveolar pressure) *and* pressure in lungs = atmospheric pressure.
(v) Thoracic cage contracts (diaphragm and intercostal muscles relax, rib cage and sternum move down and inwards) and: intrapleural pressure > atmospheric pressure.
(vi) This causes elastic recoil of the lungs and air is driven out: pressure in lungs > atmospheric pressure (intra-alveolar pressure) i.e. postive lung pressure exists.
Note that the condition in (i) has now been restored.

(i) Interval between breathing cycles   (ii) Thoracic cage expands

(iii) Lungs expand   (iv) Inspiration

(v) Thoracic cage contracts   (v) Expiration

Intra-alveolar pressure   Intrapleural pressure

Air moving into lungs

Diaphragm

Air moving out of lungs

Dalton's Law

Our discussions of the behaviour of gases so far have regarded the gases with which we are concerned as though they were one gas. This is not the case, of course, either with the air we breathe in, which we have already discussed as a mixture, or with the mixture of gases that we breathe out which contains approximately 16 per cent oxygen and 3.6 per cent carbon dioxide.

Dalton's law is a statement of the inference that can be made regarding the contribution each of the individual gases makes to normal atmospheric pressure, i.e., that normal atmospheric pressure results from the pressure contribution (or the partial pressure) of each of the component gases added together; and furthermore, that each gas exerts its own pressure, whether the other gases are present or not. Dalton's law may then be stated:

The partial pressure of a gas in a gas mixture is the pressure that this gas would exert if it alone occupied the total volume of the mixture in the absence of the other components.

$$P_{(total\ pressure)} = p_1 + p_2 + p_3 + \ldots$$

where p_1, p_2, p_3, etc., are the partial pressures of the gas mixture, which has a total pressure of P. For example,

$$P_{(air)} = p_{nitrogen} + p_{oxygen} + p_{argon} + p_{carbon\ dioxide}$$

Note: (a) The partial pressure for nitrogen in Table 7.2 may easily be calculated by multiplying the percentage of nitrogen (78.08 per cent) by the total pressure (759.9 mmHg or 101.3 kPa). Thus:

$$\frac{78.08}{100} \times 759.9 = 593.4$$

or, in kPa:

$$\frac{78.08}{100} \times 101.3 = 79.1$$

(b) If the air involved is not *dry* air, *water vapour* would be present and would also *exert a partial pressure.*

This last point is important in the lungs, where the water vapour exerts a partial pressure (at the normal body temperature of 37°C) of 47 mmHg (6.27 kPa) as a result of the *high kinetic energy of the water molecules* at this temperature – compared to the temperature of the atmosphere, which is usually less than 37°C. The consequence of this is that water is continually lost from the lungs. Conversely, atmospheric air entering the lungs is exposed to the fluids covering the surfaces of the respiratory passages and is thus humidified. The water content of the air thus decreases by dilution the partial pressures from the values given for dry air. It also reduces membrane irritation and helps to cut down on water loss from the lungs, as described under Henry's law, below.
This must be borne in mind by the practising nurse when administering gases by ventilators – particularly if these gases are bypassing the upper respiratory tract, as in a tracheostomy (the insertion of a tube in an incision in the neck and trachea to assist breathing). Obviously, higher body and/or climatic temperatures make this even more important.

Henry's Law

The concentration of a gas that will dissolve in a liquid at a given temperature is proportional to the partial pressure of the gas.
Therefore:

concentration α partial pressure (constant temp.)

This tells us that concentration is proportional to partial pressure, but to be able to connect these two quantities in an equation, we need to introduce a constant – called a proportionality constant – represented by the letter k, so that:

if C α p,
then C = kp, where k is a constant.

We will now use an equation for gas x, and, as a matter of convenience we will represent k for gas x as k_x and call it the *solubility coefficient,* which gives us an indication of the tendency or otherwise of that gas to dissolve. Carbon dioxide, for example, has a much greater tendency to dissolve in water, and thus in the plasma in the blood, than does oxygen, as can be seen from Table 7.3. This is why we have haemoglobin in our blood – if we relied on oxygen dissolving in water (and plasma) we would all be dead!
We then have:

$$C_x = k_x \times p_x,$$
where C = concentration of gas x;
k_x = a constant (called the solubility coefficient);
p_x = partial pressure of gas x.

If concentration is expressed in volume of gas x dissolved per volume of water at 0°C, the solubility coefficients for a number of important respiratory gases are as listed in Table 7.3, with partial pressures in the units indicated.
To elaborate this point further, concentration can be expressed a number of ways, but for the purposes of Table 7.3 we are using volume of gas in volume of water (mL of gas in mL of water at 0°C).

TABLE 7.3 Solubility constants

Gas	mmHg	kPa
oxygen	3.2×10^{-5}	2.4×10^{-4}
carbon dioxide	75×10^{-5}	56×10^{-4}
carbon monoxide	2.4×10^{-5}	1.8×10^{-4}
nitrogen	1.6×10^{-5}	1.2×10^{-4}
helium	1.1×10^{-5}	0.8×10^{-4}

The table shows two sets of units for partial pressures (mmHg and kPa), so that if the partial pressure for oxygen is expressed in mmHg, the value for the solubility coefficient for oxygen is 3.2×10^{-5}, but if the partial pressure is expressed in kPa, the value for the solubility coefficient of oxygen is 2.4×10^{-4}.

What does all this tell us as far as the body is concerned? Simply that a *higher partial pressure* of a particular gas will ensure that a larger quantity of that gas *will dissolve*. Since some of the gas is normally already dissolved in the body, we need to consider the difference between the partial pressures that exist, i.e. the *pressure gradient*.

Table 7.4 with p as the partial pressure (using mmHg as units) shows these values.

TABLE 7.4

Locality	pO_2	pCO_2
atmosphere	160	0.2
alveoli	105	40
pulmonary artery (i.e. pre lung)	40	45
pulmonary vein (i.e. post lung)	105	40
systemic artery (i.e. pre cell)	105	40
systemic vein (i.e. post cell)	40	45

This means that the *pressure gradient for oxygen* (Fig. 7.28) between the alveoli and the pulmonary capillary is

$$104 - 40 = 64 \, \text{mmHg}$$

which is a considerable pressure gradient. Similarly, the arteries feed into tissue capillaries and provide a pressure gradient, which is once again

$$104 - 40 = 64 \, \text{mmHg.}$$

However, while the partial pressure of oxygen builds up to 104 mmHg in the arteries, the concentration of oxygen present in simple solution (as distinct from that carried by haemoglobin) will be low, because the solubility coefficient is low. It is for this reason that only three per cent of our total oxygen requirements is carried in simple solution in the plasma. It is also true, however, that if the pressure gradient were higher, some more oxygen would dissolve, as by Henry's law.

With carbon dioxide, the pressure gradient, both at the lungs and at the tissues or cells, is

$$45 - 40 = 5 \, \text{mmHg}$$

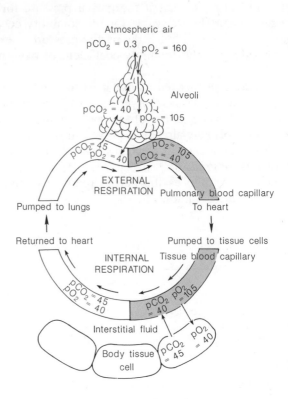

Figure 7.28. The respiration cycle. All pressures are in mm.

which is a much lower pressure gradient. If the pressure gradient were higher, more carbon dioxide would dissolve (as by Henry's law). In the case of carbon dioxide, however, the solubility coefficient is much higher (the reader might like to check this in Table 7.3) – about 22 times higher, in fact – so that much more carbon dioxide dissolves. The combination of a low pressure gradient and a high solubility coefficient results in some seven per cent of carbon dioxide being transported in simple solution in the plasma – *over twice the value for oxygen.*

It should be noted at this stage that while most blood tests are done on venous blood, the 'blood gases' test is done on arterial blood so that a true indication of oxygen uptake and carbon dioxide removal is obtained.

Another obvious illustration of Henry's law is a can or bottle of carbonated soft drink. When drink is canned or bottled, a pressure higher than atmospheric pressure ensures that the carbon dioxide gas remains dissolved in the soft drink. When the can or bottle is opened, however, the consequent reduction in pressure causes the gas to bubble out of solution.

To further illustrate Henry's law, let us consider decompression sickness, otherwise known as caisson disease, or 'the bends'. As a deep-sea diver goes deeper, the pressure on his body increases so that much more nitrogen (from his air tanks) dissolves in the blood than it would at normal atmospheric pressure. This is a rather slow process, but after several hours working at a depth of about 100 metres, for example, the body will contain about ten times the normal volume of nitrogen. If the diver then comes up too fast, bubbles of nitrogen emerge from solution in the blood. These bubbles can disrupt important pathways in the brain and spinal cord, cause severe pain by their effects on peripheral nerves, inflict permanent damage on parts of the central nervous system, lead to pulmonary oedema and cause death. This is a direct example of Henry's law, the significant factor being that a greater concentration of dissolved nitrogen in the blood is possible because of the greater pressures involved.

The bubbles we have described result from many molecules coming together, and these bubbles can form blockages. This can occur in the chambers of the heart.

The only treatment available is to place the diver into a decompression chamber, take the pressure back to that which existed at the depth he or she had reached and slowly reduce the pressure. The danger of bends is reduced by breathing a mixture of helium and oxygen (instead of air), since helium is much less soluble than nitrogen.

Partial pressures and Henry's law are very significant in determining the solubility of gases such as carbon dioxide and oxygen in the blood. The whole metabolism of the body, and indeed our very survival, depends upon the capacity of the blood to dissolve more of each of these gases under some circumstances and less under others.

It should be carefully noted that a number of different processes are involved in gaseous exchange in the lungs, but Henry's law is an important factor. The onset of altitude sickness (shortness of breath, dizziness and nausea) is then not surprising when people ascend to high altitudes. Henry's law indicates that the lower atmospheric pressure at high altitudes will result in a lower level of oxygen concentration in the blood, both in simple solution and in combination with haemoglobin. Remember that oxygen has to dissolve in the water lining the alveolar membrane before it can travel to the red blood cells.

Studies of some races show that they are particularly well adapted to life at high altitudes. The type of adaptation appropriate here is an increased concentration of red blood cells, which then increases the amount of oxygen that can be carried in the blood. A case in point is the Sherpas, a race of farming people who live in the higher country of Nepal, in the Himalayan region.

OXYGEN

We will now examine this gas in considerable detail because of its obvious importance to us. In Chapter 10 we will see that it is vital to all life processes. In addition, it is especially important in nursing, because it is used in the treatment of many conditions. It is essential, then, that nurses should know something of the properties of this gas, its uses and the precautions necessary to use it safely.

Properties

As we have already seen, oxygen is the most abundant element in the earth's crust. All living organisms, plant and animal, contain large quantities of oxygen, mainly in a combined form, such as water, carbon dioxide, carbohydrates, proteins and fats. Approximately 21 per cent of the atmosphere by volume is free molecular oxygen. It exists as diatomic molecules – molecules each of which contain two atoms of oxygen, represented by the symbol O_2. Also, small quantities of molecular oxygen can be found dissolved in certain fluids, such as blood, water, and tissue fluids, since oxygen is partially soluble in water. If this were not the case, fish would be in trouble, because they depend on dissolved oxygen for their own supply, this being extracted by their gills.

Oxygen has the following properties:

1. It is a colourless, odourless gas.
2. It is slightly heavier than air.
3. It has no taste.
4. It is transparent.
5. It is sufficiently soluble in water to diffuse from the alveoli into the bloodstream and from the bloodstream into tissue cells in animals, and to support aquatic life.
6. At ordinary temperatures, (e.g. room temperature) it is not particularly chemically active, although it will combine rapidly with certain elements such as phosphorus, sodium and potassium.
7. At higher temperatures, it is very reactive, uniting directly with most other elements.
8. It unites directly with many compounds in plant and animal tissues in the presence of enzymes (catalysts). (See Chapter 9.)

Before proceeding further, we should note that these properties, particularly 5, 7 and 8, make oxygen a very suitable gas for use in the body. In fact, it is so vital to the body in such functions as metabolism, formation of new tissues, nerve and brain function, muscle contraction (including cardiac), that no-one can live for more than a few minutes without it. Sometimes damage occurs in even less time – particularly in brain tissue.

9. Oxygen does not burn, but supports combustion. Many people think that oxygen burns, but if this were the case all the oxygen in the atmosphere would be burned whenever someone struck a match. However, oxygen is essential for combustion or burning in the usual sense of the word. When combustion occurs, oxygen is consumed to form oxides and energy is emitted in the form of heat and light (flame). In the case of burning wood, for example, heat, light, carbon dioxide and sometimes charcoal are formed as a result of the chemical reaction between oxygen, wood and heat. The greater the quantity and concentration of oxygen, the more rapidly burning occurs, as we observe when fanning a fire.

Ignition Point or Kindling Temperature

A temperature exists for all substances, below which the substance will not normally burn. This temperature is known as *the ignition point* or kindling temperature for that particular substance. With most substances, it is necessary to raise their temperatures above room temperature to this ignition point or kindling temperature to achieve burning. For example, a burning match will ignite tissue paper if the heat produced by it raises the temperature of the paper to its ignition point or kindling temperature.

Substances with low ignition points, such as many organic compounds like ether, alcohol (whether in the pure form or as methylated spirits), and paints, rags, etc., constitute a fire hazard. These substances are unfortunately sometimes labelled as being inflammable, but what does this mean? The prefix 'in' usually means 'not' as in 'flexible' and 'inflexible', in which case 'inflammable' should mean 'not flammable' – will not burn – which is not what it is meant to mean at all!

This is an unfortunate aberration of our language, which authorities are trying to overcome by avoiding the use of the term 'inflammable'. Petrol tankers and such now carry warning signs that use the word *'flammable'* to warn people of the danger of the contents and readers are strongly urged to do likewise to minimise confusion.

Some materials are capable of producing *spontaneous combustion* as a result of the build-up of heat, whereby the temperature finally reaches the ignition point and the substance catches fire. Hay is an example of this, but spontaneous combustion can occur with rags used for furniture polish, paint, etc., and then stored in a confined space.

Non-flammable substances are those whose ignition points are so high that they cannot be reached under ordinary circumstances, substances such as asbestos, rocks and most metals. Most substances have ignition points between the two extremes.

The concepts of ignition point (or kindling temperature), and of flammability and non-flammability are important considerations in the use of materials in everyday life, places of work, factories, institutions, hospitals, hotels and other buildings. Whether selecting furniture or curtains for a hospital, or choosing material for a child's winter clothing or a firefighter's uniform, consideration should be given to these important concepts in terms of safety.

Where clothing materials may be exposed to heating devices such as electric radiators, or open fires – particularly if the clothes are being worn by young children – it is necessary to consider the possible consequences. For example:

1. Flannelette nightwear, especially on young children, has resulted in some horrific burns and even deaths when it has caught fire, for instance as a result of brushing against an electric radiator. Some states now ban the sale of flannelette nightwear for young children, but overlook the fact that the smallest women's sizes fit quite young children, particularly since present-day children tend to be taller than their parents' generation. The result is that children still end up wearing flannelette nightwear.

2. Some synthetic materials such as nylon inflict shocking burns on people, not because of their flammability, but because they tend to melt and then stick to human flesh while very hot.

3. Some plastics, when subjected to heat, give off toxic gases.

Oxygen Therapy

This involves the administration of oxygen in concentrations higher than those in the normal atmosphere, for the treatment of various conditions.

1. The major use of oxygen therapy is in the correction of **hypoxia** (lack of an adequate amount of oxygen in inspired air), or in the treatment of a deficiency of oxygen in body tissues, or in **anoxia**, in which tissues are all virtually without oxygen.

These conditions may arise in such situations as high altitude flying or climbing, firefighting, pulmonary obstruction, shock, cardiac disorders, respiratory depression or failure (as a result of drugs, paralysis or severe injuries), or from pulmonary oedema.

2. It may be used in a *supportive role*, with unconscious or post-anaesthetic patients.

3. It may be administered either to displace other gases in the body as in decompression sickness ('the bends' or caisson disease), where nitrogen bubbles have formed in intracellular or extracellular spaces or to remove gases from the pleural space following pneumothoracic surgery, or from the ventricles of the brain, for example, following pneumoencephalography.

4. **Hyperbaric oxygenation.** This involves the administration of oxygen at higher than atmospheric pressure while the patient is in an airtight steel chamber (Fig. 7.29). This has proved to be a life-saving procedure for many people suffering from decompression sickness. It also has value in treating such conditions as anaerobic infections (e.g. gas gangrene), carbon monoxide poisoning, arterial insufficiency in the legs, and disorders in which hypoxia does not respond sufficiently to 100 per cent oxygen at normal atmospheric pressure, which can occur with some anaemic patients. This procedure has also been tried out as an aid in some types of cardiovascular surgery, in some types of cancer therapy and in the early treatment of spinal injuries.

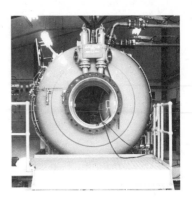

Figure 7.29 A hyperbaric chamber. (Courtesy of the Royal Australian Navy.)

Increased amounts of oxygen can be '*forced*' into the blood if the atmospheric pressure is raised. The reader will recall that normal atmospheric pressure is 101.3 kPa (760 mmHg) and that 21 per cent of oxygen in the atmosphere exerts a partial pressure of 21.3 kPa (approximately 160 mmHg). At this partial pressure, arterial partial pressure of oxygen is about 14 kPa (105 mmHg).

The partial pressure of oxygen can be increased proportionally by administering oxygen under higher pressure, two to three times normal atmospheric pressure in a hyperbaric chamber. The higher pressure 'pushes' or increases the movement of oxygen across lung tissue into the blood, thus increasing the amount of oxygen moved and raising the arterial partial pressure of oxygen. This, in turn, can promote the diffusion of more oxygen out into the body tissue.

Points to Remember When Administering Oxygen
1. Administering higher oxygen concentrations to a patient also means that there is *less humidity* in the inspired gas or gas mixture – the more oxygen and less air given, the drier the inhaled gas(es). This can lead to such problems as:

- Excessive drying of the mucosal membranes of the respiratory tract due to increased loss of surface fluid to the drier gas. This in turn leads to cracking and breakdown of tissues and even increased risk of infection.
- Thickening and drying of respiratory tract secretions, which can then form plugs and crusts in the lower tract, making it difficult to expectorate secretions and causing obstructions.

• Increasing discomfort for the patient both in terms of pain and the effort required to breathe.

2. Oxygen should be treated like a *drug* – it should be given in measured or prescribed amounts as it can be toxic or detrimental in given situations. In some instances, high concentrations of oxygen can be fatal, while lower ones are life-saving. As an example, let us look at chronic obstructive airways diseases (emphysema and chronic pulmonary disease). In some patients with these chronic disorders – which involve obstruction of bronchioles and great decreases in the total surface of the respiratory membranes available for gas exchange much of the stimulus that helps maintain ventilation in the resulting hypoxia arises from hypoxic stimulation of nerve receptors. That is, the lack of oxygen becomes a far more powerful stimulus to the respiratory centre through the nerve receptors (chemoreceptors) than is usual. Normally, it is carbon dioxide and hydrogen ion concentrations that have powerful and direct effects on respiratory centre activity.

Therefore, if oxygen is administered in these conditions to relieve hypoxia without proper consideration, it is possible for the respiration rate to fall so low that lethal levels of carbon dioxide (or hypercapnia) develops. The depressed or lowered respiration, in combination with already higher than normal levels of carbon dioxide (retention of which occurs for the same reasons as the hypoxia), may be a fatal combination in some patients. The moral of this story is – **know your hypoxia!** In other words, the nurse should understand the basic physiological principles relating to the different types of hypoxia.

Wherever possible, oxygen therapy should be administered in combination with the monitoring of blood gases so that the quantities most beneficial to the individual patient can be given.

Administration of Oxygen

Oxygen is supplied for use either in metal tanks (bottles) of various sizes or from a pipe outlet from a centralised storage supply – the outlets may be in the walls or ceilings. At all times be aware that either supply of oxygen contains oxygen gas that has been compressed into the container at very high pressures, and that the outlet will require the addition of a flow meter gauge to allow controlled release of the gas. In addition, a pressure gauge is required at the outlet of a tank or on the central supply to give an indication of the quantity of gas left in the container. Neither of these types of gauges should be regarded as accurate to the first degree. Thus a full tank should always be available as the tank in use approaches lower levels.

There are a variety of ways by which the oxygen can be delivered to the patient from the supply: nasal catheters and cannulae, masks, tents, funnels, ventilators or tracheostomy. Details concerning the types of equipment and procedures for usage can be found in specialised references and nursing texts (see Fig. 7.30).

Hazards of Oxygen Usage

As we have already pointed out, the presence of oxygen in higher than normal concentrations means that ignition of flammable substances is much easier, the rate of combustion is faster and, in addition, it may be more difficult to extinguish such fires.

Safety measures that can help to prevent the occurrence and spread of fires while oxygen is being used include:

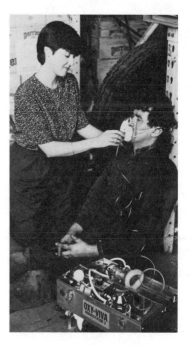

Figure 7.30. Care must always be exercised whenever oxygen is being used. (Courtesy of the Occupational Health Professionals Pty Ltd.)

1. **Do not allow smoking** by the patient, visitors or staff within the area. Post appropriate signs and remove all forms of tobacco, pipes and matches/lighters within the patient's area. Explain both to the patient and the visitors the reasons for these measures.

2. **Never use oil** on oxygen equipment or apparatus, as fuels can ignite without a spark in pure oxygen.

3. **Do not allow the use of electric razors;** in the case of oxygen tents particularly, electric call bells should be disconnected, removed and replaced with hand bells. Electric sparks can easily start fires in high oxygen areas.

4. **No open fires or flames,** frayed electrical wires or extension cords should be within the patient's area.

5. Make sure that all **electrical plugs** and equipment are properly **grounded** (earthed).

6. **Reduce the risk of static electricity.** Even sparks from static electricity can be hazardous. Items such as wool blankets which easily produce static electricity should not be used.

7. **Do not use flammable liquids or solutions,** such as alcohol, ether, antiseptic tinctures, oils (mineral oil as a lip lubricant, oily hair sprays or dressings) or greases.

8. One of the most effective and important safety measures is **communication of information,** in terms of awareness and education of the patient, visitors, staff, nursing students and aides, domestics, electricians and carpenters.

9. **If a fire occurs** in the patient's area, not only should the patient be removed and other general fire orders followed, but the oxygen supply must be turned off – and this must be done immediately if the patient's clothing or bedding is on fire.

Oxygen Toxicity

This is the other hazard *specific* to oxygen therapy. It has a greater tendency to develop at higher than normal atmospheric pressure or when oxygen is delivered in high concentrations for prolonged periods of time. Oxygen toxicity became more prevalent with the introduction of mechanical ventilators, cuffed endotracheal and tracheostomy tubes and the greater usage of hyperbaric oxygen chambers. This is because these devices make it possible to deliver higher concentrations of oxygen at higher pressures for longer periods of time.

Localities that have been damaged by oxygen toxicity include the eyes, lungs and the central nervous system.

More detailed information on this subject can be found in standard nursing texts.

To help prevent the development of oxygen toxicity it is useful to:

- Be very accurate and careful in ensuring that the correct amount of oxygen is delivered in the correct period of time.
- Alternate between air and oxygen breathing at specific intervals, as this relieves the full effect of pure oxygen, lengthening the toleration time.
- Periodically fully inflate the lungs either mechanically or by the patient's own efforts. This helps to reduce the risk of atelectasis – collapsed or airless lung.
- Monitor blood gases frequently in order to keep oxygen at the lowest concentrations necessary to achieve the desired results.

Extinguishing Fires

Everyone should receive some basic training in preventing and dealing with fires. In the case of the practising nurse, such training is imperative, quite apart from the specific policies relevant to his or her place of occupation.

Basically, one should at least know that fires can be put out by:

- *separating* burning material from its oxygen supply; and/or
- *lowering the temperature* of the burning material below its ignition point.

Some of the methods employing the principle of separation are:

- Carbon dioxide fire extinguishers. Since carbon dioxide is heavier than air, it settles down over the burning material, cutting off the air (oxygen) supply.

- Covering the burning material tightly with a non-flammable material. For example, roll the person up in a fire blanket, which is made from specially treated wool.
- Turning off the electric current in the case of electrical fires. **Do not, under any circumstances, use water for an electrical fire.** Sand, salt, or any of the special fire extinguishers designed for electrical fires may be used. Any old carbon tetrachloride fire extinguishers that may still be about should be replaced immediately. These were made at a time when people were not aware of the highly toxic nature of carbon tetrachloride. Modern BCF extinguishers may be used, but with great care. If the space where these are to be used is too confined, an alternative such as the dry powder type is preferable.
- For similar reasons, **water must NOT be used on fires where oil or fat is involved** – water might just spread the fire.

Methods involving the lowering of temperature are not as easily available and will not be discussed here.

Nebulisers

The use of nebulisers has become common in most modern treatment centres as well as in homes in some circumstances. The nebuliser is a device that injects water or a medicated solution, such as salbutamol, into a stream of oxygen or gas mixture flowing to a patient.

The nebuliser plays a very major role in respiratory therapy, since its use reduces dehydration in a patient receiving oxygen or other gases that are very dry. It also has several advantages over other methods in the delivery of certain medications to the respiratory system. These advantages are as follows:

1. It is particularly suited to those medications that are most effective in an 'aerosol' or nebulised form, e.g. salbutamol (Ventolin), orciprenaline (Alupent), terbutaline (Bricanyl), etc., all used in the treatment of asthma and chronic obstructive airways disease.

2. The dose is delivered directly to the affected area.

3. The smaller doses required by this route reduce adverse reactions.

4. The onset of drug action is usually more immediate – a very important factor in patients suffering from breathing difficulties.

In addition, nebulisers can be used with respirators, the

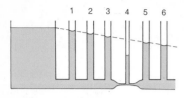

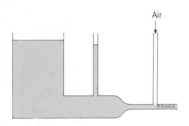

Figure 7.31. Illustration of the Bernoulli effect in tubes 1, 2, 3, 4, 5 and 6. (From Nave & Nave: *Physics for the Health Sciences*, 3rd Ed. Philadelphia. W.B. Saunders. 1985.)

intermittent positive pressure respirators in particular. This adds the advantage of delivering or pushing water and medication deeper into the respiratory system than when therapy is dependent solely on the patient's ability to inhale deeply. The patient may not have the energy or ability or take in sufficient moisture or medication and to get it deep enough into the system. Even healthy people do not use their full lung capacities without noticeable effort.

Since it is commonly the nurse's role to set up and administer or supervise the use of nebulisers, it is appropriate to examine the principles underlying their functioning.

The Bernoulli Effect in Flowing Fluids

It has been seen earlier in the chapter that when fluid flows through a uniform tube, a drop in pressure occurs. In Fig. 7.31 a drop in pressure is indicated by the progressively reduced heights of the liquid in vertical tubes or manometers 1, 2, 3, 5 and 6.

In the fourth vertical tube, a much greater drop in pressure is observed, associated with a constriction in the horizontal tube. The reason for this excessive drop is that the pressure in flowing fluids is lowest where the speed is greatest. This is referred to as the **Bernoulli effect**.

Since the constricted area of the tube is required to transport fluid at the same rate as the rest of the tube, it follows that the fluid speed through the constriction must be greater. Associated with this greater fluid speed is a greater drop in pressure. Once past the constriction, the fluid slows down and the pressure rises to some extent, as seen in Fig. 7.31, vertical tube 5.

If the constriction is severe enough, the fluid pressure may fall below atmospheric pressure. An open tube at this point would allow air to be introduced into the fluid flow, as indicated in Fig. 7.32.

Just as air may be drawn in by this pressure drop, so may other liquids. In the nebuliser, a stream of oxygen may draw a flow of liquid such as water or medicated solution into the oxygen stream to a patient's lungs. That is, the same basic concepts apply to the flow of gases as did to the liquid flow described above. The liquid drawn into the gas stream is in the form of very tiny *droplets*. This is the essential difference between a nebuliser and a humidifier, since in the latter case the liquid is in the form of a *vapour*.

Figure 7.33 illustrates one type of nebuliser utilising the Bernoulli effect.

Turn back to the beginning of this chapter and see if you can now answer the questions posed in the introduction.

Figure 7.32. The introduction of a gas into a fluid by means of the Bernoulli effect. (From Nave & Nave: *Physics for the Health Sciences*. 3rd Ed. Philadelphia. W.B. Saunders. 1985.)

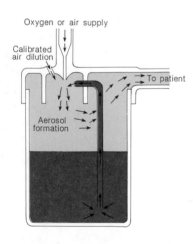

Figure 7.33. Schematic diagram of a nebuliser utilising the Bernoulli effect. (From Nave & Nave: *Physics for the Health Sciences*. 3rd Ed. Philadelphia. W.B. Saunders. 1985.)

REVIEW

1. Breathing is sometimes described as a passive process. On what basis does this description rest?.
2. In hyaline membrane disease, there is a shortage of surfactant in the lungs. What effect does this shortage have on the baby's breathing process?
3. Outline the relevance of Dalton's law to the human body.
4. Which properties of oxygen make it most suitable for use in the body?
5. List the important safety measures that must be taken when oxygen is being used.
6. What is the main effect on the heart when venous return to the heart is increased because of an increase in blood volume?
7. What effects can a disorder such as arteriosclerosis have on blood flow and pressure?
8. A newspaper carries a story of a deep-sea diver rushed to the Navy's hyperbaric chamber.
   (a) What would you surmise to be the reason?
   (b) How would this condition have developed and what effects does it have?
   (c) What part does the hyperbaric chamber play?

8

Acids and bases

OBJECTIVES

After studying this chapter the student should be able to:

1. Define an acid and a base, and outline the importance of some acids and bases in the body.
2. Distinguish between 'concentrated' and 'strong' acids and bases, and between 'dilute' and 'weak' acids and bases.
3. Describe the pH scale and define pH in terms of hydrogen ion concentration.
4. Describe the main buffering systems in the body.
5. Explain how the pH of body fluids is regulated by respiration and the kidneys.
6. List some of the causes and effects of respiratory acidosis and alkalosis, and of metabolic acidosis and alkalosis.

INTRODUCTION

Acids and bases (alkalis) are substances that we normally associate with danger in our everyday lives. It may surprise some to learn that both are not only present in the body but are also vital to its functioning. However, these substances *can* be dangerous if their concentrations are not maintained within very tight limits.

It is not uncommon for a nurse to be caring for a patient whose immediate problem may be too much or too little of one or other of these substances.

Let us take the more common problem of too high a level of acids (**acidosis**) as an example. Acidosis is a problem that may occur as a complication of a number of different diseases or disorders. The disease *diabetes mellitus* is one that can cause acidosis. This is basically a disease of the pancreatic gland causing an insufficient supply of a substance called insulin, which is essential for the processing of a sugar, glucose, to provide energy.

Acidosis can also be a complication during an acute or severe phase of chronic (long-term) bronchitis. In this case, the abnormal acid levels are occurring in association with a severe malfunctioning of the lungs.

In both these diseases, acidosis would be a critical problem requiring immediate treatment, since it can rapidly become fatal. In both cases, there may be similarities in the acidosis in terms of signs and symptoms, and even as far as some standard treatments are concerned – for example, counteracting the excess of acid with a base. However, the similarity ends there, because the acidosis has developed for completely different reasons in each case, and in completely different ways.

Therefore, to really solve this problem, to identify or anticipate it at its earliest stage, to act rapidly, to treat it comprehensively and to try to prevent a recurrence, one would have to understand what produced the acidosis and how it developed in the first place. To do this, the nurse needs to know and understand the properties of acids and bases, and the homeostatic mechanisms by which the body controls acid-base levels.

ACIDS

An acid is a species (molecule or ion) that donates a proton to another species in a reaction. A proton is a hydrogen atom that has lost an electron. (Note that this is identical to the particle described in Chapter 4 as one of the types of particles making up the nucleus of any atom.)

$$H \rightarrow H^+ + e^-$$

OR as shown in Fig. 8.1.

Since the hydrogen atom contains only one proton and no

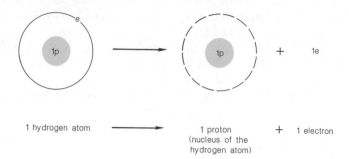

1 hydrogen atom ⟶ 1 proton   +   1 electron
                      (nucleus of the
                      hydrogen atom)

Figure 8.1. The formation of a proton from a hydrogen atom.

neutrons, the species formed when it loses an electron is called a proton.

Let us look at a few examples of acids:

1. **Hydrochloric acid.** As previously discussed in Chapter 4, hydrochloric acid exists as such *only in the presence of a solvent* – usually water. When not in a solvent, this substance exists as hydrogen chloride, which is covalently bonded and has no hydrogen ions (protons) present.

In water, hydrochloric acid exists as hydrogen ions (H^+) and chloride ions (Cl^-). Despite the tact that many textbooks of physiology and even some 'science' textbooks show something to the contrary, *there is no such thing as a molecule of hydrochloric acid.* What does exist is hydrogen chloride (HCl) in molecular form – as *molecules.* This substance is a covalently bonded gas that can exist only in the complete absence of water, because as soon as any water becomes available hydrogen chloride breaks up or 'dissociates' into hydrogen ions and chloride ions.

It is this complete dissociation in aqueous solution that leads to the description of hydrochloric acid as a *strong acid.*

Thus:

$$H-Cl \xrightarrow{\text{H}_2\text{O}} H^+_{(aq)} \quad + \quad Cl^-_{(aq)}$$

hydrogen   proton   chloride
chloride   (hydrogen ion)   ion
                 (aquated)   (aquated)

Most ions in aqueous solution (i.e. when dissolved in water) have a number of water molecules attached – hence the use of the subscript (aq). This does not affect any of the properties in which we are interested, however.

While reference will be made to this point later, the reason why hydrochloric acid is mentioned here is that it occurs in quite strong concentration in the stomach, where it plays an important part in digestive processes.

2. **Ethanoic (acetic) acid.** This is a *weak acid*, which is not completely dissociated in water, unlike hydrochloric acid.

$$CH_3COOH \quad \rightleftharpoons \quad CH_3COO^- \quad + \quad H^+$$

ethanoic   ethanoate   proton

acid   ion   (hydrogen ion)

In this case, the reaction can go both ways:

- The reaction can go to the right, in which case ethanoic acid dissociates to form ethanoate ion and a proton.
- The reaction can go to the left, in which case ethanoate ion combines with a proton to form ethanoic acid.

Hence two arrows are used to represent the reaction. However, the extent of dissociation of this acid is only of the order of seven per cent at room temperature, so that a longer arrow is used in the left direction than to the right. Another way of saying this is that only seven molecules of ethanoic acid out of every 100 break up to dissociate into ions. Thus there is a much greater tendency for the two ions to combine together to form ethanoic acid than there is for ethanoic acid to break up into ions – the reaction to the left is thus favoured.

Important Note
It must be appreciated that the term 'weak acid' refers to the extent to which the acid dissociates to yield a proton. This does not necessarily reflect the acid's ability to make a very marked impression on human flesh. Concentrated (often called 'glacial') acetic acid, for example, can inflict severe burns. Another weak acid, hydrofluoric acid, is used to etch glass. If this acid comes into contact with one's hand, by the time hospital treatment is obtained, amputation may be indicated.
The reader is well advised to treat all acidic substances with the greatest respect.

3. **Hydrogen carbonate (bicarbonate) ion.** In our definition of an acid, reference was made to the fact that an *ion can act as an acid*. One very important example of this is the hydrogen carbonate ion, which, as we shall soon see, plays a most important role in many aspects of body function. Thus:

$$HCO_3^- \quad \rightleftharpoons \quad H^+ \quad + \quad CO_3^{2-}$$

hydrogen   proton   carbonate

carbonate   (hydrogen   ion

ion   ion)

The hydrogen carbonate ion is a weak acid also, so that arrows are shown both ways. The particular conditions (for example, the concentration of hydrogen ion) prevailing at the time will determine whether this reaction will tend to move to the left or to the right. A high proton concentration will tend to send the reaction back to the left, but a low proton concentration will tend to cause the reaction to go to the right.

Acids in the Body

The first question that we might ask here is where do the acids in the body originate. They come from several sources:

1. The most important source is *metabolism*. In the next chapter, we can see the mechanism of the formation of these acids.

2. Another source is the *food* we eat, although this is much less important.

3. *Medications or drugs* are often sources of acids. One common example is aspirin, which is acetylsalicylic acid. This medication is not recommended today in an uncoated form, especially on a frequent or chronic basis, because of its irritating effects on gastric mucosa (the lining of the stomach). This can often lead to bleeding and can contribute to problems in the blood, particularly in young children. It should be noted that some of the therapeutic benefits of this same drug have only recently been realised, particularly in relation to brain function.

Other acids used as medications include ascorbic acid (vitamin C) and ethacrynic acid (a powerful diuretic).

4. Acids are often formed as a *consequence of disease*. Some examples are diabetes mellitus, severe infections, hyperthyroidism, starvation, vomiting from deep in the gastrointestinal tract, respiratory failure and chronic bronchitis.

The second question arising here concerns the general function of acids in the body. These are listed in Table 8.1. It is most important to bear in mind that, although some acids are harmful to body tissue (for example hydrochloric acid), many acids are useful in body function, and hydrochloric acid is essential in digestive processes. It should be noted that the stomach has a special lining that preserves it from attack by this acid, but other tissues are not protected. One of the authors knows an individual who claimed that it is safe to drink hydrochloric acid because it is found in the stomach! The point is that none of the tissues in the gastrointestinal tract, other than the stomach, are protected against attack by the acid, unless the acid is highly diluted.

Apart from the uses already mentioned, acids are very useful in *destroying or inactivating micro-organisms*. Examples include hydrochloric acid in the stomach, and the acidity of the vagina and perspiration.

TABLE 8.1   Acids and their functions

Acid	Function
Acetoacetic	A ketone body formed during metabolism
Acetylsalicylic	Aspirin
Amino	The group of acids which make up proteins
Ascorbic	Vitamin C
Benzoic	An antifungal agent and germicide
Carbonic	Forms part of the hydrogen carbonate ion equilibrium in respiration and renal function
Citric	Found in citrus fruits and is an intermediate in the Krebs (citric acid) cycle
Ethacrynic	A powerful diuretic
Fatty	These acids combine with glycerol to form fats
Folic	One of the vitamins of the B complex
Hydrochloric	A normal constituent of gastric juice
Lactic	A compound formed in anaerobic metabolism of carbohydrate
Nucleic	RNA and DNA – the genetic material of cells
Oleic	An unsaturated fatty acid found in animal fats
Palmitic	A saturated fatty acid found in animal fats
Pyruvic	Formed in aerobic metabolism of carbohydrate
Stearic	A saturated fatty acid found in animal fats
Uric	A metabolic by-product found in the urine

These are but a small sample of the hundreds of acids that are important in the body or that are used in some treatments.

BASES

A base (alkali) is a species that accepts a proton in a reaction. Once again, the species may be a molecule or an ion. The older definition of a base involved the production of hydroxide OH^- ions in aqueous solution.

Some examples of bases are:

1. **Sodium hydroxide.** This is a strong base in aqueous solution because it is completely dissociated into sodium ions (Na^+) and hydroxide ions (OH^-). The sodium ions are not involved in any way in the reaction of this compound as a base, since the function of accepting protons is performed by the hydroxide ion thus:

$$OH^- \quad + \quad H^+ \quad \rightleftharpoons \quad H_2O$$

| hydroxide ion | | proton (hydrogen ion) | | water |

However, the ready availability of hydroxide ions in this case and the classification of sodium hydroxide as a strong base results from the stability of the sodium ion. This means that, even in the solid state, sodium hydroxide does not exist as molecules but as an array of sodium ions and hydroxide ions. It is then already ionised even before it dissolves in water.

2. **Liquid ammonia.** This is a solution of the gas, ammonia (NH_3), dissolved in water. It is often sold as a cleansing agent known as 'cloudy ammonia' and is a weak base.

$$NH_{3(aq)} \quad + \quad H^+ \quad \rightleftharpoons \quad NH_4^+$$

ammonia	proton	ammonium
(aqueous)	(hydrogen ion)	ion

3. **Hydrogen carbonate (bicarbonate) ion.** We have already discussed the behaviour of the hydrogen carbonate ion as an acid, but this ion can also behave as a base:

$$HCO_3^- \quad + \quad H^+ \quad \rightleftharpoons \quad H_2CO_3$$

hydrogen carbonate ion	proton (hydrogen ion)	carbonic acid

Once again, this is an *equilibrium reaction*, as indicated by the arrows, that is:

- Hydrogen carbonate ion reacts with a proton to form carbonic acid.
- Carbonic acid breaks up or dissociates to form protons and hydrogen carbonate ions.
- Under particular conditions – with respect to temperature, pressure and the presence of catalysts – the reaction to the right will proceed at the *same rate* as to the left, thus maintaining a *fixed concentration* of hydrogen carbonate ions, protons and carbonic acid.

Although the concentrations of these species all remain the same, the reaction to the right and the reaction to the left do not cease but keep going at the same rate. This is what is meant by equilibrium.

However, if a change of concentration occurs in one of these species, such as H^+, the equilibrium will be upset and the reaction will then go either to the left or to the right. The direction in which the reaction will go is once again dependent on the reaction conditions. A high proton concentration will tend to send the reaction to the right, but a low proton concentration will tend to send the reaction to the left in the equation above.

Furthermore, the carbonic acid formed can then break up into water and carbon dioxide:

$$H_2CO_3 \quad \rightleftharpoons \quad H_2O \quad + \quad CO_2$$
carbonic acid \qquad water \qquad\qquad carbon
\qquad\qquad\qquad\qquad\qquad\qquad\qquad\qquad dioxide

Important Note
This reaction actually attains equilibrium very slowly. In the body, the reaction is catalysed (i.e. assisted – catalysis is discussed in Chapter 9) by *carbonic anhydrase* (one of a number of catalysts present in the body, called enzymes), without which the system simply could not operate and life as we know it would not be possible.

This equilibrium completes a series of equilibria that are most *important in terms of the transport of carbon dioxide in the body*. The complete series, may now be taken together, along with the ions that tend to make a particular reaction go one way or the other, i.e. the H^+ and OH^- ions written on top of the arrows. If an H^+ is written above (or below) an arrow, this indicates that the reaction will tend to go that way if that ion is present in increased concentration.

$$\overset{OH^-}{\underset{H^+}{CO_2 + H_2O \rightleftharpoons H_2CO_3 \rightleftharpoons}} H^+ + HCO_3^-$$

carbon \quad water \qquad carbonic \qquad proton \qquad hydrogen
dioxide \qquad\qquad\qquad acid \qquad\qquad\qquad\qquad carbonate ion

$$H^+ \updownarrow OH^-$$

$$H^+ + CO_3^{2-}$$
proton \quad carbonate

Alkalinity in the Body

This usually arises from depletion of hydrogen ion concentration. Examples include:

- Vomiting of stomach contents.
- Loss of electrolytes as a consequence of gastric suction. Such patients are not receiving adequate replacements.

Alkalinity can also arise from the direct ingestion of an alkali – especially if self-administered. One example is that of people with peptic ulcers or frequent indigestion who often take baking soda (sodium bicarbonate) or milk of magnesia, both of which are alkaline. Baking soda, in particular, if used indiscriminately, frequently causes 'acid rebound'. In this situation carbon dioxide is released, which causes the acidity to rise, and this in turn increases discomfort and causes damage to tissues, so that the patient then tends to take more baking soda. This cycle then leads to metabolic alkalosis. Patients who are vomiting or taking alkaline medications are even more vulnerable.

PROPERTIES OF ACIDS AND BASES

Acids

1. Have a sour taste (e.g. lemon – citric acid, vinegar – acetic acid).
2. Turn blue litmus red.
3. React with bases to form a salt and water (see chemical equation below).
4. Destroy body tissue.

Bases

1. Have a bitter taste (sodium bicarbonate, soap solution).
2. Turn red litmus blue.
3. React with acids to form a salt and water.
4. Destroy body tissue.

Remember that any reaction between any acid and any base can be represented as:

$$H^+ \quad + \quad OH^- \quad \longrightarrow \quad H_2O$$

proton   hydroxide   water
(hydrogen   ion
ion)

While the above is the most correct way of representing the reaction between a base and an acid, as a matter of convenience this is sometimes represented in the molecular form, or as molecules:

$$HCl_{(aq)} \quad + \quad NaOH \quad \longrightarrow \quad NaCl \quad + \quad H_2O$$

hydrochloric   sodium   sodium   water
acid   hydroxide   cloride

However, since hydrochloric acid, sodium hydroxide and sodium chloride do *not* exist as molecules but as ions, the first equation given is the more correct.

TABLE 8.2 Bases and their uses

Base	Function
Aluminium hydroxide gel	Gastric antacid
Magnesium hydroxide gel (Milk of Magnesia)	Gastric antacid
Magnesium oxide	Gastric antacid
Titanium dioxide	Sunscreen
Zinc oxide	Sunscreen

Similarly, the reaction of an acid with a bicarbonate is represented in the molecular form as:

$$NaHCO_3 \ + \ HCl_{(aq)} \ \longrightarrow \ NaCl \ + \ H_2CO_3$$

| sodium bicarbonate | hydrochloric acid | sodium chloride | carbonic acid |

$$\searrow$$
$$H_2O + CO_2$$
water   carbon
dioxide

Once again the ionic form is more correct, for the same reasons:

$$HCO_3^- \ + \ H^+ \ \rightleftharpoons \ H_2CO_3 \ \rightleftharpoons \ H_2O \ + \ CO_2$$

| hydrogen carbonate ion | hydrogen ion (proton) | carbonic acid | water | carbon dioxide |

This equation represents the reaction between excess stomach acidity and sodium bicarbonate (household baking soda), which used to be used as a home remedy, as previously discussed. The hydrogen carbonate ion reacts with the excess hydrogen ion (from hydrochloric acid) to produce carbon dioxide gas which usually manifests itself as a 'burp'.

First Aid Treatment

Having raised the question of safety, some comments should be made about first aid. Both acids and bases are extremely corrosive substances that can have a devastating effect on human tissue. The most effective first aid measure when acids or bases have come into contact with a part of the body – even an eye – is plenty of water. If sufficient water is used, all of the acid or base will be washed away, and the burn can be treated in the usual way.

Unless an appropriate solution has been provided for the purpose, no attempt should be made to neutralise the acid or base. Instances have been known where a well-meaning individual has attempted to treat a severe alkali (base) burn by pouring hydrochloric acid over the unfortunate victim! The idea was to neutralise the base with the acid, but the acid ended up causing far worse burns than the original.

The 'proper solution' to which we referred above can be made up by anyone working with these substances, as follows:

For acid burns: an almost saturated solution of sodium bicarbonate – ordinary baking soda (this substance has a 'reserve alkalinity' in that it acts as an alkali in the presence of an acid and can thus neutralise the acid).

For alkali (base) burns: an almost saturated solution of ammonium chloride, commonly known as sal ammoniac, which has a 'reserve acidity'. This should be followed in all cases by copious quantities of water.

SALTS

In passing, reference was made to the fact that an acid and a base react together to form a salt and water. Before proceeding, however, let us recapitulate some important facts:

1. A strong acid completely dissociates in water.
2. A weak acid only partly dissociates in water.
3. A strong base completely dissociates in water.
4. A weak base only partly dissociates in water.

If a strong acid and a strong base react, the salt formed is *neutral* in solution; for example, hydrochloric acid reacts with sodium hydroxide to form a solution of sodium chloride.

If a weak acid and a weak base react, the salt formed is *neutral* in solution; for example acetic acid reacts with aqueous ammonia (incorrectly called ammonium hydroxide in some texts) to form a solution of ammonium acetate.

If a strong acid and a weak base react, the salt formed is *acidic* in solution; for example, hydrochloric acid reacts with aqueous ammonia to form a solution of ammonium chloride.

If a weak acid and a strong base react, the salt formed is *basic* in solution; for example, acetic acid reacts with sodium hydroxide to form a solution of sodium acetate.

It is for this reason that sodium bicarbonate (a salt produced from a weak acid and a strong base), tends to act as a base in solution and thus react with an acid. However, it is the *hydrogen carbonate ion* that acts as a base. Furthermore, under some conditions that same hydrogen carbonate ion (HCO_3^-) can give up its proton and act as an acid.

DESCRIBING ACIDITY: pH

So far, the terms strong and weak have been applied to both acids and bases. However, we are referring to the *tendency of the acid or base to dissociate*. This should not be confused with *concentration* in the sense in which we refer to a strong or weak cup of tea.

TABLE 8.3 Salts and their uses

Salt	Function
Ammonium chloride	Treatment of alkalosis
Aluminium acetate	Astringent* – anti-perspirant
Aluminum carbonate (basic)	Gastric antacid
Aluminium chloride	Astringent* – anti-perspirant
Aluminium phosphate gel	Gastric antacid
Calcium carbonate	As an absorbent for diarrhoea
Calcium chloride	Used to restore electrolyte balance Cardiac injection associated with electric defibrillation
Calcium phosphate	Used as a source of calcium Important constituent of bones
Magnesium carbonate	Gastric antacid
Magnesium citrate	Mild laxative
Magnesium stearate	Dermatological dusting powder
Magnesium sulfate (Epsom salts)	Laxative; electrolyte replenisher
Magnesium oxide	Gastric antacid
Magnesium phosphate	Gastric antacid
Magnesium trisilicate	Gastric antacid
Mercury dichloride	Topical anti-infective agent
Potassium bicarbonate	In treatment of electrolyte depletion
Potassium chloride	In treatment of electrolyte depletion
Potassium iodide	Thyroid disorder diagnosis and treatment Management of coughing
Potassium permanganate	Topical anti-infective agent
Silver nitrate	Topical anti-infective agent
Sodium bicarbonate	In combatting acidosis; fluid electrolyte replenisher
Sodium chloride	In treatment of dehydration
Sodium sulfate (Glauber's salt)	Laxative
Sodium phosphate	Laxative
Zinc chloride	Astringent*
Zinc peroxide	Topical anti-infective agent
Zinc sulfate	Astringent*

*An astringent stops the oozing of blood, sweat, etc. **Note:** We have listed *possibilities* here. In practice, a smaller range of substances is normally utilised.

The following statements should make this point clearer.

1. The letter M means 'molar', where a 1 M solution contains one mole of solute dissolved in the solvent and made up to one litre, i.e. one mole per litre or 1 mol/L. Thus a 10 M solution contains 10 moles per litre and a 0.01 M solution contains 0.01 moles per litre. Molarity is then a measure of *concentration*. (This was discussed more fully in Chapter 6).

2. Acid (or base) *strength* is a measure of the tendency of a species to donate (or accept) a proton in a chemical reaction – to dissociate.

3. It is then possible to have:
- A *concentrated* solution of a *weak* acid: such as 10 M ethanoic acid.
- A *dilute* solution of a *weak* acid: such as 0.01 M ethanoic acid.
- A *concentrated* solution of a *strong* acid: such as 10 M hydrochloric acid.
- A *dilute* solution of a *strong* acid: such as 0.01 M hydrochloric acid.
- A wide variety of combinations of concentration and strength.

Just as we have a scale to express the concentration of an acid, it is often useful to have a scale to express the concentration of hydrogen ion. Such a scale is the **pH** scale, where pH stands for **p**otential (or **p**ower) of **H**ydrogen. Some points about the pH scale should be noted:

(a) This scale can be used to describe the concentration of hydrogen ions in *weak* acids and bases, or else *strong* acids and bases in dilute form.

(b) The pH scale is *logarithmic*, since it is based on powers of ten. By using a logarithmic scale we are able to overcome the difficulties associated with powers of a number. This means that we are able to speak in terms of a simple number rather than the power of a number.

(c) Since the concentrations with which we will be dealing are in the range 10^0 to 10^{-14}, it is useful to remove the negative sign. We achieve this by defining pH as a negative number, so that the two negatives then become a positive. This means that the normal range of the pH scale is 0 to 14. We can then define pH:

$$pH = -\log[H^+]$$

where $[H^+]$ means the molar concentration of hydrogen ions.

Then if $[H^+] = 10^{-1.0}$ M,   pH = 1.0
if $[H^+] = 10^{-5.6}$ M,   pH = 5.6
if $[H^+] = 10^{-7.0}$ M,   pH = 7.0
if $[H^+] = 10^{-12.3}$ M,   pH = 12.3

However, being a logarithmic scale, every change of one unit in pH represents a *tenfold* change in hydrogen ion concentration. Every change of two units in pH represents a *one-hundredfold* change in hydrogen ion concentration, and every change of three units in pH represents a *one-thousandfold* change in hydrogen ion concentration.

Thus, if pH = 5, $[H^+] = 10^{-5}$
if pH = 4, $[H^+] = 10^{-4}$ (a 10-fold increase)
if pH = 3, $[H^+] = 10^{-3}$ (a 100-fold increase)
if pH = 2, $[H^+] = 10^{-2}$ (a 1000-fold increase)

It can be seen that a small change in pH can represent quite a large change in hydrogen ion concentration. The implication for medical practice is that a patient's response to any change in pH as a result of intervention may be very rapid.

Looking at water, we find that at 25°C:

$$[H^+] \times [OH^-] = 10^{-14}$$

Now each molecule of water that dissociates yields one hydrogen ion and one hydroxide ion, so that the concentration of these two ions in water is always the same.

$$\text{i.e. } [H^+]^2 = 10^{-14}$$
$$\text{ie. } [H^+] = 10^{-7}$$
$$\text{and } [OH^-] = 10^{-7}$$
$$\text{so that pH} = 7$$
$$\text{and pOH} = 7$$
$$\text{where pOH} = -\log[OH^-]$$
$$\text{thus pH} + \text{pOH} = 14$$

This means that if we know that the pOH of a solution is 3, then the pH will be $14 - 3 = 11$.

Acids have a normal pH range of 0 to 7;
alkalis have a normal pH range of 7 to 14; and
pure water is neutral with a pH of 7.0.

Table 8.4 lists a number of important body fluids and their normal pH or range of pH.

TABLE 8.4   pH of important body fluids

Fluid	Where Located	pH
bile	gall bladder	7.8
blood (arterial)	circulatory system	7.35–7.45
cerebro-spinal fluid	central nervous system	7.35–7.45
gastric juice	stomach (adults)	0.9 –1.5
intracellular fluid	body cells	6.0 –7.4
pancreatic juice	pancreas	8.0 –8.3
saliva	mouth	6.0 –7.0
semen	testes	7.2 –8.0, av.7.8
urine	urinary bladder	4.6 –8.0, av.6.0

ACID-BASE BALANCE AND HOMEOSTASIS

We have seen that both acids and bases can upset a very delicate balance in the body and in physiological processes, so that it is essential that the body has a means of controlling this balance.

A balance is maintained in the body which is essentially a balance of **hydrogen ion (H^+) concentrations** in body fluids. This could just as easily be regarded as a balance of hydroxyl ion (OH^-) concentrations, but the former is much more convenient. Thus we describe the relative acidity or alkalinity of body solutions in terms of the hydrogen ion concentration, and use the pH notation as a convenient shorthand way of representing these concentrations.

Thus we have:

more $H^+ \longrightarrow$ more acidic
  less $H^+ \longrightarrow$ less acidic (i.e. more alkaline or more basic)

A reminder:

1. The *higher* the H^+ concentration (in a weak acid) – the *lower* the pH and vice versa.

2. The pH scale can be used only with *weak* acids or with *dilute* solutions of strong acids (strong acids in concentrated form are completely dissociated). Since, with the obvious exception of hydrochloric acid, all the acids in the body *are* weak acids, the concept of pH is most important.

3. It should be emphasised that the acid-base balance is very critical in living systems. The pH of the blood, for example, needs to be kept within the normal range of 7.35–7.45 if problems are not to arise. It is known that people do not normally survive if the pH of the blood is less than 7 or greater than 8.

4. Clinically a patient may be considered to be in acidosis when the pH of the blood has any value *less than 7.35*. Although this value is in fact slightly alkaline, it is still *more acidic* than the normal value of 7.35. Such a pH will usually warrant treatment, because any deviation of blood pH (or the pH of other body fluids) from the normal range is considered to be a real danger to the patient. Figure 8.2 illustrates the pH range of the extracellular fluid in various acid-base disorders.

5. Hydrogen ions have a varied role in the body:

- They must be present for proper cell function.
- They are necessary for the efficient action of enzymes.
- They are essential for the binding of oxygen by haemoglobin.

Homeostatic Mechanisms for Acid-Base Regulation

The point should be made here that while we are going to talk about various mechanisms regulating acid-base balance, it should

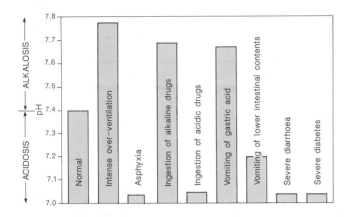

Figure 8.2. pH of the extracellular fluid in various acid-base disorders. (From Guyton: *Physiology of the Human Body*. 5th Ed. Philadelphia. Saunders College Publishing. 1979.)

be borne in mind that this is a *team effort* – the various mechanisms of the body act together to redress any imbalance upsetting the homeostasis of the body.

Before we discuss the various systems controlling body pH, some mention should be made of a minor mechanism that is capable of alleviating local excess hydrogen ion concentration. Because of a particular event in a localised area, such as the strenuous exercising of an arm, there may be a build-up of hydrogen ions in the muscles of the arm. This localised concentration excess can be diluted and removed by increased circulation and thus distributed more widely. Such a mechanism acts rapidly but is very localised in its effect.

Buffer systems
A buffer system is a chemical solution that resists a change in pH. That is:

- If extra *hydrogen ion* is added to the solution, it is able to react in such a way that the change in pH is minimised – as though the buffer is able chemically to soak up the hydrogen ions.
- If extra *hydroxyl ion* is added to the solution, it is able to react in such a way that the change in pH is minimised – as though the buffer is able chemically to soak up the hydroxyl ions.

Thus a buffer system may be regarded as having a reserve acidity and alkalinity. If an acid or an alkali is added to the buffer solution, then the pH will not change very much – within limits, of course!

This buffering means that the fluids of the body, particularly the extracellular fluid and the blood, are provided with protection against drastic changes in acidity or alkalinity (basicity). If

NON-BUFFERED SOLUTION

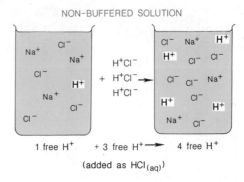

1 free H$^+$ + 3 free H$^+$ ⟶   4 free H$^+$

(added as HCl$_{(aq)}$)

Figure 8.3. Buffering (a) In this case, the beaker on the left has added buffer which can produce L$^-$ (lactate ions). These lactate ions have combined with two of the four available H$^+$ leaving only *two* free hydrogen ions in the beaker on the right, thus reducing the acidity of the solution in that beaker. (b) The beaker on the left contains one free hydrogen ion. This free hydrogen ion appears in the beaker on the right together with the free hydrogen ions added as HCl aqueous. This is a non-buffered situation where all hydrogen ions remain available in solution.

BUFFERED SOLUTION

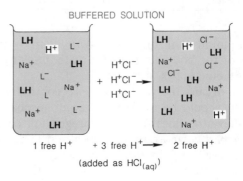

1 free H$^+$ + 3 free H$^+$ ⟶   2 free H$^+$

(added as HCl$_{(aq)}$)

we look at arterial blood, for example, the normal range of pH is from 7.35 to 7.45. A pH of much less than this gives rise to a condition called *acidosis*, and a pH of much more than this gives rise to a condition known as *alkalosis*. A pH less than about 7.0 or more than about 8.0 existing for more than a few hours is usually fatal.

The buffering concept may be illustrated by the following example, in which the buffer solution is a mixture of sodium lactate and lactic acid in water. (Many buffer solutions typically consist of a weak acid and a salt of that acid.)

The sodium lactate (see Fig. 8.3) dissociates partly into sodium ions (Na$^+$) and lactate ions which, for simplicity we will represent as L$^-$ (this is not a chemical symbol, but is rather more convenient than CH$_3$CH(OH)COO$^-$). Thus:

NaL	⇌	Na$^+$	+	L$^-$
sodium lactate		sodium ion		lactate ion

However, lactic acid is a weak acid and is dissociated only to a very limited extent:

HL	$\rightleftharpoons$	H^+	$+$	L^-
lactic acid		hydrogen ion		lactate ion

Thus we have a *higher* concentration of:
 sodium ions,
 lactate ions and
 lactic acid molecules,
and a *lower* concentration of:
 hydrogen ions.

If we now examine the lactic acid equilibrium above, we see that lactate ion is on the right-hand side of the equilibrium and thus the higher concentration of these ions (from both the lactic acid and the sodium lactate) will tend to drive the reaction back to the *left*. This will serve to decrease the hydrogen ion concentration even further. It is noteworthy that the presence of buffering systems (i.e. the compounds involved in buffering) does not present any problems to the body, since buffers act as acids and bases only when they have to. This is what is meant when it is said that buffers have *reserve acidity and alkalinity*.

The presence of buffers has two important implications:

1. If an acid (i.e. hydrogen ion) is added, the lactic acid equilibrium will be driven to the *left*, since some of the excess lactate ions (which have come from the sodium lactate) can combine with the hydrogen ions to form lactic acid, as indicated below. Thus many of the hydrogen ions are removed (or mopped up) and the pH does not change very much:

H^+	$+$	L^-	$\longrightarrow$	HL
hydrogen ions	removed by	lactate ions	to form	lactic acid

2. If an alkali (i.e. a source of hydroxide ions) is added, the lactic acid equilibrium will tend to move towards the *right* and make more hydrogen ions available:

HL	$\longrightarrow$	H^+	$+$	L^-
lactic acid (a proton donor)		proton		lactate ions

These hydrogen ions will tend to mop up the hydroxide ions to form water. Remember that an alkali or base is a proton (hydrogen ion) acceptor, and this is all that is happening here.

H^+	$+$	OH^-	$\longrightarrow$	H_2O
hydrogen ions		hydroxyl ions		water

Once again, the effect of an increase of hydroxide ions is minimised and the pH will not change very much.

$$HL \quad \overset{OH^-}{\underset{H^+}{\rightleftharpoons}} \quad H^+ \quad + \quad L^-$$

(i)   hydrogen ions drive the reaction to the left.
(ii)   hydroxyl ions drive the reaction to the right.
Mopping-up hydrogen ions:

$$H^+ \ + \ L^- \longrightarrow HL$$

Mopping-up hydroxide ions:

$$H^+ + OH^- \longrightarrow H_2O$$

So it becomes evident that the buffer system described has been able to cope with a significant increase in either hydrogen ion or hydroxide ion concentration without any marked effect on the pH of the solution.

Note that this is *not* neutralisation – we are taking advantage of the equilibria involved in weak acids and the salts of these acids to do our mopping-up for us.

Some of the most important buffer systems in the blood and extracellular fluid are the bicarbonate system, proteins (serum proteins and haemoglobin) and the phosphate system.

The Hydrogen Carbonate (Bicarbonate) Ion System
If we were going to make up a hydrogen carbonate buffer system in the laboratory, we would use some carbonic acid (which is only a weak acid but does dissociate to some extent to form the hydrogen carbonate ion) and some sodium bicarbonate. However, in the body, the hydrogen carbonate ion is already present and, as we have already seen, it is capable of acting as an acid or a base.

As an *acid* (a proton donor):

HCO_3^-	$\longrightarrow$	H^+	$+$	CO_3^{2-}
hydrogen carbonate ion		proton		carbonate ion

As a *base* (a proton acceptor):

HCO_3^-	$+$	H^+	$\longrightarrow$	H_2CO_3
hydrogen carbonate ion		proton		carbonic acid

This equilibrium, which we have already briefly discussed, is completely represented as follows:

$$CO_2 \; + \; H_2O \; \rightleftharpoons \; \overset{OH^-}{H_2CO_3} \; \rightleftharpoons \; H^+ \; + \; HCO_3^-$$

carbon   water   carbonic H^+ proton   hydrogen
dioxide   acid   carbonate ion

$$H^+ \; \updownarrow \; OH^-$$
$$H^+ \; + \; CO_3^{2-}$$

proton   carbonate

Two very important points can be made about this system:

1. Although the pH of extracellular fluid and blood is not the most favourable for this system to operate efficiently, the concentration of hydrogen carbonate ion in these fluids is quite high. This means that a ready supply of buffering agent is available. Furthermore, as we shall see, the concentration of hydrogen carbonate ion in the body is closely regulated by the kidneys.

2. The hydrogen ion concentration in these fluids is closely linked with the elimination of CO_2 from the body. If we consider the situation where hydrogen ion concentration is high, the hydrogen carbonate ion buffers this by accepting protons and forming carbonic acid, as indicated above. The carbonic acid then dissociates into carbon dioxide and water.

It would then seem likely that the increased concentration of carbon dioxide would tend to hinder this reaction and that the reaction would then slow down. In other circumstances this would indeed be true, but in the body this is not the case. In fact, the reverse tends to be true! What happens is that the high carbon dioxide concentration results in increased ventilation, which in turn leads to increased carbon dioxide elimination. Carbon dioxide then tends to be eliminated more rapidly than it is being generated. Finally, this tends to shift the equilibrium even further to the left, which removes hydrogen ions, and thus creates and maintains a very efficient and useful buffer system.

At times this system buffers up to 90 per cent of the hydrogen ions in the extracellular fluid and is consequently very important. The hydrogen ion equilibrium, as we will see, depends on the maintenance of the ratio:

$$HCO_3^- : H_2CO_3 \quad = 20{:}1$$
hydrogen carbonate ion : carbonic acid $= 20{:}1$

Protein (serum proteins and haemoglobin)
The cells of the body contain large quantities of proteins, and this makes the protein system very powerful indeed.

However, except in the case of the red blood cells, the slowness of the rate of diffusion of hydrogen and hydrogen carbonate ions through the cell membranes (from inside the cell to the extracellular fluid) means that the ability of these *intracellular* buffers to buffer *extracellular* fluids is delayed for several hours. Thus if a problem exists in the extracellular fluid, this slow rate of diffusion means that the buffers inside the cell will not be able to do much about it in the short term.

It is also interesting to note that the largest quantities of acids produced in the body are produced in the cells, so that the protein system is most important to the cells.

Since proteins, as highly complex combinations of amino acids, are many and varied, space does not permit a detailed discussion of the action of each of these. Haemoglobin will be discussed separately as an important example of a protein within the body cells, while plasma proteins (mainly serum albumin and globulins) will not be discussed further, other than to say that they act in exactly the same way as hydrogen carbonate ion and that most are excellent buffers.

Haemoglobin performs a particular function in buffering hydrogen ions that are in transit from body cells to the lungs. Let us look at this more closely.

Carbon dioxide that has been produced as a waste product of metabolism of body cells is carried from these cells to the lungs as hydrogen carbonate ion (HCO_3^-). Once again:

$$CO_2 + H_2O \rightarrow H_2CO_3 \rightarrow HCO_3^- + H^+$$

| carbon dioxide | water | carbonic acid | hydrogen carbonate ion | proton |

As blood passes through the lungs and gaseous exchange takes place, the above reactions all reverse, lowering the hydrogen carbonate ion and hydrogen ion concentrations and producing carbon dioxide gas, which is then exchanged in the lungs and removed by breathing. However, the hydrogen ions involved must be buffered while in transit from the cells to the lungs and haemoglobin performs this function very effectively. The reason lies in the fact that reduced haemoglobin (or haemoglobin that is not combined with oxygen and represented as Hb) has a much greater affinity for hydrogen ion than does oxyhaemoglobin (represented as HbO_2), thus:

$$HbO_2 \rightarrow Hb(+O_2) \xrightarrow{H^+} HHb^+$$

| oxyhaemoglobin | haemoglobin | acidic haemoglobin (very weakly acidic) |

By buffering these hydrogen ions (by chemical combination), haemoglobin has temporarily removed them from solution so that the pH of the blood is not markedly disturbed.

Note that the reactions above occur *in the red blood cells and*

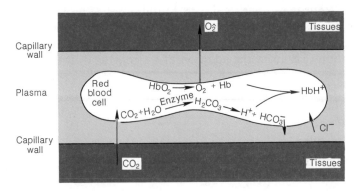

Figure 8.4. Buffering in the red blood cell. HbO_2 = oxyhaemoglobin, Hb = haemoglobin, HbH^+ = acid haemoglobin, E = enzyme (carbonic anhydrase).

all cells of the body where carbon dioxide is being exchanged for oxygen (as distinct from the alveoli of the lungs, the other part of the body where gaseous exchange takes place). When the blood reaches the alveoli, these reactions are all reversed: hydrogen ions are released and haemoglobin combines with oxygen ready to transport it to the cells. The hydrogen ions then combine with hydrogen carbonate ion to effect the release of carbon dioxide as described above.

The reactions at the cellular level are summarised in Fig. 8.4. The hydrogen carbonate ion then moves into the plasma, where it acts as a carrier of carbon dioxide to the lungs (70% of the carbon dioxide produced by body cells is transported as hydrogen carbonate ions). However, the movement of hydrogen carbonate ions into the plasma from the red cells in the blood upsets the electrical balance in these cells, so chloride ions move into the red blood cells to restore the balance. This exchange, and a similar one in the opposite direction at the lungs is called the *chloride shift* or *hamburger shift*.

The phosphate system

This system acts in a similar way to the bicarbonate system. It consists of ions that are derived from the dissociation of phosphoric acid:

$$H_3PO_4 \rightleftharpoons H^+ + H_2PO_4^- \rightleftharpoons 2H^+ + HPO_4^{2-} \rightleftharpoons 3H^+ PO_4^{3-}$$

| phosphoric acid | dihydrogen phosphate ion | monohydrogen phosphate ion | phosphate ion |

In each step, a hydrogen ion is produced, and as each proton is lost, the remaining ion becomes more highly charged. It is then more difficult to remove another hydrogen ion (with its positive charge) from the highly negative ion. The ions with which we are concerned are **(a)** the dihydrogen phosphate ion ($H_2PO_4^-$) which is a *weak* acid (pK_a 7.2), and **(b)** the monohydrogen phosphate ion (HPO_4^{2-}), which is a very weak acid (pK_a 12.4). The prefix 'di-' means 'two' and 'mono-' means 'one'.

Both these ions, however, can also act as proton acceptors, that is as bases, which is why the double arrows are used.

This system copes with an increase in hydrogen ion concentration (e.g. from the addition of a strong acid) thus:

$$HPO_4^{2-} \quad + \quad H^+ \quad \longrightarrow \quad H_2PO_4^-$$

monohydrogen   dihydrogen
phosphate   phosphate
ion   ion

and an increase in hydroxide (e.g. from the addition of a strong alkali) thus:

$$H_2PO_4^- \quad + \quad OH^- \quad \longrightarrow \quad HPO_4^{2-} \quad + \quad H_2O$$

dihydrogen   hydroxide   monohydrogen   water
phosphate   ion   phosphate
ion   ion

giving an overall equilibrium reaction of:

$$H_2PO_4^- \quad \overset{OH^-}{\underset{H^+}{\rightleftharpoons}} \quad HPO_4^{2-}$$

dihydrogen   monohydrogen
phosphate   phosphate
ion   ion

This system operates near its maximum buffering power in body fluids, but its concentration in extracellular fluid, for example, is only about one-twelfth that of the hydrogen carbonate ion. Thus its total buffering contribution in *extracellular fluids* is very limited. However, it is most important *in the tubular fluids of the kidneys*. There are two reasons for this, which the reader is asked to note at this stage, prior to a full treatment of these issues in regard to the kidneys, which will follow shortly.

Firstly, the phosphate concentration in the kidney tubules is very much higher than in extracellular fluid and so the phosphate system becomes an effective buffer system. Secondly, the tubular fluid becomes more acidic than extracellular fluid, bringing the pH into the most effective range of operation of the phosphate system.

For exactly the same reasons, the *phosphate buffer system is very important in intracellular fluids*.

Important Note
These various buffer systems do *not* remove hydrogen ions from the body. This function is performed by the lungs and kidneys. What the buffer systems are able to do is to compensate for any situation that tends to alter the normal pH of body fluids, and thus maintain homeostasis. This is achieved by all the buffer systems of the body working together to bind or 'lock up' hydrogen ions and remove them from solution.

Buffers do this quickly – since they are already on the scene – and efficiently, within limits (as previously indicated), since the supply of buffers in the body is not endless. It follows that other systems in the body are required when the body's total buffering capacity is being utilised.

Respiratory Regulation of Body Fluid pH

To understand this section fully, we really need to look at the implications of a relationship called the Henderson-Hasselbalch equation. However, it may be left out at an initial stage of studying acid-base regulation. Before we apply this equation, it is necessary to define some terms.

1. **pK_a**. This is a term used to describe the strength of weak acids. Let us first look at the dissociation of a hypothetical weak acid with the formula HA:

$$HA \rightleftharpoons H^+ + A^-$$

Since it is a weak acid, which is only slightly dissociated, the equilibrium position will be well to the left, i.e. the reaction towards the left will occur much more readily than the reaction towards the right, as indicated by the arrows.

One quantitative way of expressing this is in terms of a dissociation constant (K), which, because it is an acid in this case, is usually given the symbol K_a, which is called the **acid dissociation constant** and is a measure of the *tendency of an acid to dissociate*.

$$\text{i.e. } K_a \quad \frac{[H^+].[A^-]}{[HA]}$$

The K_a for acetic acid, for example, is 1.76×10^{-5}. Since this type of number is rather clumsy, we use the term pK_a, defined as follows (note the similarity to the definition of pH):

$$pK_a = -\log K_a$$

In the case of acetic acid:

$$
\begin{aligned}
pK_a &= -\log K_a \\
&= -\log(1.76 \times 10^{-5}) \\
&= -(0.25 + [-5]) \\
&= -(-4.75) \\
pK_a &= 4.75
\end{aligned}
$$

Table 8.5 lists a number of weak acids that are important in the body and their pK_a values.

TABLE 8.5   Selected pK_a values

Acid	pK_a
carbonic acid H_2CO_3	6.1
hydrogen carbonate ion HCO_3^-	10.3
dihydrogen phosphate ion $H_2PO_4^-$	7.2
monohydrogen phosphate ion HPO_4^{2-}	12.4
ammonium ion NH_4^+	9.3

Note that acids with a *lower* pK_a value are *stronger* acids than those with a higher pK_a value.

2. **The Henderson-Hasselbalch equation.** In the hydrogen carbonate ion/carbonic acid equilibrium it is found that, at 37°C, the ratio $[HCO_3^-]/[H_2CO_3]$ is numerically equal to 20. This will be applied now in the equation below.

In general, for the reaction

$$HA \rightleftharpoons H^+ + A^-,$$
$$pH = pK_a + \log \frac{[A^-]}{[HA]}$$

and for the carbonic acid/hydrogen carbonate system,

$$pH = pK_a + \log \frac{[HCO_3^-]}{H_2CO_3}$$
$$= 6.1 + \log 20 \text{ (from above)}$$
$$= 6.1 + 1.3$$
$$= 7.4.$$

Since this is the normal pH of the blood, it follows that the maintenance of the hydrogen carbonate ion/carbonic acid ratio at 20 (or 20:1) is most desirable, so that the pH of the blood may be maintained at, or very close to, 7.4.

Plasma hydrogen carbonate levels are regulated by the kidneys, and carbonic acid levels (and thus carbon dioxide levels) in the blood are maintained by the respiratory system. It follows that the lungs and the kidneys thus provide 'physiological buffering' against significant changes in blood pH.

The work of the lungs is normally maintained at such a rate that elimination of carbon dioxide at the lungs is equal to the rate of production of this gas in the cells of the body. However, if the lungs are not removing carbon dioxide fast enough, we see from the hydrogen carbonate equilibrium that this *increases* the hydrogen ion concentration, which then *lowers* the pH of the blood and the extracellular fluid.

It has been found that chemoreceptors in the aorta and carotid arteries are sensitive to changes in blood pH and that chemoreceptors in the medulla are even more sensitive to changes of pH of the cerebro-spinal fluid (CSF). The rate of ventilation will then be altered by the respiratory centre in the medulla to compensate for this change, i.e. it will increase. This increase of ventilation rate removes carbon dioxide more rapidly than before, which drives the equilibrium back so as to decrease hydrogen ion concentration and restore normal blood pH levels, i.e. to restore homeostasis.

This whole mechanism is extremely sensitive and restoration of homeostasis is normally very rapid. A similar, but opposite, response occurs if the hydrogen ion concentration decreases and pH increases – the rate of ventilation slows.

It should be noted that while temporary acid-base stress (departure from homeostasis) may be rapidly rectified by these respiratory mechanisms, species such as hydrogen ions and hydrogen carbonate ions cannot be removed by such mechanisms to cope with chronic problems. However, some degree of adaptation is possible. In the case of emphysema, for example, the body is able to adapt itself to restore the pH of the blood in minutes from, say, 7.0 to about 7.2 or 7.3, but not necessarily right back to 7.4.

Furthermore, this mechanism deals with hydrogen ions formed from the carbonic acid equilibrium, but cannot do anything about other acids in the body – metabolic acids, for example.

However, the kidneys are also able to regulate and control the concentrations of hydrogen ions and hydrogen carbonate ions (among others). The kidneys, while slower in response, are able to cope with chronic acid-base imbalance much more effectively.

Renal Regulation of Body Fluid pH

The great strength of the kidneys in maintaining homeostasis is that they have the capability to *selectively* remove or return ions and substances from or to the blood and thus exercise very effective control over the concentrations of various acids and bases in the blood. This means that blood pH can be closely controlled. Most importantly, the kidneys do not adapt to a situation in the same way as respiratory mechanisms, nor do quantity restraints exist as is the case with buffers. It is noticed that the efficiency of removal tends to increase with time, for example, over a half-day period. However, the kidneys are slower in action than the lungs.

Fig. 8.5 shows the general structure of the kidney and Fig. 8.6 shows the detailed structure of a nephron, the remarkable filtering unit of the kidney, of which each kidney has some one million.

Filtration of all the ions and substances the blood carries, other than the blood cells and large protein molecules, occurs within the glomerulus of the nephron. Subsequently, reabsorption of useful components of the filtered solution (for example,

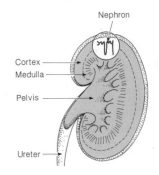

Figure 8.5. General structure of the kidney. (From Arms & Camp: *Biology*. 2nd Ed. Philadelphia. Saunders College Publishing. 1982.)

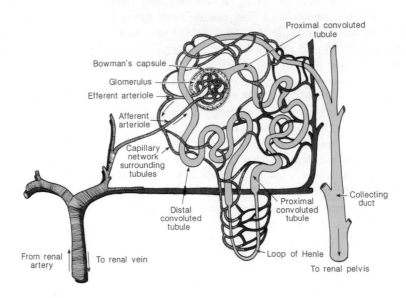

Figure 8.6. A typical cortical nephron.

glucose, some amino acids, vitamins, ions) occurs in the tubules. Any ions or substances that are in excess, or are waste products, will not be reabsorbed, but will be passed down into the urine for eventual elimination from the body.

Renal control mechanisms
If the pH of arterial blood is *decreased*, the kidneys respond by:

- Secreting hydrogen ions into the kidney tubules which then cause the concentration of hydrogen ions to fall and the pH of the blood to rise (see Fig. 8.7).
- Transporting hydrogen carbonate ions to the blood, which will tend to send the hydrogen carbonate equilibrium back towards increased carbonic acid production. This, in turn, uses up more hydrogen ions and causes blood pH to rise.

Alternatively, when arterial blood pH is *higher* than normal, the kidneys are able to remove hydrogen carbonate ions from the blood and decrease hydrogen ion secretion, which brings the hydrogen carbonate equilibrium back towards the production of more hydrogen ions. This increase in hydrogen ion concentration lowers pH and restores homeostasis.

Secretion in the Renal Tubules
In addition to reabsorption, the tubular cells are capable of secreting substances to assist in the maintenance of homeostasis

in the extracellular fluid. Secretion is a process whereby cells release substances into the body fluids. In the kidney tubules, substances secreted by the cells into the tubules to pass out in the urine include hydrogen ions, ammonia and potassium ions.

Secretion of hydrogen ions. It is believed that the hydrogen ions secreted by the tubular cells arise from the reaction of CO_2 (entering the cells from the blood and from the fluid in the tubules) with water, resulting in the formation of hydrogen carbonate and hydrogen ions. The hydrogen ions are then secreted into the tubules to pass eventually into the urine. The hydrogen carbonate ions are transported into the blood (see Fig. 8.7). An important point here is that hydrogen ion secretion will be directly affected by CO_2 concentrations in the extracellular fluids and so their concentration can be altered in accordance with the concentration of CO_2 and thus the resultant pH.

Transport of hydrogen carbonate ions. The supply of hydrogen carbonate ions to the blood is believed to arise from the reaction described above. While hydrogen carbonate ions are present in renal filtrate (fluid in tubules), they are not readily reabsorbed into the tubular cells because of size and charge. The ion undergoes a process of reabsorption in times of need, after first being converted to CO_2. The hydrogen carbonate ion can react with the hydrogen ions being secreted into the tubules, to form carbonic acid. This acid dissociates into CO_2 and H_2O. The H_2O is excreted in urine, thus removing hydrogen ions. The CO_2 diffuses rapidly into tubular cells to go through a reaction with H_2O, as discussed previously. In addition, some CO_2 moves directly into the blood to react with water, forming hydrogen carbonate ions (see Fig. 8.7).

Buffering in the Renal Tubules

In acidosis, the number of hydrogen ions being secreted is greater than the number of hydrogen carbonate ions available in the tubules to react with the hydrogen ions to produce water and carbon dioxide. The result is a more acidic tubule fluid and a need to raise the pH level of this fluid to prevent problems inside the tubules (tissues affected). The excess H^+ are usually buffered by the following means:

1. Within the kidney, the phosphate buffer system is most important because:

- the ions of the phosphate system become greatly concentrated in the tubules, which increase their buffering capacity; and
- the tubular fluid usually becomes more acidic than the extracellular fluid and brings the buffer into the range of pH where it functions most effectively.

Figure 8.7. Chemical reactions for (1) hydrogen ion secretion, (2) sodium ion absorption in exchange for a hydrogen ion, and (3) combination of hydrogen ions with hydrogen carbonate ions in the tubules. (From Guyton: *Textbook of Medical Physiology*. 6th Ed. Philadelphia. W.B. Saunders. 1981.)

Secretion of ammonia by the tubular epithelial cells, and reaction of the ammonia with hydrogen ions in the tubules.

Chemical reactions in the tubules involving hydrogen ions, sodium ions, and the phosphate buffer system.

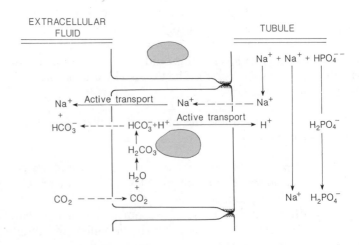

2. The ammonia buffer system is also most important in the kidneys. Ammonia (NH_3) is synthesised in the tubular cells and secreted into the tubules. It combines with a hydrogen ion to form the ammonium ion (NH_4^+), which is then passed into the urine.

$$NH_3 \quad + \quad H^+ \quad \longrightarrow \quad NH_4^+$$

ammonia   proton   ammonium
                                                 ion

Note that the sodium ion tends to be involved in many of the reactions described in the preceding sections, in that it is invariably present in all the body fluids. It is able to combine with anions, such as the phosphate anions, and form salts, which can then be removed by the kidneys. Sodium ions are also sometimes exchanged for the secreted hydrogen ions, which in turn can lead to high Na^+ levels in some of the body fluids such as the extracellular fluids.

Thus buffers are able to play a significant role as part of a 'team effort' to maintain homeostasis with respect to acid-base balance in the body.

We will now go on to examine the acid-base stress conditions to which we have already referred – acidosis and alkalosis. Since each of these conditions may arise from either respiratory or metabolic causes, each will be treated separately.

Respiratory Acidosis

Any factor that decreases the depth or rate of pulmonary ventilation will increase the concentration of *dissolved carbon dioxide* in the extracellular fluid. This leads to a shift of the equilibrium position, which in turn leads to an increase in hydrogen ion concentration, a drop in pH and an acidosis condition.

This normally arises from a pathological condition, for example, damage to the respiratory centre in the medulla causing breathing problems, obstruction of the respiratory tract passageways, pneumonia, or any factor that impairs the normal diffusion of gases or pulmonary circulation, such as emphysema, tuberculosis, fibrosis, embolisms or hypoxia (low oxygen content of the blood).

Some drugs depress the activity of the respiratory centre as part of their action, for example morphine sulfate and pethidine (narcotics). This does not happen with barbiturates to any extent unless very large doses are being taken or in an overdose situation.

However, narcotics, when used in the clinical situation on a regulated basis, such as every four hours for 24 hours would be unlikely to lead to acidosis unless there was a contributing pulmonary disorder.

The activity of the respiratory centre is also depressed by anaesthetics and indirectly by such afflictions as polio, which affects the nerves. This nerve malfunction or paralysis can also render the chest muscles inoperative. It follows that the nurse should be aware of these possibilities and be prepared to act quickly.

The symptoms of respiratory acidosis are tachypnoea (abnormal rapidity of respiration) whilst at rest, rapid pulse, sweating, small pupils and rise in blood pressure and, if severe, may also include cyanosis and disorientation. If not treated, further changes will occur to respiration: shallow and rapid to severe dyspnoea (difficulty in breathing), to laboured or suprasternal retraction. Laboured or difficult breathing will often be evident.

This problem is frequently alleviated in the first instance by the body itself through:

- the action of buffers as previously described, particularly those within body cells, such as haemoglobin;
- increased respiration in response to the fall in blood and extracellular fluid pH;
- the kidneys eliminating excess hydrogen ions into the urine.

Respiratory Alkalosis

Only rarely do pathological conditions cause respiratory alkalosis, although severe anxiety can sometimes lead to this condition. At high altitudes, ventilation is increased in response to hypoxia (see above), which can lead to respiratory alkalosis.

The cause of this condition is the opposite to respiratory acidosis, i.e. in this case, pulmonary ventilation is excessive, causing hydrogen ion concentration to decrease. Compensation for this condition is normally achieved by:

- the buffer system previously discussed;
- restriction of hyperventilation by the increase in blood pH;
- the action of the kidneys in excreting hydrogen carbonate ions into the urine. This tends to push the bicarbonate equilibrium towards producing more hydrogen carbonate ions, and thus more hydrogen ions, which then lowers the pH.

The major effect of alkalosis on the body is *over excitability of the nervous system*. Although it occurs in both parts of the nervous system, the peripheral nerves are usually affected before the central nervous system. The nerves repeatedly fire even without stimuli, causing the muscles to fully contract (to go into a state of tetany), starting in most cases in the forearm, then the face, followed by the rest of the body. In extreme cases, tetany of the muscles associated with respiration can be fatal.

In some cases, alkalosis may lead to excitability of the central nervous system, which is manifested as extreme nervousness or possibly convulsions.

Note: Fig. 8.8 illustrates the relationship between H^+ and CO_2 concentration.

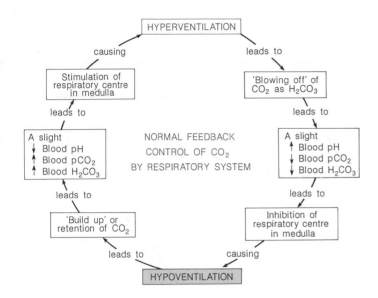

Figure 8.8. Feedback control of H^+ concentration and the elimination of CO_2. (From Luckmann & Sorenson: *Medical-Surgical Nursing*. 2nd Ed. Philadelphia. W.B. Saunders. 1980.)

Metabolic Acidosis

This term refers to an excess of hydrogen ions, which in turn is caused by an excess of acids *other than those resulting from carbon dioxide* (which is often referred to as a 'respiratory acid') in the body fluids. It can result from:

- failure of the kidneys to excrete the metabolic acids (where the term 'metabolic acids' refers to those acids formed by metabolism or simply by ingestion);
- formation of excessive quantities of metabolic acids in the body;
- intravenous administration of metabolic acids;
- ingestion of metabolic acids;
- loss of alkali from the body fluids.

These effects can be brought about by the following:

1. *Diarrhoea.* If severe, this is a very frequent cause of acidosis, since a large loss of hydrogen carbonate-rich gastrointestinal secretions occurs. This has the same effects as those previously described, and the shift in the hydrogen carbonate equilibrium towards the acid side to replace the lost hydrogen carbonate results in a build-up of hydrogen ion concentration and thus acidosis. This condition is one of the most common causes of death in young children.

2. *Vomiting* of the contents of the deeper parts of the gastrointestinal tract (as distinct from the stomach contents alone), which frequently occurs, causes loss of alkali and thus acidosis.

3. *Uremia.* This is the failure of the kidneys to excrete metabolic acids as a result of severe renal disease.

4. *Diabetes mellitus.* As described in the introduction to this chapter, this condition results from the failure of the pancreas to secrete sufficient quantities of insulin. This means that glucose is not utilised by normal metabolic processes but is replaced by fat for energy production. This results in large concentrations of acetoacetic acid being formed, and despite the fact that large quantities of this compound are removed by the kidneys, acidosis results.

5. *Other causes.* These include the administration of drugs such as Diamox (acetazolamide), which is a carbonic anhydrase inhibitor. This can lead to the loss of hydrogen carbonate ions and consequent acidosis. Similarly, an excess of potassium ions can inhibit the removal of hydrogen ions, with the same result.

Symptoms include increased rate and depth of respiration, and depression of the central nervous system.

Metabolic Alkalosis

This condition results from loss of hydrogen ions (other than those associated with high carbon dioxide concentrations in the blood) or inappropriate addition of a base such as hydrogen carbonate ion or lactate. Some common causes are listed below.

1. *Administration of some diuretics.* These compounds lead to increased flow of fluid through the tubules of the kidneys, which can lead to loss of hydrogen ions and thus to alkalosis.

2. *Excessive ingestion of alkaline drugs.* If an alkali such as sodium hydrogen carbonate or milk of magnesia is ingested in excessive quantities for the treatment of gastritis or a peptic ulcer, alkalosis can result.

3. *Loss of aqueous hydrogen chloride and thus loss of*

hydrogen ions. Excessive vomiting of the contents of the stomach can lead to a loss of hydrogen ions and thus alkalosis.

4. *Excess aldosterone.* If excess quantities of aldosterone are secreted by the adrenal glands, the extracellular fluid can become slightly alkaline.

Symptoms are opposite to those arising from metabolic acidosis.

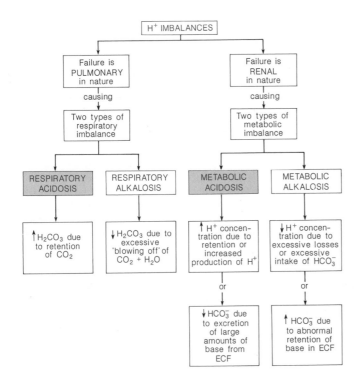

Figure 8.9. Summary of the four major H^+ imbalances. (Adapted from Luckmann & Sorenson: *Medical-Surgical Nursing*, 2nd Ed. Philadelphia. W.B. Saunders. 1980.)

Supplementary Note: Sodium hydrogen carbonate is quite alkaline and is thus likely to cause unfortunate interactions with many drugs. It is therefore best to operate on the assumption that this substance must *not* be administered with any other drug, unless a pharmacist advises to the contrary.

Summary
The above has been summarised in Fig. 8.9.

The reader cannot fail to realise that the fluids of the body represent a most important study. The implications for nursing should be equally obvious and it follows that the professional nurse cannot perform his/her functions satisfactorily without a clear understanding of the matters discussed. One of the most important of these is the concept of chemical equilibrium, particularly as applied to the hydrogen carbonate ion/carbonic acid system – one which is absolutely critical to our own survival and that of our patients.

REVIEW

1. Show how the hydrogen carbonate (bicarbonate) ion can act both as a base and as an acid.
2. Distinguish between (a) a concentrated acid and a strong acid; and (b) a weak acid and a dilute acid.
3. A patient was admitted to an emergency unit in a state of acidosis. A provisional diagnosis of metabolic acidosis resulting from diabetes mellitus was made.
   (a) Why is it important to know the type of acidosis?
   (b) Describe in detail the methods by which the body would have endeavoured to restore homeostasis as the acidosis developed.
   (c) Why didn't the body succeed in restoring homeostasis?
4. Following a major road accident, a man was admitted with extensive and severe chest injuries. One of the potential complications of which you should be aware is respiratory acidosis.
   (a) What deviations from the norm would warn you of the development of such a complication?
   (b) In what ways would the body attempt to correct such a situation?
5. A urine specimen is found to contain a high level of ammonium ions. Give a reason for this.
6. (a) A patient with an arterial blood pH of 7.50 could be described as being in what state?
   (b) What symptoms might one expect to observe in this case?
   (c) Discuss the various mechanisms which would be activated to restore homeostasis.

9

Biological chemistry

OBJECTIVES

After studying this chapter the student should be able to:

1. Utilise basic biological chemistry to understand the fundamentals of metabolism and genetic structures.
2. Forge links between this biological chemistry and relevant applications in the human body.
3. Apply knowledge of this chemistry towards an understanding of metabolism that may be applied in professional situations.
4. Give some examples of monosaccharides, disaccharides and polysaccharides, and distinguish between them in terms of structure.

INTRODUCTION

In previous chapters, atoms, together with ions and simple molecules which are formed from these, have been described as entities of which the body consists. However, many of the molecules in the body and those which are used by it are much more complex. For example, the three major food groups that we consume to keep us alive, i.e. carbohydrates, fats and proteins, contain molecules which range from the comparatively simple to very complex, some with atomic arrangements containing many hundreds of atoms.

The genetic materials which make up our body cells are extremely complex substances consisting of many thousands of atoms arranged as complex molecules of various types linked together.

To be able to understand the range and extent of the difficult task which the body has in building and maintaining itself, a brief examination of some of the structures with which it works will increase our appreciation of these functions. Furthermore, some of the following chapters (such as those on energy production and genetics) will be easier to follow with more background in the chemistry of the substances involved.

Nevertheless, one should realise that the information presented here is but a small portion of a highly specialised study and is offered only as a means of increasing understanding of highly complex processes of particular interest to nursing students.

A number of specific groupings of atoms are commonly found in biological chemistry. For example, many fats contain long hydrocarbon chains, many biological molecules contain methyl and ethyl groups, alcohol (−OH) groups are found in carbohydrates and amino acids, many carbohydrates contain the aldehyde (−CHO) group of atoms, the carboxylic acid group has biological significance in carbohydrates, proteins and nucleic acids, and amino groups are found in proteins and nucleic acids (DNA and RNA).

Furthermore, the phosphate group is a constituent of many nucleic acids, carbohydrates and lipids in living systems and is very important in energy storage compounds and energy transfer reactions. Ester linkages join many molecules together to form nucleic acids, fats and many other larger compounds. Finally, many biologically important molecules and pharmaceuticals contain the benzene ring.

The practice of medicine has in fact been revolutionised by developments in pharmacology. Steroids, antibiotics, sulfa drugs and tranquilisers are some examples of compounds of these types which have been synthesised (prepared in laboratories) in the last few decades.

Our first step is to become familiar with some basic chemical principles and types of compounds which are used in biological chemistry so that we can later grasp some of the rather complex biochemical reactions which occur in metabolic processes.

HYDROCARBONS

This is the simplest group of biologically relevant compounds. Each compound consists of carbon and hydrogen atoms only. Those of interest at this stage are saturated, unsaturated and aromatic hydrocarbons. These are the compounds from which many other compounds are derived.

Saturated Hydrocarbons (Alkanes)

These are hydrocarbons in which only **single** bonds are present in the compound. They may be 'straight-chain' or branched compounds. We will be concerned only with the former, which, at the atomic level are 'zig-zagged', but which overall have a straight arrangement of carbon atoms. They have the general formula C_nH_{2n+2}.

Thus, if the number of carbon atoms is 5, so that n is 5, the number of hydrogen atoms is 2n + 2 or (2 × 5 + 2), which is 12. Thus the formula for this hydrocarbon, pentane, is C_5H_{12}.

Some examples are shown in Fig. 9.1:

Name	Molecular Formula
methane	CH_4
ethane	C_2H_6
propane	C_3H_8
butane	C_4H_{10}
pentane	C_5H_{12}

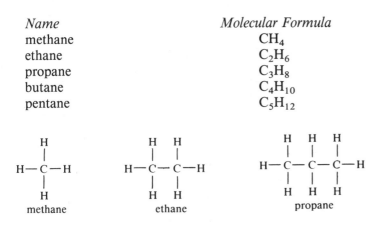

Figure 9.1.

In the case of methane, the carbon atom has a valency of four and shares a total of eight electrons:

    — four from the outermost energy level of the carbon atom;
and
    — four from the hydrogen atoms, one electron from each.

In the case of ethane and propane, as well as other similar compounds, we see that once again each carbon atom has a valency of four and shares a total of eight electrons:

    — four from the outermost energy level of the carbon atom;
and

    — four other electrons, each of which has come from either a hydrogen atom or a carbon atom.

These compounds form the basis of many of the long chains found in foods such as carbohydrates, fats and proteins (for example, those illustrated on p 278–281), as well as many other molecules found in the body (such as cholesterol), many amino acids, acetylcholine, dipalmitoyl licithin (the surfactant in the lungs), cholic acid (one of the bile acids), etc.

Readers will have noticed that the name of all these *saturated* hydrocarbons ends in '-ane'. In contrast, we will soon see that the names of *unsaturated* compounds end in either '-ene' or '-yne'.

Also, the prefixes in each case indicate the number of carbon atoms:

meth-	1	hex-	6
eth-	2	hept-	7
prop-	3	oct-	8
but-	4	non-	9
pent-	5	dec-	10

Alkanes are somewhat unreactive and find their chief use as fuels. However many of their derivatives are of interest.

Unsaturated Hydrocarbons

A hydrocarbon is **unsaturated** if at least one of the carbon-carbon bonds in its molecule is a **multiple** bond.

Two examples of types of unsaturated hydrocarbons are:

1. **Alkenes**. These hydrocarbons have at least one carbon-carbon *double* bond per molecule (Fig. 9.2).

ethene　　　　　　　　　　　　　propene

Figure 9.2.

They have the general formula $C_{2n}H_{2n}$. Once again, the octet rule is satisfied, each carbon atom having four bonds, each of which represents an electron pair, giving a total of eight electrons around and shared by each carbon atom. Similarly, each hydrogen atom is able to share two electrons.

2. **Alkynes**. These hydrocarbons have at least one carbon-carbon *triple* bond per molecule (Fig. 9.3).

ethyne　　　　　　　　　　　　　propyne

Figure 9.3.

The general formula for the alkynes is C_nH_{2n-2} and once again the octet rule is satisfied.

Unsaturated hydrocarbons are much more reactive than alkanes, since substances such as hydrogen and chlorine can *add* across the double bond in alkenes to form *saturated* compounds. Such reactions occur much more readily than the substitution reactions characteristic of alkanes (Fig. 9.4).

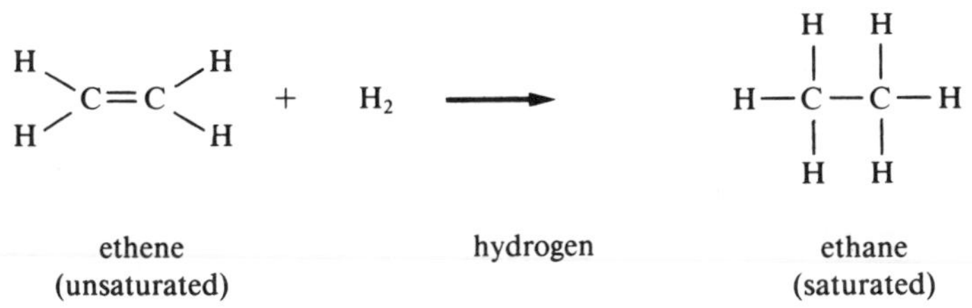

| ethene | hydrogen | ethane | |
| (unsaturated) | | (saturated) | Figure 9.4. |

This is a typical addition reaction in which an atom of hydrogen has been added to each of the carbon atoms, across a double bond, thus changing the double bond into a single bond. Thus an unsaturated compound (having a double or triple carbon-carbon bond present) is changed to a saturated compound (not having any carbon-carbon double or triple bonds present). Because hydrogen has been added, it is called a **hydrogenation** reaction. If chlorine had been added across the double bond it would be called a **chlorination** reaction, etc.

With alkanes, however, no double bond is present across which other atoms can be added. In such cases, *substitution* reactions occur in which existing hydrogen atoms are replaced by other atoms. Addition reactions occur more readily than substitution reactions because one of the bonds in a double bond (and two in a triple bond) is more easily broken than the single carbon- carbon bond in alkanes. The following reaction is typical of the substitution reactions undergone by alkanes (Fig. 9.5).

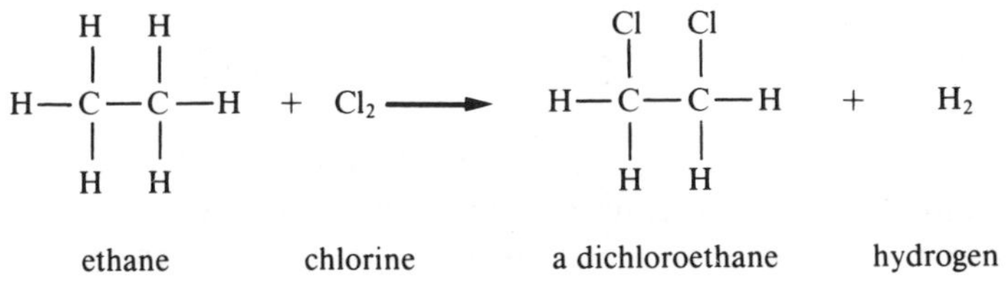

| ethane | chlorine | a dichloroethane | hydrogen | |
| | | | | Figure 9.5. |

Saturated hydrocarbons can undergo substitution reactions and unsaturated hydrocarbons can undergo addition reactions to form compounds such as shown in Figs 9.6 and 9.7.

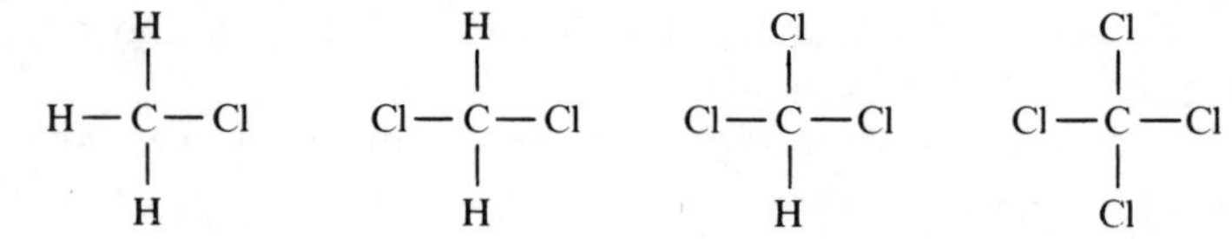

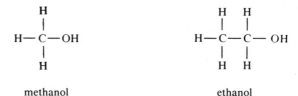

Figure 9.6.

monochloromethane dichloromethane trichloromethane tetrachloromethane
(chloroform) (carbon tetrachloride)

Figure 9.7.

methanol   ethanol

Polyunsaturated Fats

Many fats are formed from two components, glycerol and one or more fatty acids. Saturated fatty acids contain no double bonds between the carbon atoms, whereas unsaturated fatty acids (which do not contain all the hydrogen atoms which could be bonded) do contain double bonds. Polyunsaturated fats contain more than one double bond in each molecule (see Fig. 9.8).

Figure 9.8.

unsaturated fatty acid   saturated fatty acid

Although fats are one of the major food groups required for optimum body functioning, they have been linked in the past decade to heart and blood vessel disease. The fat, cholesterol, has been particularly vilified. However, it is now known that a number of factors are related to or associated with heart and blood vessel diseases.

Research knowledge regarding fats indicates that:

1. Eating unsaturated fats instead of saturated fats lowers the blood cholesterol concentration (for reasons which are not known), which in turn seems to be associated with the prevention of atherosclerosis. Some foodstuffs, such as table margarine, have a P:S ratio of 2:1. This is the ratio of polyunsaturated fats to saturated fats, and does not mean that one can consume vast quantities of this food with impunity! Obviously, such food does

contain saturated fats, but they form only one-third of the total fat content.

2. A high fat diet increases one's chances of developing atherosclerosis – a form of arteriosclerosis, in which fatty deposits form in, or on, the lining of the arteries. Atherosclerosis is responsible for almost half of all deaths of human beings in western societies.

Aromatic Hydrocarbons

This is the family of compounds derived from the compound benzene C_6H_6. Benzene is still a hydrocarbon, but because of its cyclic structure and arrangement of electrons, it does not behave as a normal saturated or unsaturated hydrocarbon.

The structure of this compound is usually represented as in Fig. 9.9.

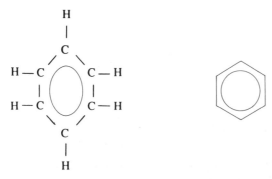

Figure 9.9.

In this case the circle in the centre indicates three pairs of electrons which are not *localised*, so that they are free to move around within the circle. This results in a 'ring of electron density'. This means that this family of compounds has some unique properties, with which we are not going to be directly concerned here. Suffice it to say that many of the compounds found in the body and used as drugs are derivatives of benzene or are similar compounds.

Some examples are shown below:

1. Phenanthrene. This compound is used in the synthesis of drugs (Fig. 9.10).

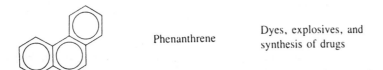

Phenanthrene   Dyes, explosives, and
                      synthesis of drugs

Figure 9.10.

2. 3,4-Benzpyrene. This compound is a potent carcinogen, which has been detected in cigarette smoke and smog (Fig. 9. 11).

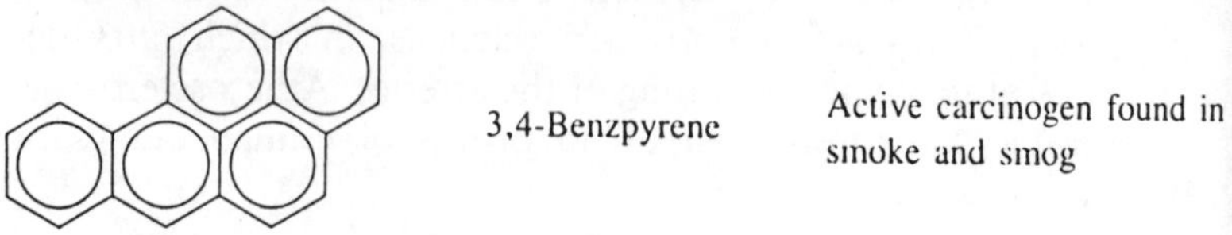

3,4-Benzpyrene

Active carcinogen found in smoke and smog

Figure 9.11.

3. Cholesterol. This steroid is the starting material for the formation of bile acids, steroid hormones and vitamin D, and has been implicated in the formation of plaque in the walls of arteries (atherosclerosis), which can lead to partial or complete blockage. Cholesterol is synthesised by liver cells as one of the products of the metabolism of fats in the body (Fig. 9.12).

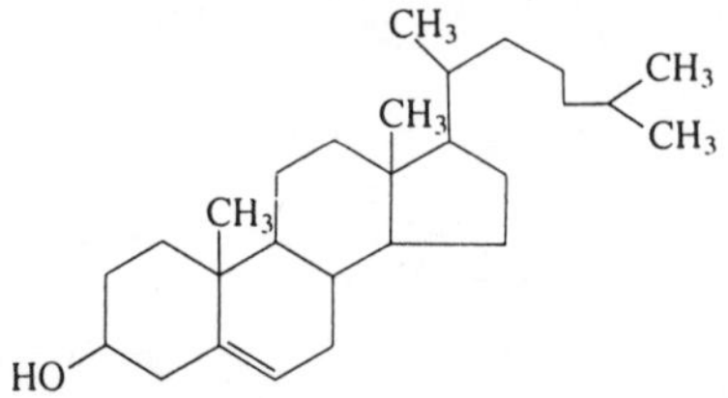

Figure 9.12.

4. Vitamin D. This is a substance from which the body manufactures a hormone called 1,25-dihydroxyvitamin D_3 (or 1, 25-$(OH)_2D_3$), which stimulates active calcium absorption by the intestine (Fig. 9.13).

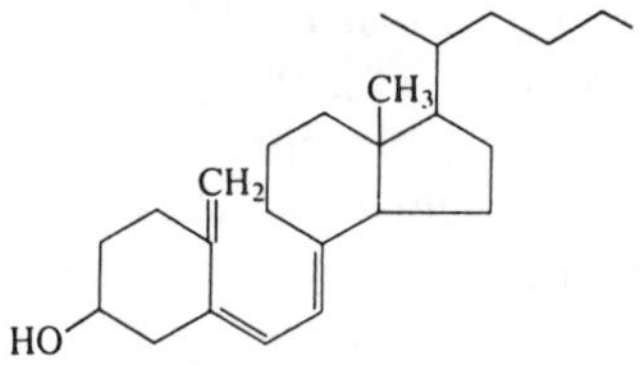

Figure 9.13.

5. Testosterone. This is a steroid and the most important of the male hormones (Fig. 9.14).

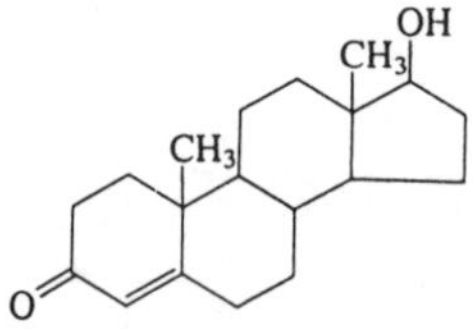

Figure 9.14.

6. Progesterone. This is also a steroid and one of the most important female hormones (Fig. 9.15).

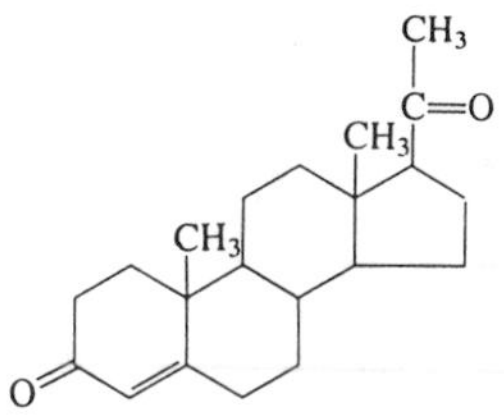

Figure 9.15.

These structures are shown only for interest to indicate their complexity. It should be remembered that any point where lines (chemical bonds) intersect, represents a carbon atom, with the appropriate number of hydrogen atoms attached.

FUNCTIONAL GROUPS

Compounds which contain a particular **functional group**, such as −OH (e.g. methanol and ethanol, as shown on p. 252) are found to have similar chemical properties as a result of the presence of these functional groups.

Some functional groups are listed in Table 9.1. These functional groups may replace a hydrogen atom in an alkane to form a compound of a particular type. For example, if we replace one hydrogen atom in methane (CH_4) with an −OH, we get CH_3OH (methanol).

$$CH_3-H \qquad \text{becomes} \qquad CH_3OH \text{ (methanol)}$$

Similarly, ethane (C_2H_6) becomes ethanol (C_2H_5OH). It follows that the '-ol' suffix indicates the type of compound) – in these cases they are alcohols. These compounds then all have a number of similar properties because of the presence of the alcohol functional group.

In any one compound it is possible to have more than one functional group present. However, these different functional groups will normally be attached to *different carbon atoms.* Hence when we look at the ethanoic acid in the dehydration reactions described below, it would appear that we have both a ketone and a carboxylic acid, because of the presence of both of the −C=O and the −OH groups respectively. Since these are both attached to the same carbon atom, however, we in fact have a carboxylic acid group, i.e. −COOH or

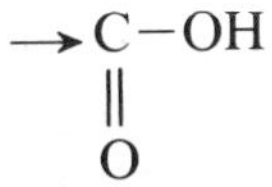

$$\longrightarrow C-OH$$
$$\overset{\|}{O}$$

TABLE 9.1 Common classes of organic compounds

Class	Functional group of the class	Examples of the compound	
Alcohols	—OH	CH_3OH methanol	$C_3H_5(OH)_3$ glycerol
Ethers	—O—	CH_3OCH_3 dimethyl ether	Acetylcholine
Aldehydes	$\overset{O}{\underset{/}{\overset{\backslash\backslash}{C}}}$ —H	HCHO methanal (formaldehyde)	$C_6H_3OHOCH_3CHO$ vanilla
Ketones	$-\overset{O}{\overset{\|}{C}}-$	CH_3COCH_3 (acetone*)	cortisol and progesterone
Carboxylic acids	$-\overset{O}{\overset{\|}{C}}-OH$	CH_3COOH ethanoic acid	$C_{17}H_{35}COOH$ stearic acid
Esters	$-\underset{O}{\overset{}{C}}-O-$	CH_3COOCH_3 methyl acetate	animal fats and vegetable oils
Amines	$-NH_2$	CH_3NH_2 aminomethane (methylamine)	$C_5N_2H_7NH_2-H^+$ histamine (dimethylamine)
Amino acids	$NH_2CRHCOOH$ (where R may be CH_3-, C_2H_5-, etc)	$NH_2CH_3CHCOOH$ alanine	NH_2CH_2COOH glycine (both form proteins)

*Acetone is produced in uncontrolled diabetes mellitus and is often observed on the breath of the patient.

In this case, in general terms, the compound will exhibit some of the characteristics of each type of functional group. It will also undergo many of the reactions which are normal for that functional group.

Consider now the ketone functional group $-C=O$ which is present in acetone (Fig. 9.16) or in progesterone, as shown on p. 255. It must be remembered here that the hexagonal (and any other) 'rings' in this structure contain carbon atoms. The ketone group is identified in the lower left 'corner' in the structure.

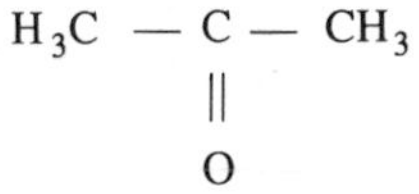

$$H_3C - C - CH_3$$
$$\|$$
$$O$$

Figure 9.16.

Other examples are: glucocorticoids such as cortisol; mineralocorticoids such as aldosterone; testosterone; and acetyl-choline.

These ketones, along with other compounds which contain the ketone group, undergo particular reactions, including, for example, addition reactions. One of these is the addition of water to form alcohols containing two $-OH$ groups, called diols (Fig. 9.17).

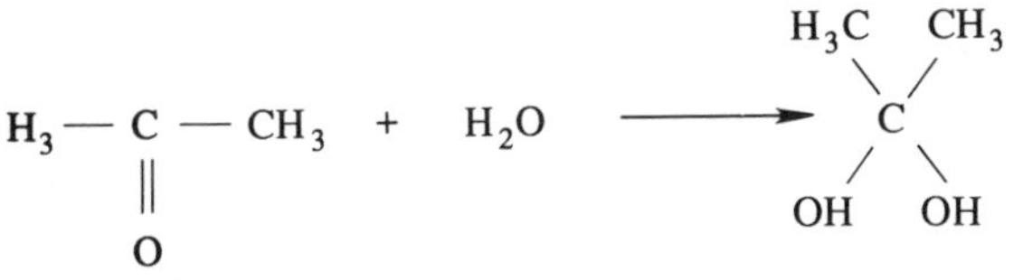

$$H_3 - C - CH_3 \;+\; H_2O \longrightarrow$$

a diol

Figure 9.17.

This is but one example of one of the characteristics of just one functional group. Even when a chemical formula looks complicated, the reader should practise looking for, and identi-fying, various functional groups. This may give some clues to enable the reader to understand some of the behaviour of that compound in the body.

CHEMICAL EQUILIBRIUM

Before we proceed to examine some important chemical reac-tions which occur in the body, it is important that we consider the concept of chemical equilibrium, so that we might under-stand better some of these reactions.

If we have a reaction as follows (note that for simplicity the letters A, B, C and D are used to represent some chemical compounds):

$$A + B \longrightarrow C + D$$

we are saying that the two substances A and B react together to give the two substances C and D.

However, since the reactions with which we are concerned are **equilibrium reactions**, the following reaction also occurs:

$$C + D \longrightarrow A + B$$

Thus we have the overall reaction:

$$A + B \rightleftharpoons C + D$$

This is an *equilibrium reaction*. This means that the rate of the forward reaction (the left-to-right reaction) is *the same* as the rate of the backward reaction (the right-to-left reaction), under the prevailing conditions.

If we have a fixed set of conditions with respect to temperature and pressure (and in the body these are normally 37°C and atmospheric pressure), an equilibrium position will be reached at which:

1. A and B react to give C and D.
2. At the same time, C and D react to give A and B, *at the same rate.*
3. The two reactions proceed at such a rate that the **actual concentrations of the four reactants is always the same**, even though the reactions are continually proceeding in both directions.
4. This occurs whether we start with A and B *or* C and D.
5. If one of the products is continually being removed, the reaction will tend to keep going in that direction. If C is constantly being removed, for example, A and B will keep on reacting (i.e. the equilibrium position will shift to the right, so that more C and D is formed). This has special relevance to the body in many of the reactions with which we are concerned, such as digestive reactions, in which the shift in the equilibrium position is complete and all food is digested.

Chemical equilibrium can take time, since many chemical reactions, particularly those which occur at body temperature, are *very slow*.

The statements above outline what is meant when the term *chemical equilibrium* is used. Chemical equilibrium might then be defined as *an equilibrium in which the rates of simultaneous forward and reverse chemical reactions are the same and the amounts of those species which are present do not change with time.*

Let us now examine chemical equilibrium in more detail,

since the maintenance of homeostasis depends very much on this. We have made statements about chemical equilibrium under certain conditions of temperature, pressure, etc. It is found that if we change these conditions, it is possible to predict what will happen. Such predictions are based on a statement first proposed by a French chemist named Le Chatelier, in 1888:

When a system in equilibrium is subjected to stress or a change in conditions, the system shifts to compensate for the effects of that change or stress.

Before proceeding further, it is instructive to compare this to the concept of homeostasis. If, for example, parts of the body are not getting sufficient blood, the heart will respond by increasing its output. The heart has thus compensated for a change in conditions (i.e. stress) by shifting an equilibrium position, i.e. by increasing cardiac output.

If we follow this principle we will see that it is possible to understand chemical equilibrium the same way, as we now examine some of the changes which can occur.

1. Effects of concentration changes on chemical equilibrium: Of all the changes to which chemical equilibria are subjected, concentration changes are the most important in physiological systems, since most of the reactions in our bodies usually take place at constant temperature and pressure. In normal circumstances, changes of temperature and pressure are rather small but changes in concentration are much more significant.

For example, consider the reaction between haemoglobin (shown as Hb) and oxygen. This is a rather complex reaction, but for our purposes it can be represented in Fig. 9.18 as follows:

$$Hb \quad + \quad O_2 \quad \rightleftharpoons \quad HbO_2$$

haemoglobin   oxygen   oxyhaemoglobin

Figure 9.18.

If the concentration of oxygen is *increased*, the equilibrium position will change to compensate for this and the forward reaction (left-to-right) will *increase* its rate relative to the backward reaction (right-to-left). This will produce an *increase* in the equilibrium concentration of oxyhaemoglobin.

Similarly, if the concentration of oxygen is *decreased*, the equilibrium position will change to compensate for this and the forward reaction will *decrease* its rate relative to the backward reaction. This will produce a *decrease* in the equilibrium concentration of oxyhaemoglobin.

Also, if the concentration of oxyhaemoglobin is *decreased*, the equilibrium position will change to compensate for this, the forward reaction will *increase* its rate relative to the backward reaction, thus producing an *increase* in the equilibrium concentration of oxyhaemoglobin.

It then follows that an *increase* in the concentration of oxygen has the same effect as a *decrease* in the concentration of oxyhaemoglobin.

2. *Effects of temperature changes on chemical equilibrium:* Any change in temperature is a stress on a system which is in equilibrium, causing a change in the rates of *both* reactions.

As an example, consider the reaction discussed on p. 293 (and on p. 291, but note that the 12 molecules of water becomes six molecules when the six molecules of water on the right hand side are deducted). This is the reaction between glucose and oxygen to produce carbon dioxide and water, with the release of energy (Fig. 9.19):

$$C_6 H_{12} O + 6O_2 \rightleftharpoons 6CO_2 + 6H_2O + \text{ENERGY}$$

glucose   oxygen   carbon   water
                                                      dioxide

Figure 9.19.

When energy is *supplied*, as in photosynthesis, the reaction to the *left* is favoured. When energy is *used*, as in cellular respiration, the reaction to the *right* is favoured. These responses to a form of stress are once again consistent in concept with that of homeostasis.

3. Since pressure changes are inconsequential in the human body, these will not be discussed, but the principles remain the same.

4. *Catalysts* play a big part in chemical reactions and those catalysts which are present in the human body, i.e. enzymes are superb performers. These are discussed on p. 293ff.

In summary, a basic understanding of chemical equilibrium will be of great value in understanding body function and will be facilitated by drawing a parallel with the concept of homeostasis, the maintenance of which so often depends on equilibrium systems.

The attainment of equilibrium can be speeded up using a *catalyst*. We can then define a catalyst as *a substance which hastens the attainment of equilibrium*. In some books, a catalyst is defined as a substance which speeds up a reaction, but this does not tell us *which* reaction is speeded up, the forward reaction or the backward reaction, i.e. in the example above, is it the reaction between A and B to give C and D or the reaction between C and D to give A and B? What we are saying is that *both* reactions are speeded up where necessary to attain equilibrium more quickly. The world 'equilibrium' means that the reaction between A and B is proceeding at the *same* rate as the reaction between C and D, so that, for a given temperature and pressure, the concentrations of A, B, C and D are all *constant*.

This attainment of equilibrium is achieved by decreasing the amount of energy needed to initiate the reaction. For more details, see Box 9.1.

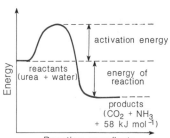

Figure 9.20. Energy diagram for the reaction between urea and water. (From Cree & Webb: *Biology Outlines*. Sydney. Pergamon Press. 1984.)

BIOCHEMICAL REACTIONS

The following biochemical reactions are of importance at this stage.

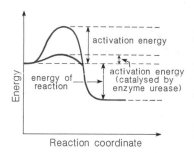

Figure 9.21. A comparison of activation energies, catalysed and uncatalysed, between urea and water. Note that the energy of reaction is unaltered. (From Cree & Webb: *Biology Outlines*. Sydney. Pergamon Press. 1984.)

1. Hydration

This is also an addition reaction, in which a hydrogen atom and an $-OH$ group from a molecule of water add across a double bond, forming an alcohol (Fig 9.22).

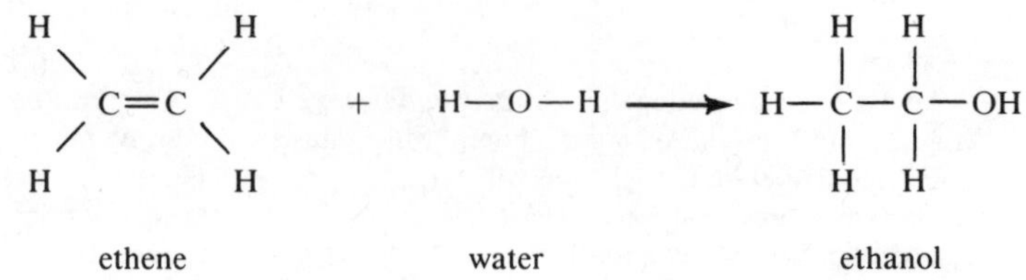

Figure 9.22.

ethene   water   ethanol

2. Dehydration

The opposite of hydration. In these reactions, compounds have water removed, with one compound contributing a hydrogen atom and the other contributing an $-OH$ group, as indicated by the 'lasso' (Fig 9.23). This reaction is of the same type as that shown for the reaction between a fatty acid and glycerol.

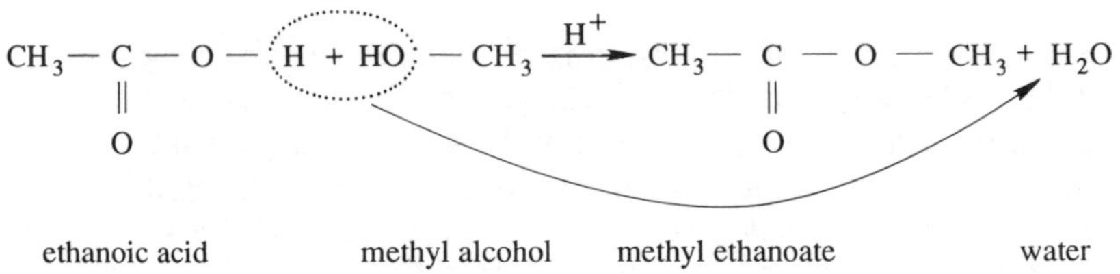

Figure 9.23.   ethanoic acid   methyl alcohol   methyl ethanoate   water

3. Hydrolysis

This is similar to hydration in that water is involved, but in this case the water *decomposes* other molecules (Fig. 9.24).

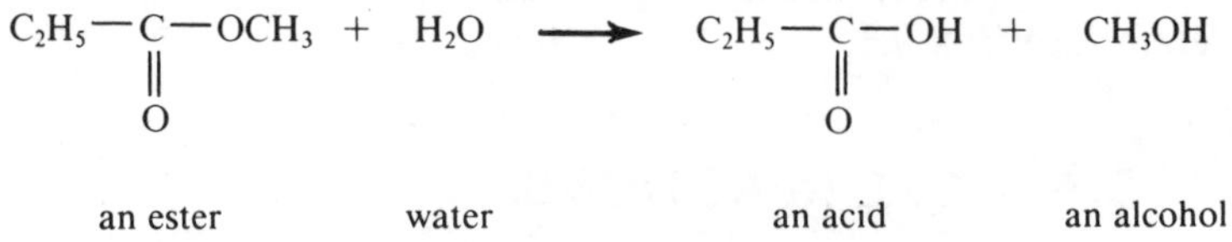

Figure 9.24.   an ester   water   an acid   an alcohol

4. Synthesis

This is the formation of a compound from its constituent elements or other compounds. The hydrolysis reaction above may be regarded as a synthesis reaction, together with some of the reactions shown later in this chapter in Figs. 9.36, 9.37, 9.38 and 9.41.

5. Oxidation and Reduction

Many of the chemical reactions which we will be discussing in relation to the carbon-oxygen cycle, the nitrogen cycle and under 'Energy Release', are called **oxidation and reduction** reactions (collectively, 'redox' reactions).

In the section which follows, biochemical reactions of the type discussed above are important, as may soon be seen.

Oxidation
Oxidation is any chemical reaction in which a substance has gained oxygen or lost hydrogen (see Fig. 9.25).

All of these reactions are **oxidation** reactions.

Figure 9.25.

(a)

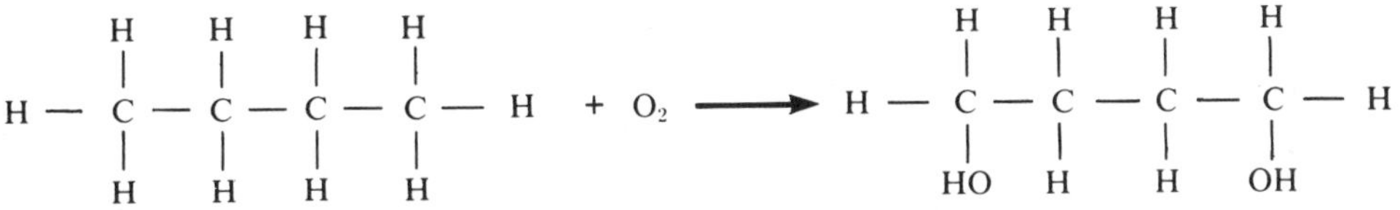

$$H - \underset{\underset{H}{|}}{\overset{\overset{H}{|}}{C}} - \underset{\underset{H}{|}}{\overset{\overset{H}{|}}{C}} - \underset{\underset{H}{|}}{\overset{\overset{H}{|}}{C}} - \underset{\underset{H}{|}}{\overset{\overset{H}{|}}{C}} - H \ + \ O_2 \longrightarrow H - \underset{\underset{HO}{|}}{\overset{\overset{H}{|}}{C}} - \underset{\underset{H}{|}}{\overset{\overset{H}{|}}{C}} - \underset{\underset{H}{|}}{\overset{\overset{H}{|}}{C}} - \underset{\underset{OH}{|}}{\overset{\overset{H}{|}}{C}} - H$$

(no oxygen present)   (2 oxygen atoms present per molecule)

i.e. *the oxygen content has* **increased**.

(b)

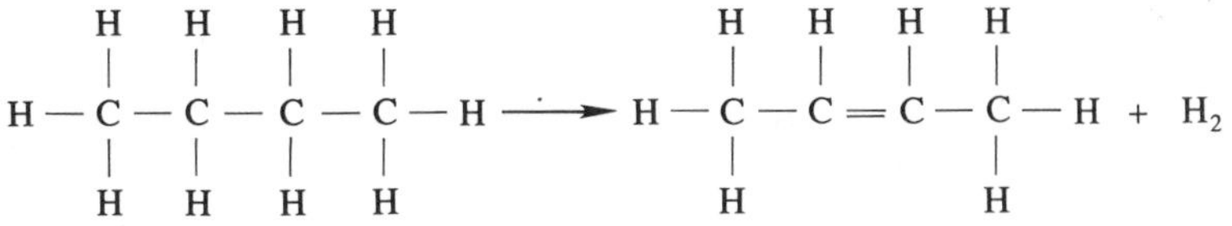

$$H - \underset{\underset{H}{|}}{\overset{\overset{H}{|}}{C}} - \underset{\underset{H}{|}}{\overset{\overset{H}{|}}{C}} - \underset{\underset{H}{|}}{\overset{\overset{H}{|}}{C}} - \underset{\underset{H}{|}}{\overset{\overset{H}{|}}{C}} - H \longrightarrow H - \underset{\underset{H}{|}}{\overset{\overset{H}{|}}{C}} - \underset{H}{\overset{H}{C}} = \underset{H}{\overset{H}{C}} - \underset{\underset{H}{|}}{\overset{\overset{H}{|}}{C}} - H \ + \ H_2$$

(10 hydrogen atoms present per molecule)   (8 hydrogen atoms present per molecule)

i.e. *the hydrogen content has* **decreased**.

(c)

$$2\{H - \overset{\overset{O}{\|}}{C} - O - H\} + O_2 \rightarrow 2CO_2 + 2H_2O$$

(two hydrogen atoms present per molecule)   (no hydrogen)

i.e. *the hydrogen content has* **decreased**.

(d)

$$C \ + \ O_2 \longrightarrow CO_2$$

(no oxygen)   (2 oxygen atoms per molecule)

i.e. *the oxygen content has* **increased**.

Reduction

Reduction is any chemical reaction in which a substance has lost oxygen or gained hydrogen. Since reduction is the opposite of oxidation, it follows that each of the reactions in Fig. 9.25, if reversed, would be a reduction. For example, if we take reaction (b) we have the situation shown in Fig. 9.26.

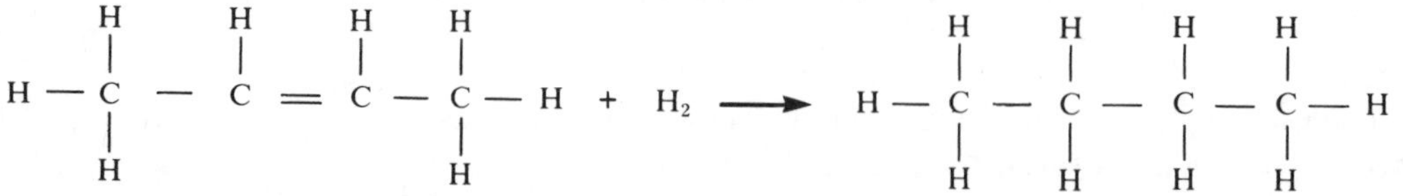

$$H - \overset{\displaystyle H}{\underset{\displaystyle H}{C}} - \overset{\displaystyle H}{C} = \overset{\displaystyle H}{C} - \overset{\displaystyle H}{\underset{\displaystyle H}{C}} - H \; + \; H_2 \; \longrightarrow \; H - \overset{\displaystyle H}{\underset{\displaystyle H}{C}} - \overset{\displaystyle H}{\underset{\displaystyle H}{C}} - \overset{\displaystyle H}{\underset{\displaystyle H}{C}} - \overset{\displaystyle H}{\underset{\displaystyle H}{C}} - H$$

(8 atoms of hydrogen per molecule) (10 atoms of hydrogen per molecule)

i.e. *the hydrogen content has **increased**.*

Figure 9.26.

Electron Transfer or Redox Reactions

These are reactions in which electrons are lost *and* gained. One cannot occur without the other.

Oxidation is a *loss* of electrons.

Reduction is a *gain* in electrons.

Thus when oxidation/reduction or redox reactions occur, one ion (for example) loses one or more electrons and another ion gains the same number of electrons. One ion gives up electrons and the other receives them – so it is that both reactions must occur together and neither reaction can proceed without the other. For example:

$$Fe^{3+,} + Cu^+ \longrightarrow Fe^{2+} + Cu^{2+}$$

We can represent this reaction in two parts as shown in Fig. 9.27.

$$Cu^+ \longrightarrow Cu^{2+} + \text{electron} \quad \text{(LOSS of an electron - OXIDATION)}$$

$$\underline{Fe^{3+} + \text{electron} \longrightarrow Fe^{2+}} \qquad \text{(GAIN of an electron - REDUCTION)}$$

$$Fe^3 + Cu^+ \longrightarrow Fe^{2+} + Cu^{2+}$$

Figure 9.27.

In this case, the electron that has been lost by the copper ion is gained by the iron ion.

The above reaction is given so that the reader may appreciate the important principles involved, which show up more clearly in this type of reaction. However, in the body this type of reaction is exemplified in the **electron transport chain**, in which use is made of both electron transfer reactions and hydrogen transfer reactions (discussed in the next chapter).

Many cellular reactions are **oxidation** reactions, since the oxygen content of the compounds involved increases and, in the process, oxygen is consumed.

These reactions are all burning or **combustion** reactions, since, despite the fact that no flames are present, oxygen is consumed, oxidation occurs and heat is given out, as is the case with other burning or combustion.

As we have seen, any oxidation reaction must be accompanied by a corresponding reduction reaction. That is, as one substance is oxidised, another must be reduced. Since many oxidation reactions occur in the body, what substances are being reduced? In many oxidation steps, **Cofactors** (see full discussion in the next chapter) are involved. One very important example is the vitamin niacin (or nicotinamide adenine dinucleotide), normally represented as NAD^+.

The reduction reaction for NAD^+ may be represented thus:

$$NAD^+ + 2H \longrightarrow NADH + H^+$$

Many of the reactions which will be discussed in the next chapter, showing the metabolism of foods, are oxidation reactions in which hydrogen is lost. This hydrogen may not be lost, however, since a cofactor may well pick it up and transport it elsewhere.

Thus if we represent these compounds by the notation 'RH_2', we could write such an oxidation reaction as

$$RH_2 \longrightarrow R + 2H$$

If the two equations above are then added:

$$NAD^+ + 2H \longrightarrow NADH + H^+$$

$$RH_2 \longrightarrow R + 2H$$

we obtain:

$$RH_2 + NAD^+ \longrightarrow R + NADH + H^+$$

This is often written as:

$$RH_2 \longrightarrow R$$
$$NAD^+ \qquad NADH + H^+$$

that is, as various substances are *oxidised* NAD^+ is *reduced* to form NADH.

Flavine adenine dinucleotide (or FAD), which is obtained from riboflavin, behaves in a similar way to NAD.

NUCLEIC ACIDS

Another set of organic compounds of major importance to the development, reproduction and functioning of the human body are the nucleic acids. These substances literally hold the key to all life. One, **deoxyribonucleic acid** (or **DNA**) is able to store and transmit genetic information, and is a huge molecule with a formula mass as high as several thousands of millions.

Working with other similar nucleic acids called the **ribonucleic acids** (RNA), DNA is involved in the synthesis of the various proteins needed by the cell to carry out its life functions. RNA molecules have formula masses which are smaller than those of DNA and are of the order of 20 000 to 40 000.

The fundamental structural unit (or **monomer**) of the nucleic acids is called a **nucleotide** and is composed of three distinct parts:

1. A *five-carbon sugar*, deoxyribose in DNA and ribose in RNA, as shown in Fig. 9.28.

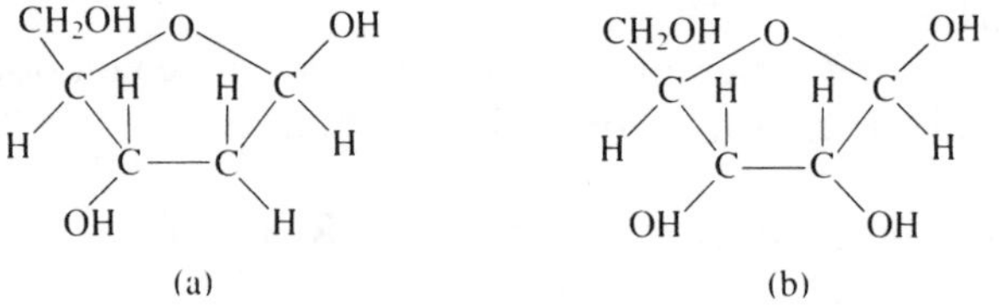

Figure 9.28. The sugars deoxyribose (a) and ribose (b).

2. A *nitrogen-containing organic base* of the type shown in Fig. 9.29.

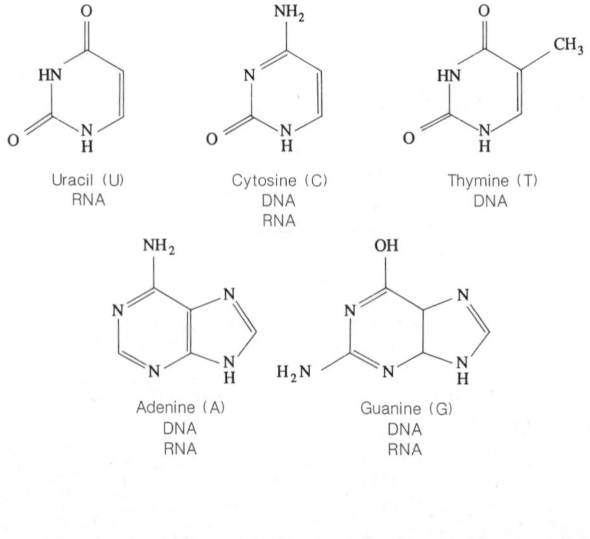

Figure 9.29. The organic bases found in DNA and RNA.

3. A *phosphoric acid molecule* (H_3PO_4).

The five-carbon sugar and the nitrogen base combine as shown in Fig. 9.30(a) to form a compound which then reacts with phosphoric acid to form a nucleotide, Fig. 9.30(b). Note that these are both *dehydration* reactions. A further series of dehydration reactions then produces a structure consisting of many monomers linked together (and thus called a polymer – 'poly' means many) of the type shown in Fig. 9.31. Such polymers can have thousands of millions of monomer units.

RNA is formed as a single chain polymer.

DNA is formed as a double chain polymer in the form of a **helix**. DNA is thus a double helical structure (Fig. 9.32) with the two twisted strands held together by hydrogen bonds between the bases from each strand. The bases involved are shown in Fig. 9.33.

The importance of these compounds is becoming more and more obvious as research unravels the way in which these substances are able to transmit coded information from one generation to the next in genes (the units of heredity). Such genes also control the overall function of the cell.

Little is known about the actual functioning of genes in human beings. This is still a frontier area of research, but research and development in such fields as in-vitro fertilisation and monoclonal antibodies is helping to provide us with more information about them.

Figure 9.30. Adenosine formed by the reaction of adenine and ribose, in (a). This compound reacts with phosphoric acid to form a nucleotide, in (b).

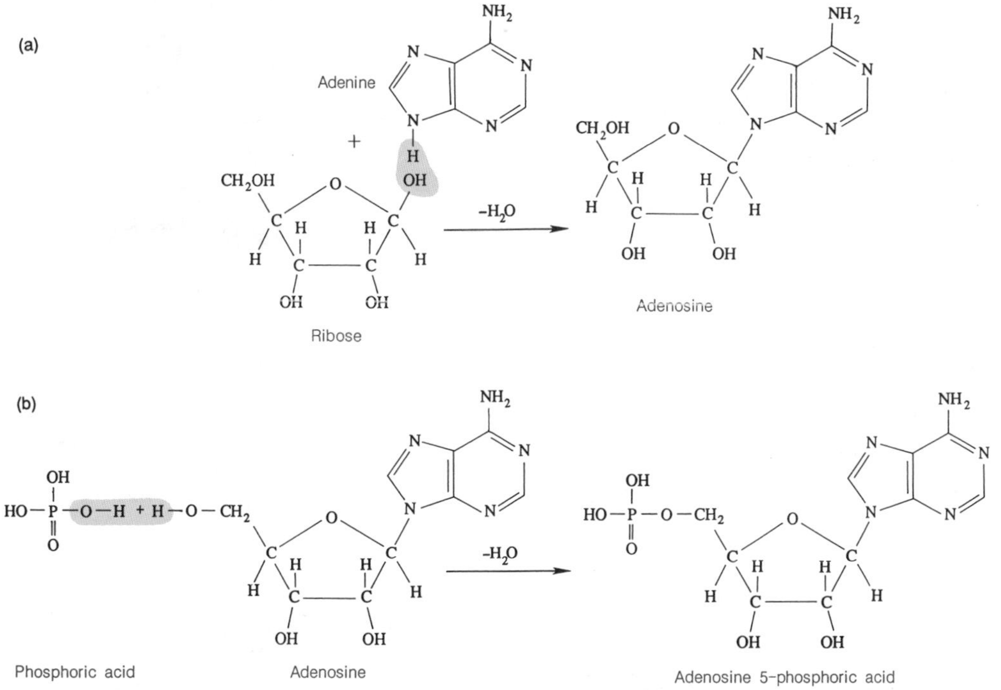

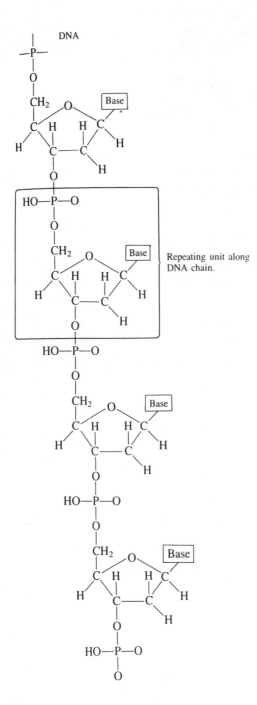

Figure 9.31. A portion of a typical nucleic acid chain.

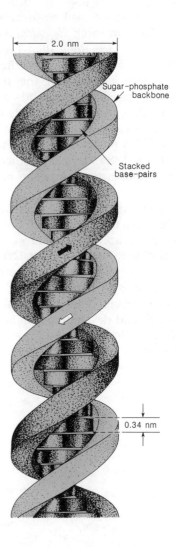

Figure 9.32. DNA is composed of two polynucleotide strands running in opposite directions that twist into a double helix so as to bring the bases into contact in the centre. The sugar phosphate ester backbones of the strands are exposed on the outside of the helix. Ten pairs of nucleotide residues, with their associated paired bases in the centre, form one complete turn of the helix. (From McGilvery & Goldstein: *Biochemistry A Functional Approach.* 3rd Ed. Philadelphia. W.B. Saunders. 1983.)

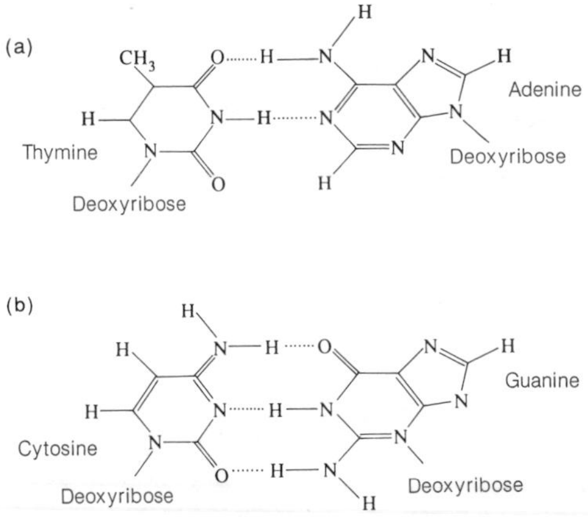

Figure 9.33. The complementary bases on the two strands of DNA's double structure. The structure of (a) thymine-adenine and (b) cytosine-guanine form hydrogen-bonding pairs.

The transmission of information from one generation to the next will be considered more fully in Chapter 16.

We are now in a position to extend our researches into the actual use of some of the compounds mentioned above in the day to day functioning of the body, as well as the conversion of energy, the origin of energy for life and the way in which various food types are able to release the energy which our bodies require. This is the subject of the next chapter.

ORGANIC COMPOUNDS IMPORTANT TO THE BODY

The term 'organic' is now taken to mean compounds containing carbon, but it had its origin as a description of a class of compounds derived from living material.

We have already discussed the elements that are important in the human body. It will be recalled that most compounds in the body (with some obvious exceptions such as water) contain the elements carbon, hydrogen and oxygen. Other elements are present in some types of compounds, e.g. nitrogen is present in proteins (Fig. 9.34).

These types of compounds will now be examined more closely, in particular, carbohydrates, lipids, proteins and amino acids.

CARBOHYDRATES

Chemical Structure

Carbohydrates are compounds of carbon, hydrogen and oxygen, with the hydrogen to oxygen ratio normally 2:1.

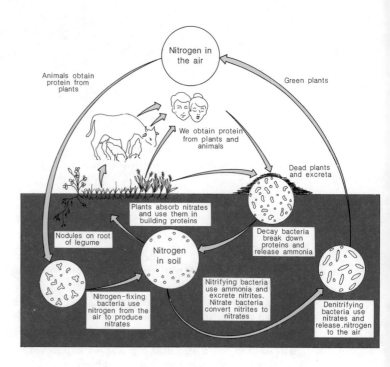

Figure 9.34. The nitrogen cycle.

These compounds consist of a central chain of three to seven carbon atoms with hydrogen and oxygen atoms attached, either singly or in groups.

Major Sources

The major sources of carbohydrate in the normal human diet are sucrose (cane sugar) and lactose (milk sugar) – both of which are represented by the formula $C_{12}H_{22}O_{11}$ – and starches, which are complex molecules present in all foods, particularly grains and foods prepared from grains, such as bread, cakes and cereal. Other carbohydrates that are ingested (to a very limited extent) include glycogen, pectins, and dextrins. Some other compounds that do not have an H:O ratio of 2:1 and are also ingested to a limited extent include alcohol, lactic acid and pyruvic acid.

Classes

The classes of carbohydrate in which we are most interested include:

1. Monosaccharides
'Mono' means 'one' and the word 'saccharide' refers to sugar, so

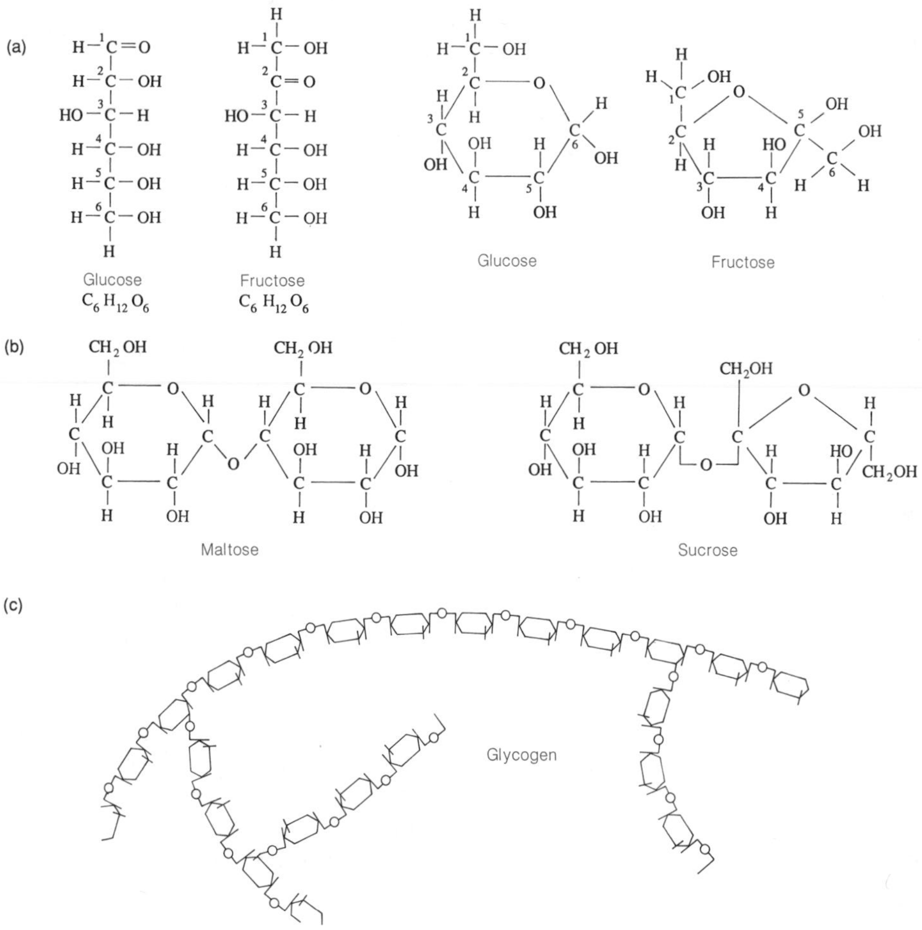

Figure 9.35. (a) Stick formulae and ring formulae for glucose and fructose. (b) Maltose and sucrose as examples of disaccharides. (c) Glycogen as an example of a polysaccharide, where each small ring represents a structure similar to the two rings in maltose and sucrose, i.e. a glucose unit. (From Solomon & Davis: *Human Anatomy & Physiology.* Philadelphia. Saunders College Publishing. 1983.)

that a monosaccharide is a simple sugar with *one* sugar unit per molecule. Monosaccharides are the only forms of carbohydrate that can be absorbed directly across the wall of the GI (gastro-intestinal) tract. All other carbohydrates are broken down to one or more of the three major monosaccharides (listed below) for absorption:

(a) glucose (dextrose) (Fig. 9.35(a)), which is natural in foods, can be formed by the body and is the form that is the pre-ferred energy source for the body;

(b) fructose (Fig. 9.35(a)), obtained from fruits and honey; and

(c) galactose, which is not found free in foods but is produced from lactose.

2. Disaccharides

These have *two* sugar units per molecule.

The three main disaccharides are:

(a) sucrose (cane sugar), which is made from one glucose and one fructose

(b) lactose (milk sugar), which is made from one glucose and one galactose; and

(c) maltose (malt sugar) (Fig. 9.35(b)), which is made from two glucoses.

3. Polysaccharides

'Poly' means 'many'. It follows that these are more complex carbohydrates than those above and may contain very large numbers of units. They include long-chain carbohydrates such as:

(a) starch, consisting of long chains of glucose units, which makes up a large proportion of the diet in the Western world and as much as 50 per cent of the carbohydrate intake in America;

(b) cellulose, which comes from plants (e.g. cotton) but cannot be digested by humans, although it is important in providing bulk for proper bowel functioning;

(c) glycogen (Fig. 9.35(b)), the complex form in which energy is stored in the liver and, to a lesser extent, in the muscles; and

(d) inulin, which is insignificant from the dietary point of view, but provides the basis for a test for renal function. It can be filtered through the glomerulus of the kidneys, but is neither secreted nor reabsorbed by the tubules and is therefore used in some patients to measure glomerular filtration rate. This is known as the inulin clearance test.

Functions of Carbohydrates

1. Energy production

The prime function of carbohydrates is to produce energy. Each gram of carbohydrate can yield 16 kilojoules of energy and all cells take in monosaccharides, which they can process to provide this energy. However, with the important exception of the brain, cells require assistance from the hormone insulin to facilitate the movement of glucose into the cells. In the case of the brain cells do not require the presence of insulin, but neither do they store glucose (or glycogen) and are therefore dependent upon a minute-by-minute supply of glucose via the blood. It is then obviously most important that blood sugar levels are maintained by the body to avoid brain damage.

Glycogen in heart muscle is a very important source of

contractile energy (though not the most important source), especially where the demand on the heart is suddenly increased. If a heart is damaged, glycogen stores may be low and sudden increased demands may be hard to meet, giving rise to severe problems, as in patients with angina.

2. Protective action
Carbohydrates function in exerting protective action by participating in specific detoxifying metabolic pathways in the liver, which reduce the toxicity of some drugs and break down poisons. Derivatives of carbohydrates or intermediate products of carbohydrate metabolism are used to help reduce the toxicity of some drugs by breaking them down and combining with them to form a new compound. For example, phenol compounds, female sex hormones and sulfa drugs can be combined with glucuronic acid to reduce toxicity.

3. Protein-sparing action
The presence of carbohydrates prevents too much protein being used for energy (as happens in starvation and diabetes mellitus) and allows major amounts to be used for tissue repair and building.

4. Anti-ketogenic effect
The presence of carbohydrates prevents the use of a lot of fat to meet the energy needs of the body, which prevents the build-up of a damaging excess of acids.

5. Compound synthesis
Carbohydrates combine with other food compounds to form new compounds essential for various processes in the body, such as the nucleic acids used to build DNA and RNA, which transmit genetic codes. Other examples include the formation of lactose in lactation, mucopolysaccharides, which are involved in the production of mucus, and compounds such as heparin, which prevents blood clotting.

Important Reactions and Properties

In the normal diet, the final products of carbohydrate digestion are about 80 per cent glucose and 10 per cent each of galactose and fructose. The equation below illustrates the breakdown or **hydrolysis** (because water is involved), of a complex carbohydrate (sucrose) to the simple sugars glucose and fructose:

$$C_{12}H_{22}O_{11} \quad + \quad H_2O \quad \rightarrow \quad C_6H_{12}O_6 \quad + \quad C_6H_{12}O_6$$

sucrose   water   glucose   fructose

This is the opposite reaction to the **dehydration synthesis** reaction – that in which sucrose is made or synthesised by the removal of water:

$$C_6H_{12}O_6 \ + \ C_6H_{12}O_6 \ \rightarrow \ C_6H_{22}O_{11} \ + \ H_2O$$

These reactions are shown in structural form in Fig. 9.36. Glucose can:

1. be converted to glycogen for storage in the muscles and liver;

2. be converted to fat (i.e. triglycerides, as described later); and

3. undergo glycolysis and the other reactions described under cellular respiration to produce energy in the form of ATP. Some of these compounds are illustrated in Fig. 9.36.

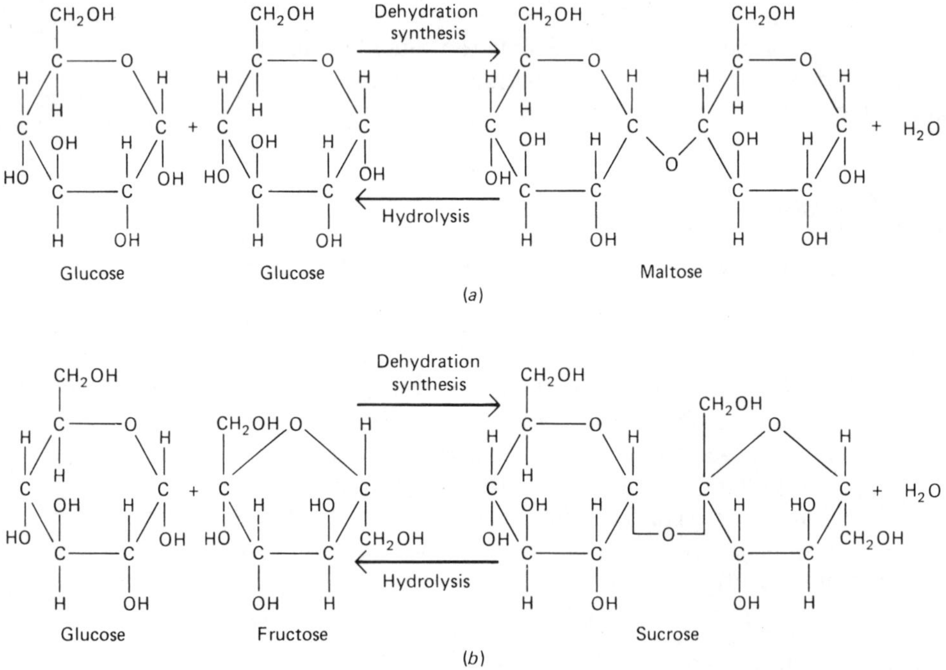

Figure 9.36. (a) Synthesis of maltose from two glucose molecules. (b) Synthesis of surcose and fructose. Note that in each case an ⁻OH and a ⁻H have been removed to form water and to leave the two rings or glucose units bonded by a single oxygen atom. (From Solomon & Davis: *Human Anatomy & Physiology*. Philadelphia. Saunders College Publishing. 1983.)

LIPIDS

Sometimes referred to by the simpler term, fats, these are the waxy, greasy and oily compounds of the body. They are ingested into the body in such foods as butter, margarine, meat, eggs, milk, nuts and chocolate.

If they are liquid at room temperature, they tend to be regarded as oils, and if solid, as wax. Ear wax is an example of the latter. They repel water, i.e. they are **hydrophobic** (meaning fear of water), and this property is important in the way in which some of these compounds function in the body, as in membrane formation.

While they are not soluble in water, lipids are soluble in solvents such as alcohols, including ethanol (common alcohol). They are also compounds of carbon, hydrogen and oxygen, but with a lower oxygen content per molecule than carbohydrates.

The lipids that are most significant as far as the human body is concerned are neutral fats, phospholipids, steroids and waxes. No more will be said of the waxes, but the other types will be discussed in more detail.

Types of Lipids

1. Neutral Fats – also known as Simple Fats
These compounds are the richest sources (by weight) of fuel energy in the body, being more than twice as rich as carbohydrates. They are stored in the body as **adipose** tissue.

The two chemical building blocks of a neutral fat are **glycerol** (otherwise known as glycerine) and one or more **fatty acids**. These are also the basic chemical building blocks of other lipids, which are built up with a number of variations and additions to this basic structure.

Glycerol is an alcohol with three carbon atoms in its chain, to each one of which is attached an – OH or hydroxyl group. A fatty acid is a compound with a straight chain of carbon atoms to which other atoms are attached, usually hydrogen atoms, with a carboxylic acid group ($-COOH$) at one end. The length of the chain varies, as does the number of double bonds (to some extent) to give a very large number of different kinds of fatty acids.

If a glycerol molecule combines chemically with *one* fatty acid molecule, then a **monoglyceride** is formed, as shown in Fig. 9.37.

If a glycerol molecule combines chemically with *two* fatty acid molecules, a **diglyceride** is formed.

Figure 9.37.

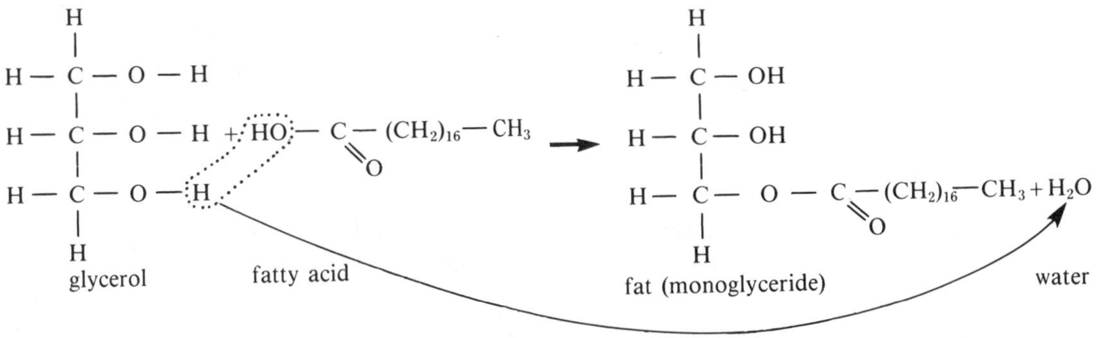

glycerol   fatty acid   fat (monoglyceride)   water

If a glycerol molecule combines chemically with *three* fatty acid molecules, a **triglyceride** is formed, as shown in Fig. 9.38.

As a matter of interest, the fatty acid shown in the figure is stearic acid, commonly used to make soap, and the triglyceride formed is tristearin.

The fatty acids most commonly present in neutral fat in the human body are:

(a) stearic acid, which is a saturated acid with an 18-carbon chain;

(b) oleic acid, which also has an 18-carbon chain but has one double bond in the middle of the chain and is thus unsaturated; and

(c) palmitic acid, which is a saturated acid with a 16-carbon chain.

These and other very similar fatty acids are also the major constituents of fats in food – other than those in milk products, which have shorter chains. Glycerol combines chemically with these fatty acids to form triglycerides, which are the fats with which we will be chiefly concerned.

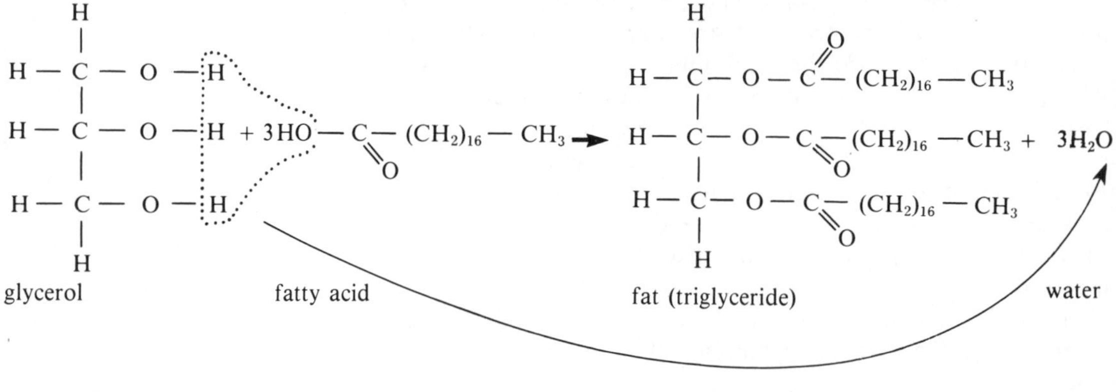

Figure 9.38.

2. Compound Lipids

The compound lipids consist of a combination of neutral fat and other components. Examples are the phospholipids (which originate from a neutral fat and such compounds as phosphoric acid and a nitrogenous base) and glycolipids (which originate from fatty acids, carbohydrate and nitrogen, and are found chiefly in the brain).

Another example is the lipoproteins, which, as their name suggests, contain lipids and proteins. One example is the combination of lipids found in the plasma, with certain parts of plasma protein. This provides the chief transport mechanism for lipid substances in the blood.

Plasma lipoproteins contain such substances as cholesterol, phospholipids, neutral fat, free fatty acids, fat-soluble vitamins, steroid hormones and protein elements. Thus fat-related and/or fat-soluble substances are transported through the body via the blood to various areas. It can be seen at this stage that the various nutrients that we discuss separately are often interrelated.

As mentioned earlier, phospholipids are important components of cell membranes and have several other vital functions in the body. However, they have no direct role in energy production.

They are similar in structure to the triglycerides, but at least one of the fatty acids is replaced by a phosphoric acid radical, and a nitrogen-containing group is usually present. It should be noted that neither phosphorus nor nitrogen are present in neutral fats.

One very intriguing feature of the structure of all phospholipids is that they have a **hydrophobic** (water-fearing or water-hating) end and a **hydrophilic** (water-loving) end. Because these lipid molecules are polarised in this way, they tend to arrange themselves in a double layer in a cell membrane so that the hydrophobic ends are together and the hydrophilic ends point towards the water in the inside and on the outside of a cell (as shown in Fig. 9.39). The membrane actually contains lumps of protein embedded in the lipid bilayer.

Figure 9.39. (a) A phospholipid. The fatty acid portions form the two long chains to the right of the oxygen atoms which link the chains to the remainder of the molecules. (b) A lipid bilayer. The fatty acid (hydrophobic – 'water-fearing') ends form the centre portion of the diagram. (From Solomon & Davis: *Human Anatomy & Physiology*. Philadelphia. Saunders College Publishing. 1983.)

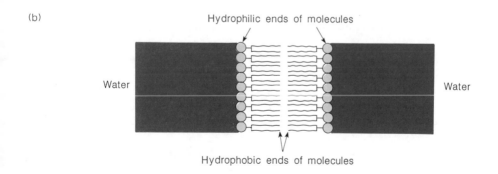

3. Derived Lipids

These are fat substances derived from simple and compound fats. One example is glycerol, the water-soluble components of triglycerides (discussed above under neutral fats), which may be readily converted to carbohydrates and therefore contributes to the total available glucose in the diet.

While this group of compounds is classified as a type of lipid, their structure is quite different from that of other lipids. It is of interest to observe that the female and male hormones, oestrogen and testosterone respectively, are steroids, Steroids consist of four interlocking rings, three containing six carbon atoms and the fourth with five carbon atoms in the ring. Different side-chains extend out from the rings, and the nature of these determines the properties of that particular steroid.

Another steroid of particular importance is cholesterol, which is used to form cholic acid in the liver, which, with other substances forms bile salts. These bile salts are very important in digestive processes, particularly the digestion and absorption of fats.

Other examples of steroids are ergosterol, a Vitamin D precursor, and cortical adrenal hormones such as cortisone.

Functions of Lipids

1. Lipids are the most energy-rich foods of all, yielding 37 kJ for each gram of fat – compared to 16 kJ per gram for carbohydrates.

2. They provide protection for the entire body, as well as protection for individual vital organs and structures such as the kidneys and nerves.

3. They act as a heat insulator for the whole body and as an electrical insulator in some nerves.

4. They play a role in the formation of new compounds in the body, such as lipoproteins, phospholipids and cholesterol.

5. They assist in the transport of fat-soluble substances such as vitamins.

PROTEINS

Proteins make up about three-quarters of the solid parts of the body. Included in these are:

- structural proteins, e.g. cell membranes;
- enzymes, e.g. pepsin (found in stomach);
- parts of genes;
- proteins that transport oxygen, e.g. haemoglobin;
- muscle proteins; and
- many others such as antibodies and hormones, e.g. insulin.

Proteins consist essentially of amino acids, which contain the elements C,H,O,N and frequently other elements such as S. About 20 of these occur in the body in significant quantities, but their structures are very varied and complex. They are all alpha amino acids, i.e. the two important functional groups (the acid group ($-COOH$) and the amino group ($-NH_2$)) are both attached to the same carbon atom. We thus have the general structure given in Fig. 9.40.

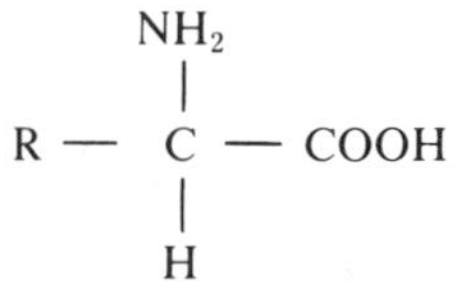

$$\begin{array}{c} NH_2 \\ | \\ R - C - COOH \\ | \\ H \end{array}$$

Figure 9.40.

The 'R' group shown here can represent anything from a simple methyl group ($-CH_3$) to a highly substituted benzene ring (C_6H_6) or another acid ($-COOH$) group.

It is important to note here that although the four bonds have been represented as being at right angles to each other, this is only a matter of convenience in representing a three dimensional structure in two dimensions. In fact, the angle between these four bonds is about 110 deg. This means that the acid group and the amino group are more separated than it would appear in the formula above. This is significant in the formation of peptide bonds.

It should also be noted that, since the amino group is a derivative of ammonia, it is basic in nature. Thus this type of compound has an acidic end and a basic end. It follows that the basic end of one amino acid can combine chemically with the acidic end of another, and that this process can be repeated to form a very long chain of amino acids, i.e. a protein molecule. Furthermore, the number of possible combinations of 20 or so amino acids in very long chains means that an almost infinite variety of compounds can be formed. Some proteins have as many as a hundred thousand amino acid molecules, and even the smaller ones have more than 20 amino acid molecules. For example, insulin has 51 amino acids.

When the acid group in one molecule combines with the amino group in another molecule, a **peptide** link or bond is formed, as illustrated in Fig. 9.41.

If you examine this figure, you will notice:

1. In the second amino acid, the $-NH_2$, group has been opened up so that the lasso can be shown encircling an H atom and an OH group, which then combine chemically to form water.

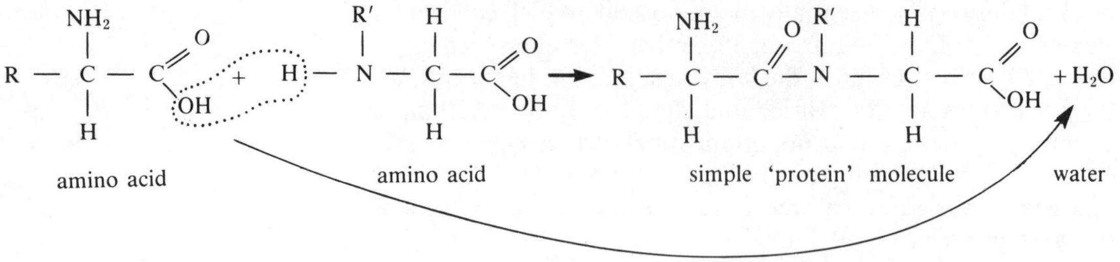

Figure 9.41.

The two R groups may be the same or they may be different, as indicated.

2. The new compound resulting from the formation of a peptide link still has an acid group at one end and an amino group at the other, enabling more peptide links to be formed.

3. A number of other types of link can also be formed between amino acids, but these will not be dealt with here.

Protein Types

1. Globular Proteins

Most of the proteins in the body (excepting the fibrous proteins, discussed below) have either a globular or an elliptical shape and are called globular proteins. These proteins are generally soluble in water or saline solutions and perform thousands of different functions in the body. Some important examples of globular proteins are the albumin, globulins and fibrinogen that make up the plasma proteins, as well as haemoglobin, the cytochromes and most of the cellular enzymes.

It should be noted at this point that proteins contain groups of atoms that can become polar, because of a greater tendency of some atoms to attract electrons. The tendency to form polar bonds is an important property of some proteins and gives rise to their role in establishing osmolarity of fluids, for example.

2. Fibrous Proteins

These make up many of the highly complex proteins in the human body. They consist of long peptide-linked chains running parallel to each other, many of which are held together by cross-linkages. The main types are:

(a) collagens, which are the basic structural proteins of connective tissue, tendons, cartilage and bone;

(b) elastins, which are the elastic fibres of tendons, arteries and connective tissue;

(c) keratins, which are the essential proteins of hair and nails; and

(d) actin and myosin, the contractile proteins of muscle.

All of these protein fibres are very strong, and are capable of being stretched and then return to their original length.

3. Conjugated Proteins
Many proteins combine with substances that are not proteins to form conjugated proteins. Examples of these are listed here:

(a) Nucleoproteins These are combinations of simple proteins and nucleic acid (this may be DNA or RNA, which are compounds consisting of C, O, H, N and P) and are found in chromosomes, for example.

(b) Proteoglycans. These are the major components of all tissues, serve as lubricants in joints and occur in the vitreous humour of the eyes. They are glycoproteins and are formed from long polysaccharide chains containing amino groups linked to a protein core, like bristles on a bottle brush.

(c) Others. These include several other types of protein (many of which contain the elements Mg, Cu, Fe, and Zn) such as lipoproteins, glycoproteins, metalloproteins (many enzymes), chromoproteins (such as haemoglobins) and mucoproteins. It can be observed that the names and categories of many of these substances give a clue as to their origin and composition.

Functions of Proteins

Some reference has been made already to some of these. The following is a list of functions, with examples:

1. Structural   – collagen, cell membranes.
2. Contractile   – muscle.
3. Regulatory   – hormones.
4. Transport   – haemoglobin, which transports oxygen.
5. Protective   – antibodies, gamma globulins
                        – fibrinogen, which is involved in blood clotting.
                        – mucus formation.
6. Fluid balance – establishing the osmolarity of fluids, such as blood (albumin, etc.)
7. Building   – forms compounds with other substances such as lipids and carbohydrates (phospholipids, muco-polysaccharides).
8. Facilitatory   – enzymes. These assist many chemical reactions in the body – pepsin aids the breakdown of peptide bonds; carbonic anhydrase facilitates the equilibrium reaction between CO_2 and H_2O in the red blood cells.

Amino Acids

At the beginning of our discussion on the structure of proteins, reference was made to amino acids as the building blocks of

SCIENCE IN NURSING

Figure 9.42. The amino acids, showing the ten essential amino acids, which cannot be synthesised at all or in sufficient quantity in the body. (From Guyton: *Textbook of Medical Physiology*. 6th Ed. Philadelphia. W.B. Saunders. 1981.)

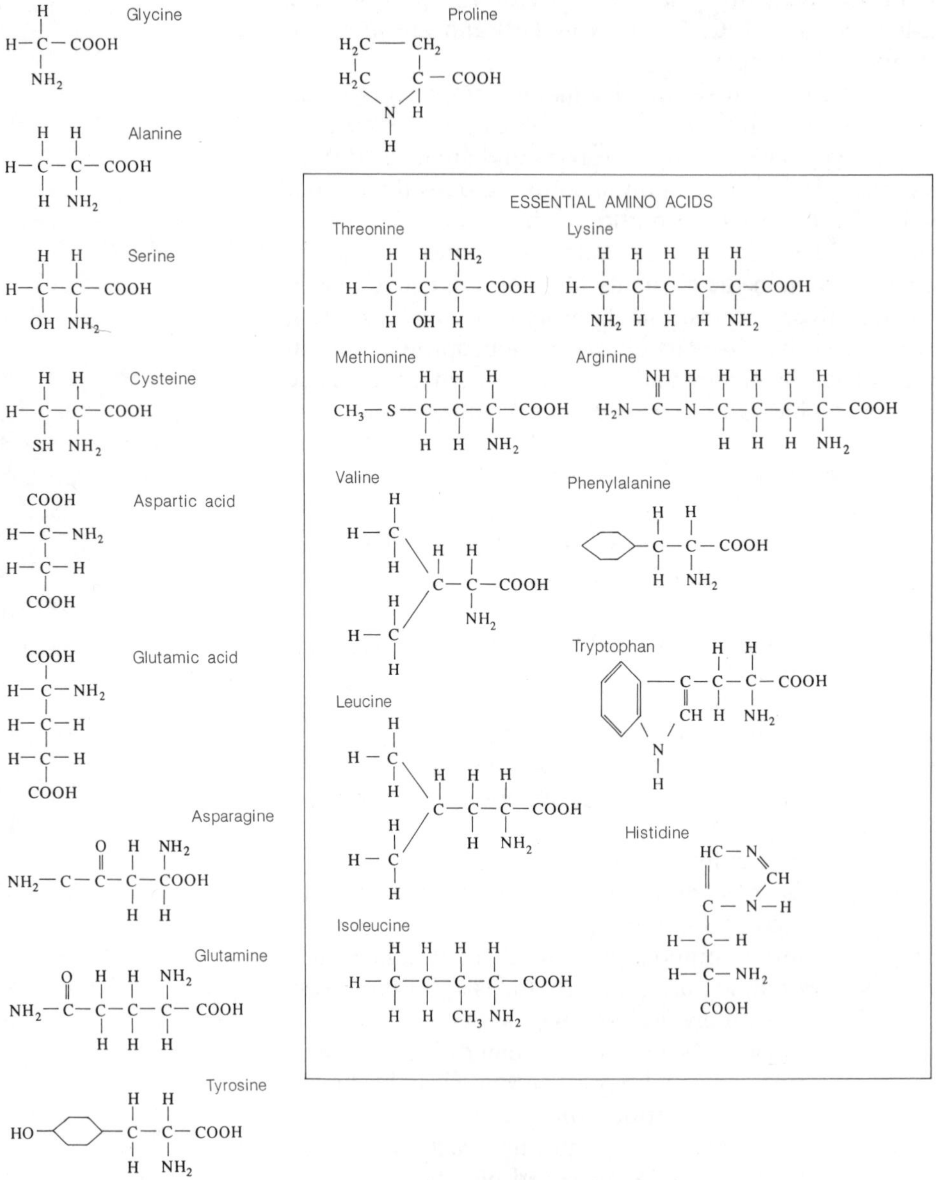

Glycine

$$H-\underset{\underset{NH_2}{|}}{\overset{\overset{H}{|}}{C}}-COOH$$

Alanine

$$H-\underset{\underset{H}{|}}{\overset{\overset{H}{|}}{C}}-\underset{\underset{NH_2}{|}}{\overset{\overset{H}{|}}{C}}-COOH$$

Serine

$$H-\underset{\underset{OH}{|}}{\overset{\overset{H}{|}}{C}}-\underset{\underset{NH_2}{|}}{\overset{\overset{H}{|}}{C}}-COOH$$

Cysteine

$$H-\underset{\underset{SH}{|}}{\overset{\overset{H}{|}}{C}}-\underset{\underset{NH_2}{|}}{\overset{\overset{H}{|}}{C}}-COOH$$

Aspartic acid

$$H-\overset{\overset{COOH}{|}}{C}-NH_2$$
$$H-\overset{|}{C}-H$$
$$\underset{COOH}{|}$$

Glutamic acid

$$H-\overset{\overset{COOH}{|}}{C}-NH_2$$
$$H-\overset{|}{C}-H$$
$$H-\overset{|}{C}-H$$
$$\underset{COOH}{|}$$

Asparagine

$$NH_2-\overset{\overset{O}{\|}}{C}-\underset{\underset{H}{|}}{\overset{\overset{H}{|}}{C}}-\underset{\underset{H}{|}}{\overset{\overset{NH_2}{|}}{C}}-COOH$$

Glutamine

$$NH_2-\overset{\overset{O}{\|}}{C}-\underset{\underset{H}{|}}{\overset{\overset{H}{|}}{C}}-\underset{\underset{H}{|}}{\overset{\overset{H}{|}}{C}}-\underset{\underset{H}{|}}{\overset{\overset{NH_2}{|}}{C}}-COOH$$

Tyrosine

$$HO-\bigcirc-\underset{\underset{H}{|}}{\overset{\overset{H}{|}}{C}}-\underset{\underset{NH_2}{|}}{\overset{\overset{H}{|}}{C}}-COOH$$

Proline

$$H_2C - CH_2$$
$$H_2C \quad C-COOH$$
$$\underset{H}{\overset{N}{|}}$$

ESSENTIAL AMINO ACIDS

Threonine

$$H-\underset{\underset{H}{|}}{\overset{\overset{H}{|}}{C}}-\underset{\underset{OH}{|}}{\overset{\overset{H}{|}}{C}}-\underset{\underset{H}{|}}{\overset{\overset{NH_2}{|}}{C}}-COOH$$

Methionine

$$CH_3-S-\underset{\underset{H}{|}}{\overset{\overset{H}{|}}{C}}-\underset{\underset{H}{|}}{\overset{\overset{H}{|}}{C}}-\underset{\underset{NH_2}{|}}{\overset{\overset{H}{|}}{C}}-COOH$$

Valine

$$\overset{\overset{H}{|}}{\underset{\underset{H}{|}}{H-C}}$$
$$\overset{\overset{H}{|}}{\underset{\underset{H}{|}}{H-C}} \underset{\underset{NH_2}{|}}{\overset{\overset{H\ \ H}{|\ \ |}}{C-C}}-COOH$$

Leucine

$$\overset{\overset{H}{|}}{\underset{\underset{H}{|}}{H-C}}$$
$$\overset{\overset{H}{|}}{\underset{\underset{H}{|}}{H-C}} \underset{\underset{NH_2}{|}}{\overset{\overset{H\ H\ H}{|\ |\ |}}{C-C-C}}-COOH$$

Isoleucine

$$H-\underset{\underset{H}{|}}{\overset{\overset{H}{|}}{C}}-\underset{\underset{H}{|}}{\overset{\overset{H}{|}}{C}}-\underset{\underset{CH_3}{|}}{\overset{\overset{H}{|}}{C}}-\underset{\underset{NH_2}{|}}{\overset{\overset{H}{|}}{C}}-COOH$$

Lysine

$$H-\underset{\underset{NH_2}{|}}{\overset{\overset{H}{|}}{C}}-\underset{\underset{H}{|}}{\overset{\overset{H}{|}}{C}}-\underset{\underset{H}{|}}{\overset{\overset{H}{|}}{C}}-\underset{\underset{H}{|}}{\overset{\overset{H}{|}}{C}}-\underset{\underset{NH_2}{|}}{\overset{\overset{H}{|}}{C}}-COOH$$

Arginine

$$H_2N-\overset{\overset{NH}{\|}}{C}-\underset{\underset{H}{|}}{\overset{\overset{H}{|}}{N}}-\underset{\underset{H}{|}}{\overset{\overset{H}{|}}{C}}-\underset{\underset{H}{|}}{\overset{\overset{H}{|}}{C}}-\underset{\underset{NH_2}{|}}{\overset{\overset{H}{|}}{C}}-COOH$$

Phenylalanine

$$\bigcirc-\underset{\underset{H}{|}}{\overset{\overset{H}{|}}{C}}-\underset{\underset{NH_2}{|}}{\overset{\overset{H}{|}}{C}}-COOH$$

Tryptophan

$$\bigcirc\hspace{-0.3em}\bigcirc-\underset{\underset{CH}{|}}{\overset{}{C}}-\underset{\underset{H}{|}}{\overset{\overset{H}{|}}{C}}-\underset{\underset{NH_2}{|}}{\overset{\overset{H}{|}}{C}}-COOH$$
$$\underset{\underset{H}{|}}{N}$$

Histidine

$$HC-N$$
$$\| \qquad CH$$
$$C-N-H$$
$$|$$
$$H-\overset{|}{C}-H$$
$$H-\underset{\underset{COOH}{|}}{\overset{|}{C}}-NH_2$$

protein molecules. As a matter of interest, these amino acids are listed in Fig. 9.42 so that the reader can see the variation in structure that he or she is otherwise called upon to imagine. They are divided into essential and non-essential amino acids. **Essen-**

tial amino acids cannot be synthesised in the body (or, in some cases in sufficient quantities to meet the body's needs) and so must be present in the diet. The so-called non-essential amino acids are just as essential as the essential amino acids, but the former can be synthesised in the cells of the body.

Some comments need to be made about Fig. 9.42. It shows ten essential amino acids. In some other literature, nine essential amino acids are shown, but the one that is left out varies! Sometimes it is tryptophan (despite the fact that tryptophan deficiency can lead to the protein-deficiency syndrome known as *kwashiorkor*) and in other cases it is arginine. The situation is further complicated by the fact that two of these amino acids are regarded as essential for children and those who are still growing, but non-essential for adults.

The principle of the existence of essential amino acids, and the implications of this for diet planning, are what is significant here.

The protein content of diets also raises the question of complete and incomplete proteins. *Complete proteins are those that provide the essential amino acids in the proportions required by the body, and are of animal origin. Incomplete or partial proteins have ratios of amino acids different from the body's requirements*, and may also be deficient in one or more of the essential amino acids and are therefore not as nutritionally valuable as complete proteins. These are of plant origin and include grains, legumes and nuts.

Examples of complete proteins include lean meat, eggs, fish, cheese and milk. A nutritionally balanced diet can easily be obtained by using foods from both groups to provide a mixed source of proteins. A diet with the required essential amino acids can also be obtained through a vegetarian diet by careful selection and planning of plant foods so that they will supple- ment and com- plement each other to obtain the correct quantities and ratios.

DIGESTION OF FOOD

Apart from minerals, vitamins and water, the three major food types are carbohydrates, proteins and fats.

It is interesting to note that in the formation of each of these food types, molecules of water have been removed, as explained below. Thus, the process of digestion seeks to reverse the chemical reactions involved and, by supplying water, furnish the hydrogen atoms (H) and hydroxyl radicals (OH) needed to resynthesise the original compounds or original basic units from which the compound was formed. Examples include glucose, fructose and galactose in the case of carbohydrates; amino acids in the case of proteins; and glycerol and fatty acids in the case of fats.

This process is called *hydrolysis*, and each of the reactions involved in breaking down these food types is a hydrolysis reaction, which may be represented thus:

$$G - G' + H_2O \xrightarrow[\text{enzyme}]{\text{digestive}} G - OH + G' - H$$

where G and G' represent two groups of atoms, as described below.

Carbohydrates

If we consider disaccharides, for example, we can regard these as having been formed from two monosaccharides (simple sugars) by a **dehydration synthesis** or condensation reaction, as below:

$$C_6H_{12}O_6 \quad + \quad C_6H_{12}O_6 \quad \rightarrow \quad C_{12}H_{22}O_{11} \quad + \quad H_2O$$

| glucose | fructose | sucrose | water |

Thus the digestive reaction is the opposite to this, e.g. the breakdown of sucrose by water into glucose and fructose, as shown

$$C_{12}H_{22}O_{11} \quad + \quad H_2O \quad \rightarrow \quad C_6H_{12}O_6 \quad + \quad C_6H_{12}O_6$$

| sucrose | water | glucose | fructose |

See Fig. 9.36 where these reactions are shown in structural form.

The reactions involving polysaccharides are very similar in principle, although the complexity of some of these molecules (e.g. starch) means that the reactions are much more complex.

These hydrolysis reactions depend upon the action of enzymes, however, as we shall soon see.

Proteins

In this reaction we see the formation of a simple protein molecule as discussed on p. 278. An H atom and an OH radical have been removed, one each from two amino acids shown, to form a simple protein molecule. The proteins in the body are formed in the same way from amino acids, i.e. by the elimination of a water molecule (R and R' are alkyl groups which may or may not be the same). Digestion of proteins is thus the reverse of the reaction above. Although the proteins involved are much more complex, they are broken down in a series of steps represented by the reverse of the reaction above.

$$
\begin{array}{cccccc}
& \text{H} & & & \text{O} & \\
& | & & & \parallel & \\
\text{H} - & \text{C} & - \text{O} - & \text{C} & - (CH_2)_{16} - CH_3 & \\
& | & & & & \\
\text{H} - & \text{C} & - \text{O} - & \text{C} & - (CH_2)_{16} - CH_3 & + 3H_2O \\
& | & & & & \\
\text{H} - & \text{C} & - \text{O} - & \text{C} & - (CH_2)_{16} - CH_3 & \\
& | & & & & \\
& \text{H} & & & &
\end{array}
$$

fat (triglyceride)   water

$$
\longrightarrow
$$

$$
\begin{array}{cccc}
& \text{H} & & \\
& | & & \\
\text{H} - & \text{C} & - \text{O} - \text{H} \\
& | & & \\
\text{H} - & \text{C} & - \text{O} - \text{H} \\
& | & & \\
\text{H} - & \text{C} & - \text{O} - \text{H} \\
& | & & \\
& \text{H} & &
\end{array}
$$

glycerol

$$
+ 3HO - \overset{O}{\underset{\parallel}{C}} - (CH_2)_{16} - CH_3
$$

fatty acid

Fats

Most of the fat portion of our diets consists of triglycerides (neutral fats) which are formed (as shown on p. 276) by the reaction between glycerol and three fatty acid molecules, with the elimination of three molecules of water (Fig. 9.43). Thus digestion of triglycerides is effected by their reaction with water to form three fatty acid molecules and glycerol. This is once again a hydrolysis reaction.

Thus we see that digestion really boils down to a series of hydrolysis reactions in which the part played by enzymes is vital and, as explained later, different enzymes are able to catalyse different reactions. It is interesting to note that all the enzymes involved are themselves proteins.

Figure 9.43. Hydrolysis of triglycerides (fats), as occurs in digestion, to form glycerol and fatty acids.

REVIEW

1. Give a word equation for the hydrolysis of sucrose and state why this is important.
2. What effect does a shortage of oxygen have on the energy-producing process in the cell?
3. Discuss the reasons why the cell uses mainly glucose as an energy source rather than proteins or fats.
4. Using a simple flow diagram, illustrate the relationship between fat and glucose in terms of energy production.
5. Glucose and ATP may both be regarded as sources of energy. In what ways do they differ in this regard?
6. The nucleus of the cell controls all cell functioning either directly or indirectly. What agents, produced through genetic coding, are utilised in this control? Describe their nature and role in the cell.
7. What is cellular respiration?

10

Energy in the body

OBJECTIVES

After studying this chapter, the student should be able to:

1. Define energy, distinguish between different types of energy and describe how one form of energy may be converted to another.
2. Distinguish between food types and list the major sources of each type.
3. Discuss the functions of various lipids in the body and the relative importance of saturated and unsaturated fats in the diet.
4. List some of the important amino acids in the body, describe peptide links and relate how amino acids are used to construct protein molecules.
5. Discuss cellular respiration and describe how each food type is involved in metabolism.
6. Discuss enzymes and their importance in the body as organic catalysts.
7. Distinguish between aerobic and anaerobic respiration and discuss the involvement of oxygen in these.

INTRODUCTION

'What you eat today walks and talks tomorrow.' This baker's slogan makes a fitting introduction to any discussion on energy in the body. While it does not convey the whole story (the food we eat is essential for us to maintain our body temperatures), it reminds us of the link between our energy intake and our capacity to carry out the tasks that form part of our daily existence. Let us not overlook the fact that all the activities of our bodies – be it exercise, sleeping, breathing, nerve transmission, cell activity, even thinking – require energy.

The concept of energy is a very broad one and while it is possible to give a definition that makes sense to the physicist, a working definition embracing all the senses in which the term energy is used is not easy to formulate. The usual scientific definition of energy is *the capacity to do work*. If we lift an object from a table or walk upstairs or move any muscle, work is done. It should be noted that the term work is used here in the scientific sense, where work is defined as *the force applied multiplied by the distance moved*. This is not entirely consistent with our everyday definition of work, of course, since we certainly feel that we are working when we try to move a heavy object that will not budge. In terms of our definition, however, this does not constitute work, because the object has not moved.

CONVERSION OF ENERGY

Energy exists in a number of different forms:

1. heat
2. chemical
3. electrical
4. mechanical
5. kinetic
6. potential
7. nuclear
8. electromagnetic (e.g. light)
9. sound

Those which concern us most in the body include:

- chemical energy, e.g. manufacture of new compounds in the cells,
- electrical energy, e.g. conduction of signals in nerves,
- mechanical energy, e.g. movement
- heat energy, e.g. maintenance of body temperature.

Energy can be converted from one form to another. In fact, an important law called the **principle of conservation of energy** states that *energy cannot be created or destroyed in an ordinary chemical reaction, but it can be changed from one form to another*. Note that the definition is stated in this way because, under certain circumstances, energy can be changed into mass and vice versa.

However, we are much more concerned with changes of energy from one form to another. Let us look at this question in general before moving on to more clinical applications. Table 10.1 lists a number of examples of conversion from one energy form to another.

TABLE 10.1

Energy conversion	Examples
mechanical → electrical	generator, alternator
electrical → mechanical	electric motor
heat → electrical	thermocouple
electrical → heat	radiator, toaster, jug, iron
chemical → electrical	car battery
electrical → chemical	electroplating
chemical → heat	fuels such as gas, oil
mechanical → heat	friction
heat → mechanical	steam engine
electrical → light	light bulb
etc.	

The types of energy conversions in which we are particularly interested include:

- food (chemical energy) → heat and mechanical energy (in the cells);
- light energy → electrical energy in the eye;
- sound energy → mechanical energy → electrical energy in the ear;
- heat energy → electrical energy in the skin;
- light energy → chemical energy, which occurs in the leaves of plants (photosynthesis) and without which we would have no food.

Kinetic and Potential Energy

Kinetic energy is the energy a body possesses by virtue of its **motion**. We have already spoken of the motion of particles that make up a gas and the fact that the pressure exerted by a gas is due to the kinetic energy of the gas particles. Furthermore, as temperature increases, the average kinetic energy of the gas particles increases proportionately.

Potential energy is energy possessed by an object by virtue of its position or state. Potential energy of **position** is the easier concept of the two, and refers to the energy a body possesses as a result of its height above a given reference point. Thus, a weight in a traction apparatus has potential energy because it is higher than the floor or ground. A rock at the top of a cliff has greater potential energy than one at the bottom, and so forth.

Potential energy of **state** is the energy possessed by a wound-up clock spring; a compressed coil spring; a stretched elastic band; or a bow that has been pulled back ready to fire an arrow. In all these circumstances, work can be done by the potential energy that is present. In a similar way, the elasticity of a number of types of body tissue contributes to mechanical movement.

Potential energy of state also refers to the *storage of energy in a chemical form* in the chemical bonds of compounds. Energy can be transferred from the processes involved in the breakdown of one type of molecule to the processes involved in the manufacture of another by means of 'coupled reactions' – reactions that operate in concert, as it were. An example of this will be discussed in detail later in the chapter.

Each of these two forms of energy (kinetic energy and potential energy) can be converted to the other form. If a traction weight (which has no kinetic energy) is suddenly released, the potential energy possessed by the weight is continually changed to kinetic energy as the weight travels towards the floor. At the point of impact, the weight has its maximum *kinetic* energy and no longer possesses any *potential* energy.

Similarly, if a ball is thrown up on to a root, the kinetic energy imparted to the ball when it is thrown upwards is changed into potential energy as the ball moves upwards and then lands on the roof.

The above examples serve to convey the general idea of these types of energy conversions, but are oversimplified, since some of the energy involved is changed into heat and sound energy, some is used to overcome air resistance, and so on.

WHERE DOES ENERGY IN THE BODY ORIGINATE?

The major source of energy for the human body is the food we consume. In fact human beings are not capable of manufacturing their own food as do plants. Our primary sources of food are carbohydrates, proteins and fats. Without these food types, and water, vitamins and minerals, together with the oxygen needed for the processing or metabolism of these foods, we simply would not survive.

In recent times people have become increasingly aware of the vital role that the sources of these foods (plants and animals) play in our lives. However, no community can protect, maintain, promote and develop its sources of food (whether on a local or a worldwide basis) unless individuals become more aware of some vital interrelationships existing in nature. Some knowledge of the interrelationships between human beings, plants, animals and the environment is crucial to the continuation of life on earth. Since nurses can play a particularly important (and increasingly significant) role in the health of a community, we must have a look at some of these interrelationships and the primary sources of these essential compounds and molecules.

Photosynthesis and Energy for Life

The word photosynthesis consists of **photo**, meaning 'light', and **synthesis**, meaning to 'make'. Thus we have a chemical reaction that makes carbohydrates, using light as a source of energy. This is a most important reaction. For convenience, this reaction is described below in point form:

1. Plants take in carbon dioxide from the atmosphere through their leaves by gaseous diffusion.
2. The diffusion process occurs through the **stomates**, which are openings in the upper and lower epidermis of the leaf, formed by the **guard cells** (Fig. 10.1).
3. Carbon dioxide and water combine chemically under the influence of light energy to produce stored chemical energy in the form of carbohydrates. This reaction cannot occur unless chlorophyll is present, and really consists of a series of reactions that are summarised in Fig. 10.2.
4. In Fig. 10.2, arrows are used to show the fate of the individual reactants and to account for the fact that water occurs on both sides of the equation – we cannot just cancel out some of the water to simplify the equation, because we would then not have the correct equation for the reaction.
5. The final product of this reaction is glucose (a carbohydrate), which is stored as starch (another carbohydrate) in all the cells of the plant. However, some structures of plants are

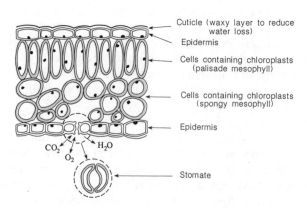

Figure 10.1. Section through a leaf.

particularly adapted to function for food storage purposes. These include grains such as corn, wheat, rice and barley, tubers such as potatoes, and modified taproots such as carrots and parsnips.

6. We should bear in mind that the capacity of plants to synthesise (or make) their own food is critical for our own survival, as has already been pointed out. Indeed, if scientists were to learn how to reproduce commercially the photosynthesis reaction performed by even the most humble plant, the world's food problems would be solved.

7. Furthermore, the human body is not able to digest the cellulose that makes up a significant proportion of the weight of any plant. However:

(a) this cellulose provides dietary fibre, which is now regarded by dietary experts as being very important in providing necessary roughage in our diets;

(b) animals such as ruminants (cattle, sheep, goats, etc.) are able to digest cellulose and assimilate the products into their bodies. We make use of this by eating the animals.

8. In summary, then, *photosynthesis acts as a chemical and energy bridge* between the inorganic (non-living) world and the organic (living world), as shown in Fig. 10.3. Note that a monosaccharide is a simple sugar and a disaccharide is a sugar made from two monosaccharide molecules.

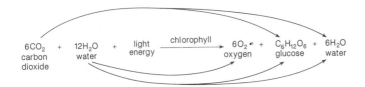

Figure 10.2. Chemical equation for photosynthesis.

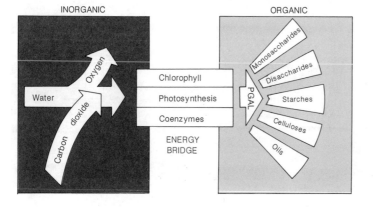

Figure 10.3. Photosynthesis acts as a chemical and energy bridge between the in-organic (non-living) world and the organic (living) world.

The Flow of Energy

The ultimate source of all of the energy that we use in this way is the sun, and much of this energy is finally released in one way or another to the atmosphere, as shown below.

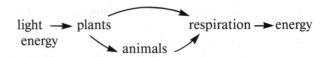

light → plants   respiration → energy
energy   ↘ animals ↗

Associated with this are the cycles of carbon and nitrogen, as shown in Figs 9.34 and 10.4.

These cycles demonstrate the original sources of the elements so vital to our existence – carbon, hydrogen, oxygen and nitrogen.

ENERGY IN THE BODY

We will look at this very large topic under five main headings:

1. Energy exchange
2. Catalysts – enzymes
3. Hormones
4. Storage of energy
5. Energy production – cellular respiration

Figure 10.4. The carbon-oxygen cycle.

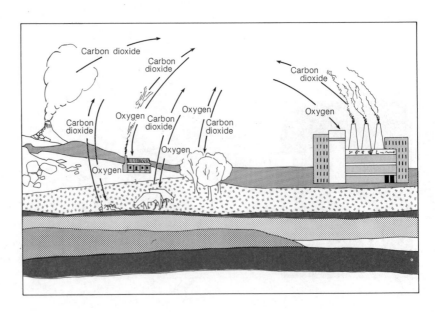

Energy Exchange

The cells of the body require energy. Without energy they are not able to function, i.e. they are not able to:

1. Synthesise large molecules, for example proteins, from smaller ones (this is called **anabolism**);
2. Act together to cause muscles to contract;
3. Support the electrical activity of nerves;
4. Effect active transport; or
5. Supply heat.

All of these activities come under the general term *endergonic* (energy-requiring) reactions.

The energy for such activities is supplied by *exergonic* (energy-releasing) reactions, cellular respiration being the significant exergonic reaction in the human body. This is the process by which fuels such as glucose are utilised by means of an involved series of chemical reactions to produce energy. Oxygen is required, and water and carbon dioxide are released as by-products.

$$C_6H_{12}O_6 \ + \ 6O_2 \ \longrightarrow \ 6CO_2 \ + \ 6H_2O \ + ENERGY$$

glucose   oxygen   carbon   water

                                    dioxide

This reaction is the opposite of the photosynthesis reaction, already discussed.

In general terms, the energy produced in this reaction, and others such as catabolism, is used for some of the reactions listed. This may then be regarded as an *energy exchange*.

Catalysts – Enzymes

Most of the chemical reactions in the body will not progress at an appreciable rate at body temperature without the assistance of catalysts. The body's catalysts are the enzymes, a group of proteins which perform brilliantly – much better than any that are used in industry.

The student is strongly advised to revise the section on chemical equilibrium (p. 257) before proceeding further.

Characteristics of Enzymes
1. The functioning of enzymes depends upon:

(a) **pH.** Enzymes normally function within a very narrow range of pH, although the pH is different for different enzymes.

Pepsin, a protein-digesting enzyme, operates at a pH of 1-2 in the stomach, but *trypsin*, another protein-digester, cannot function at that pH and operates at a pH of 8, in the small intestine.

(b) **Temperature.** This is an important factor, since enzymes function best at normal body temperatures. In hypothermic situations, it follows that enzyme activity, and thus metabolism, is decreased. As temperatures rise, enzymes do not function as effectively and will soon denature (break down chemically).

2. Frequently, the action of enzymes depends upon *co-factors* (see below).

3. Enzymes are usually very *specific* in their action – they generally each tend to catalyse one reaction only. This is consistent with our 'lock and key' model for the operation of enzymes (described below).

4. Enzymes can be *inhibited,* i.e. some substances are capable of interfering with the action of enzymes, particularly if they have very similar structures to that of the substrate (the substance being acted upon). This probably explains the drastic effects that minute quantities of poisons have on people. A typical cell requires only a minute amount of each enzyme and has about 1000 separate chemical reactions occurring within it. Thus very tiny quantities of poisons have the capacity to interfere with these reactions and can have very pronounced effects.

5. Some enzymes have to be stored in an *inactive* form. For example, if pepsin (the active form) were not stored as pepsinogen (the inactive form) until required, it would digest the protein in the stomach wall.

6. Enzymes, like the rest of our bodies, don't last for ever!

7. Enzymes are considered to operate by forming a complex substance with one of the reacting molecules, called the **substrate**. The enzyme and the substrate must fit together perfectly for reaction to occur, just like a jigsaw, as shown in Fig. 10.5.

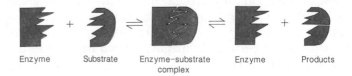

Enzyme   Substrate   Enzyme–substrate   Enzyme   Products
complex

Figure 10.5. A model for the action of enzymes. (From Cree & Webb: *Biology Outlines*. Sydney. Pergamon Press. 1984.)

The diagram shows an enzyme and a substrate forming a complex intermediate 'molecule', which then breaks up to release the enzyme to go and do the same again, at the same time forming the reaction products.

An example of the marked effect of an enzyme deficiency is that of phenylketonuria (PKU). This results from the deficiency of a liver enzyme, which reduces the effective processing of the amino acid phenylalanine. The patient may show moderate to severe mental retardation and other neurological disturbances. If diagnosed in early infancy, this can be corrected by dietary measures.

Co-factors

These are entities which assist enzymes to function and are of two types:

1. Ions such as Zn^{2+}, Cu^{2+}, Mg^{2+}, Mn^{2+}, K^+, Cl^-, Fe^{2+}, and Na^+. For example, salivary amylase requires the presence of Cl^- to function.
2. Small organic molecules called **co-enzymes** which have several functions in the body.

Firstly, they act as hydrogen and electron carriers and thus perform a vital role in metabolism. Examples are NAD^+, $NADP^+$, and FAD^+, the function of which was described in the last chapter and is reiterated later in this chapter. Such substances are not proteins and thus cannot be inactivated by heat, unfavourable pH conditions, etc., as enzymes are.

Secondly, they assist enzymes in their action. Most vitamins, of which NAD^+, $NADP^+$ and FAD^+ are derivatives, are thought to be involved in metabolism in this way. Vitamins cannot be synthesised in adequate amounts in the body and hence must be present in the diet. If these are not available in the diet, problems may soon arise.

Examples of these are the B vitamins such as B_1 (thiamine), B_2 (riboflavin) and niacin (nicotinamide). This is probably the most important role of many vitamins, which are described below. **Vitamins** are organic compounds that are essential for homeostasis – for normal functioning of the body. They are not manufactured in the body and so must form part of our normal diet. Tables 10.2 and 10.3 list the presently known vitamins, their function in the body, the results of deficiencies in these vitamins, the food sources of each and some comments, along with the recommended dietary allowance in Australia.

The fat-soluble vitamins, such as A, D, E and K are absorbed together with fats as part of the process of fat digestion and absorption.

The water-soluble vitamins, such as C and the B group (except B_{12}), are absorbed by passive diffusion in the intestine. Vitamin B_{12} combines with a glycoprotein substance called 'intrinsic factor' in the stomach and is then absorbed by active transport through the intestinal wall.

TABLE 10.2   The vitamins

Vitamins and U.S. RDA*	Actions	Effect of Deficiency	Sources	Comments
Fat soluble				
A 5000 IU†	Component of retinal pigments essential for normal vision. Essential for normal growth and integrity of epithelial tissue. Promotes normal growth of bones and teeth by regulating activity of osteoblasts and osteoclasts	Failure of growth; night blindness; atrophy of epithelium; epithelium subject to infection; scaly skin	Liver, fish-liver oils, egg; yellow and green vegetables	Can be formed from provitamin carotene (a yellow or red pigment). Sometimes called anti-infection vitamin because it helps maintain epithelial membranes; excessive amounts harmful
D 400 IU	Promotes calcium absorption from digestive tract; essential to normal growth and maintenance of bone	Bone deformities; rickets in children; osteomalacia in adults	Liver, fish-liver oils, egg yolk, fortified milk, butter, margarine	Two types: D_2 (calciferol), a synthetic form; D_3, formed by action of ultraviolet rays from sun upon a cholesterol compound in the skin; excessive amounts harmful
E 30 IU	Inhibits oxidation of unsaturated fatty acids and vitamin A that help form cell and organelle membranes; precise biochemical role not known	Increased catabolism of unsaturated fatty acids, so that not enough are available for maintenance of cell membranes and other membranous organelles; prevents normal growth	Oils made from cereal seeds, liver, eggs, fish	
K	Essential for blood clotting	Prolonged blood-clotting time	Normally supplied by intestinal bacteria; green leafy vegetables	Antibiotics may kill bacteria; then supplements needed in surgical patients
Water soluble C (ascorbic acid) (30 mg)**	Needed for collagen synthesis and for other intercellular substances; formation of bone matrix and tooth dentin, intercellular cement; needed for metabolism of several amino acids. May help body withstand injury from burns and bacterial toxins	Scurvy (wounds heal very slowly and scars become weak and split open; capillaries become fragile; bone does not grow or heal properly)	Citrus fruits, strawberries, tomatoes	Possible role in preventing common cold or in the develoment of acquired immunity? Very excessive dose is harmful

TABLE 10.2 The vitamins (continued)

Vitamins and U.S. RDA*	Actions	Effect of Deficiency	Sources	Comments
Water soluble B Complex				
Thiamine (B$_1$) (1.0 mg)**	Acts as coenzyme in many different enzyme systems; important in carbohydrate and amino acid metabolism	Beriberi (weakened heart muscle, enlarged right side of heart, nervous system and digestive tract disorders)	Liver, yeast, cereals, meat, green leafy vegetables	Deficiency common in alcoholics
Riboflavin (1.2 mg)**	Used to make co-enzymes (FAD) essential in cellular respiration	Dermatitis, inflammation and cracking at corners of mouth; mental depression	Liver, cheese, milk, eggs, green leafy vegetables	
Niacin (nicotinic acid) (16 mg)**	Component of important co-enzymes (NAD and NADP) essential to cellular respiration	Pellagra (dermatitis, diarrhoea, mental symptoms, muscular weakness, fatigue)	Liver, meat, fish, cereals, legumes, whole grain and enriched breads	
Pyridoxine (B$_6$) (1.5 mg)**	Co-enzyme needed for amino acid synthesis and protein metabolism	Dermatitis, digestive tract disturbances, convulsions	Liver, meat, cereals, legumes	
Pantothenic acid 10 mg	Constituent of co-enzyme A (a compound important in cellular metabolism)	Deficiency is extremely rare	Widespread in foods	
Folic acid 0.4 mg	Co-enzyme needed for nucleic acid synthesis and for maturation of red blood cells	A type of anaemia	Produced by intestinal bacteria; liver, cereals, dark green, leafy vegetables	
Biotin	Co-enzyme needed for cellular metabolism	Deficiency unknown	Produced by intestinal bacteria; liver, chocolate, egg yolk	
B$_{12}$ (2.0 mg)**	Co-enzyme important in nucleic acid metabolism	Pernicious anaemia	Liver, meat, fish	Contains cobalt; intrinsic factor secreted by gastric mucosa needed for absorption of B$_{12}$

*RDA is the recommended dietary allowance, established by the Food and Nutrition Board of the U.S. National Research Council to maintain good nutrition for healthy persons.
**The values in brackets are the 1970 dietary allowance for use in Australia (average values for an adult male), as determined by the Nutrition Committee of the National Health & Medical Research Council.
† International Unit: the amount that produces a specified biological effect and is internationally accepted as a measure of the activity of the substance. (Adapted from Solomon & Davis: *Human Anatomy & Physiology*. Philadelphia. Saunders College Publishing. 1983.)

TABLE 10.3 Recommended dietary intakes (expressed as mean daily intake)

Subject	Age	VitaminA (retinol equivalents) µgRE	Thiamin mg	Riboflavin mg	Niacin (niacin equivalents) mg NE	Vitamin B-6 mg	Total Folate µg	Vitamin B-12 µg
Infants	0-6 months							
	— breast-fed	425	0,15	0.4	4	0.25	50	0.3
	— formula-led	425	0.25	0.4	4	0.25	50	0.3
	7–12 months	300	0.35	0.6	7	0.45	75	0.7
Children	1–3 years	300	0.5	0.8	9–10	0.6–0.9	100	1.0
(male & female)	4–7 years	350	0.7	1.1	11–13	0.8–1.3	100	1.5
Boys	8–11 years	500	0.9	1.4	14–16	1.1–1.6	150	1.5
	12–15 years	725	1.2	1.8	19–21	1.4–2.1	200	2.0
	16–18 years	750	1.2	1.9	20–22	1.5–2.2	150	2.0
Girls	8–11 years	500	0.8	1.3	14–16	1.0–1.5	150	1.5
	12–15 years	750	1.0	1.6	17–19	1.2–1.8	200	2.0
	16–18 years	750	0.9	1.4	15–17	1.1–1.6	200	2.0
Men	19–64 years	750	1.1	1.7	18–20	1.3–1.9	200	2.0
	65+ years	750	0.9	1.3	14–17	1.0–1.5	200	2.0
Women	19–54 years	750	0.8	1.2	12–14	0.9–1.4	200	2.0
	55+ years	750	0.7	1.0	10–12	0.8–1.1	200	2.0
Pregnancy		750 (+0)	1.0 (+0.2)	1.5 (+0.3)	14–16 (+2)	1.0–1.5 (+0.1)	400 (+200)	3.0 (+1.0)
Lactation		1200 (+450)	1.2 (+0.4)	2.0 (+0.8)	17–19 (+5)	1.6–2.2 (+0.7–0.8)	350 (+150)	3.5 (+1.5)

Subject	Iodine µg	Zinc mg	Iron mg	Magnesium mg	Calcium mg	Sodium mmol	Sodium (mg)	Potassium mmol	Potassium (mg)
Infants	50	3–6	0.5	40	300	6–12	(140–280)	10–15	(390–580)
	50	3–6	3.0	40	500	6–12	(140–280)	10–15	(390–580)
	60	4.5–6	9	60	550	14–25	(320–580)	12–35	(470–1370)
Children	70	4.5–6	6–8	80	700	14–50	(320–1150)	25–70	(980–2730)
(male & female)	90	6–9	6–8	110	800	20–75	(460–1730)	40–100	(1560–3900)
Boys	120	9–14	6–8	180	800	26–100	(600–2300)	50–140	(1950–5460)
	150	12–18	10–13	260	1200	40–100	(920–2300)	50–140	(1950–5460)
	150	12–18	10–13	320	1000	40–100	(920–2300)	50–140	(1950–5460)
Girls	120	9–14	6–8	160	900	26–100	(600–2300)	50–140	(1950–5460)
	120	12–18	10–13	270	1000	40–100	(920–2300)	50–140	(1950–5460)
	120	12–18	10–13	270	800	40–100	(920–2300)	50–140	(1950–5460)
Men	150	12–16	7	320	800	40–100	(920–2300)	50–140	(1950–5460)
	150	12–16	7	320	800	40–100	(920–2300)	50–140	(1950–5460)
Women	120	12–16	12–16	270	800	40–100	(920–2300)	50–140	(1950–5460)
	120	12–16	5–7	270	1000	40–100	(920–2300)	50–140	(1950–5460)
Pregnancy	150 (+30)	16–21 (+4–5)	22–36 (+10) (2nd & 3rd trimester)	300 (+30)	1100 (+300) (3rd trimester)	40–100	(920–2300)	50–140	(1950–5460) (+0)
Lactation	200 (+50)	18–22 (+6)	12–16 (+0)	340 (+70)	1200 (+400)	40–100 (+0)	(920–2300)	65–140 (+0)	(2540–5460)

These recommended dietary intakes are for use in Australia. Material reproduced by kind permission of the National Health and Medical Research Council.

Hormones

Hormones are essentially chemical messengers. They may:

1. Trigger and control the action of enzymes, for example, thyroxine.

The effects of thyroxine are many and varied in the body and many of these result from the action of this hormone on enzyme systems. In the case of cellular enzyme systems, if thyroid hormones are administered to a patient, within about a week, the concentration of at least 100 intracellular enzymes increases, some as much as six-fold. This leads to much more rapid utilisation of carbohydrates and generally increased efficiency of mitochondria.

One of these enzymes is *Na-K ATPase*, which increases the rate of transport of sodium and potassium ions through the cell membranes of some tissues. This may be one of the mechanisms by which thyroid hormone increases the body's metabolic rate.

2. Act indirectly by altering the levels of particular compounds in the blood or cells, which in turn affects the attainment of equilibrium of various reactions and also the production of energy. Examples include insulin, glucagon and adrenalin (called epinephrine in United States books).

There is a surprising number of hormones involved in the metabolism of all three food types in the body. They are secreted from a wide variety of regions in the body by either endocrine glands or endocrine tissue within organs other than endocrine glands. A brief examination of their effects on organic metabolism, particularly energy balance, will clearly demonstrate that energy production in cells would become inefficient, inadequate or inflexible, or all of these, without the availability of these hormones. For a more detailed general discussion of these hormones per se, the reader is referred to a physiology text, since that which follows will focus only on a specific role of these hormones.

Insulin

This hormone is the single most important controller of organic metabolism. It is synthesised in the Islets of Langerhans in the pancreas and transported in the blood to its target cells.

Insulin acts in two major ways to influence metabolism. Firstly, it may act on the process of transport of the substance across the cell membrane, as in the case of glucose. It acts to increase the movement of glucose into many cells, particularly muscle and adipose tissue. Two significant major exceptions to this influence are the brain cells and liver cells.

Secondly, it is also able to alter the activities or concentrations of many intracellular enzymes involved in the metabolic pathways of carbohydrates, fats and proteins. It thus has a powerful effect not only on energy production but on metabolism as a whole.

Insulin acts in

1. Carbohydrate metabolism to:

- stimulate

(a) glucose uptake by many cells

(b) glycogen anabolism or synthesis (glycogenesis)

(c) glycolysis

- inhibit

(a) glycogen catabolism or breakdown

(b) gluconeogenesis (formation of glucose in the liver from substances other than carbohydrates, such as glycerol and amino acids).

The *overall effect* of all of this is a decrease in the glucose level in the plasma and an increase in glucose utilisation and storage (as glycogen).

2. Fat metabolism to:

- stimulate

fat synthesis (two of the major sources of fatty acids for this synthesis are: glucose which has been broken down during glycolysis in the liver, and secondly, glucose which directly enters adipose cells).

- inhibit

fat catabolism.

The *overall effect* of this is a decrease in glycerol and fatty acid levels in the plasma.

3. Protein metabolism to:

- stimulate

(a) amino acid uptake by cells

(b) protein anabolism

- inhibit

protein catabolism.

The *overall effect* of this is a decrease in amino acid levels in the plasma and an increase in protein synthesis.

In summary, insulin promotes glucose storage as glycogen and particularly as fat, promotes fat storage and the decreased use of fat for energy production and promotes protein synthesis (anabolism). The source of energy most favoured by insulin is glucose. A severe shortage or absence of insulin would produce the opposite effects to those described. One can deduce from the above that insulin is particularly active during eating, when the three major foodstuffs are usually most readily available.

Question for thought: What are the implications of all this for an insulin-dependent patient being prepared for surgery and thus nil-by-mouth?

Glucagon

This hormone is also produced in the Islets of Langerhans of the pancreas, but by a different type of cell to those which produce insulin, and is secreted into the blood for transport and distribution. It activates enzymes which in turn alter the metabolism of carbohydrates, fats and proteins in such a way that the effects are opposed to those caused by insulin.

Glucagon acts in

1. Carbohydrate metabolism to:
- stimulate
(a) glycogen catabolism (glycogenolysis) in the liver (but not in another major area of glycogen storage-skeletal muscle)
(b) the rate of gluconeogenesis in the liver (formation of glucose from other substances as described above).

The *overall effect* is an increase in glucose levels in the plasma and a decrease in glucose stores in the liver.

2. Fat metabolism to:
- stimulate
(a) ketone synthesis in the liver (ketones are compounds formed from fatty acids and are an important energy source for those tissues in the body which are capable of using them as such)
(b) lipolysis (the catabolism of fats in adipose tissue which release glycerol and fatty acids into the blood, thus making them available as an energy source for other cells).

The *overall effect* is an increase in fatty acid, glycerol and ketone levels in the plasma.

In summary, since glucagon increases plasma levels of glucose, it can effectively raise blood glucose concentration when it drops below normal. Glucagon does this both by increasing the release of glucose itself from the liver and also through its glucose-sparing actions, i.e. by providing other sources of energy for body cells such as ketones, glycerol and fatty acids, which are capable of releasing more energy per gram than glucose. The maintenance of a normal plasma glucose level is essential to the functioning of the nervous system, since the brain normally uses only glucose as its source of energy.

Adrenalin (epinephrine)
This is the major hormone secreted by the medulla of each adrenal gland. It would appear that its most important role in metabolism is to:
- stimulate
(a) glucagon secretion when plasma glucose levels drop below normal
(b) gluconeogenesis directly
(c) glycogenolysis (glycogen breakdown) in the liver and muscles
(d) lipolysis in adipose tissue

- inhibit

(a) insulin secretion

(b) glucose uptake by skeletal muscle, a major user of glucose.

Thus this hormone has effects opposite to those of insulin and similar to those of glucagon. As a result of this the chief source of energy for most cells is shifted to fat products.

The *overall effect* is an increase in plasma concentrations of glucose, glycerol and fatty acids. This response is once again important in maintaining the energy source of glucose to the brain. Adrenalin is a hormone secreted especially in times of stress, when more energy is normally needed.

Cortisol (hydrocortisone)

This is a major hormone secreted by the cortex of each of the adrenal glands. It also acts to influence various enzymes to alter the state of metabolism of organic compounds and to mobilise amino acids.

Cortisol can act in

1. Carbohydrate metabolism to:

- stimulate

(a) gluconeogenesis by the liver, often increasing the rate of gluconeogenesis as much as six to tenfold

(b) glycogen storage by the liver

- inhibit

(a) (slightly) the uptake of glucose by cells

(b) (moderately) glucose utilisation by most of the cells in the body.

The *overall effect* is an increase in the level of glucose in the plasma.

2. Fat metabolism to:

- stimulate

(a) lipolysis (breakdown of fats) in adipose tissue

(b) (moderately) the oxidation of fatty acids in cells for energy.

The *overall effect* is an increase in the levels of fatty acids in the plasma.

3. Protein metabolism to:

- stimulate

(a) protein catabolism in most cells

(b) amino acid transport into liver cells

(c) protein anabolism in the liver

- inhibit

(a) amino acid transport into extrahepatic tissues

(b) protein anabolism in most cells.

The *overall effect* is an increase in the levels of amino acids in the plasma and a depletion of protein stores in all body cells other than those of the liver.

In summary, cortisol reduces glucose usage for energy production in most cells, once again ensuring an adequate supply of glucose for the nervous system. It effectively shifts the energy production source in most cells to fat products. Exceptions to this are the liver, which has a plentiful supply of both amino acids and fats and the brain, which utilises the 'spare' glucose.

Thyroid Hormones

The two most significant hormones produced by the thyroid gland as far as metabolism is concerned are thyroxine and triiodo-thyronine. These hormones are the single most important deter-minant of the basal metabolic rate of the body at any given size, age and sex. The *basal metabolic rate* is the energy expenditure of an individual under basal conditions (please refer to the discussion of BMR towards the end of this chapter). In other words, thyroid hormones can increase the metabolic activities of almost all tissues of the body, with a few noteworthy exceptions, viz. the brain, lungs, spleen, retina and testes. The basic mechanism(s) by which these hormones function is not fully understood, but it is known that they act to influence many intracellular enzymes in terms of quantity available and rate of action.

Thyroxine and triiodothyronine can act in

1. *Carbohydrate metabolism* (all aspects) to:
 • stimulate
 (a) uptake of glucose by cells
 (b) glycolysis
 (c) gluconeogenesis
 (d) absorption by the gastrointestinal tract
 (e) insulin secretion.
 The *overall effect* is a decrease in the level of glucose in the plasma.

2. *Fat metabolism* (all aspects) to:
 • stimulate
 (a) lipolysis, mobilising lipids from adipose tissue
 (b) oxidation of free fatty acids by cells for energy production.
 The *overall effect* is an increase in the levels of free fatty acids in the plasma.

3. *Protein metabolism* (depending on the type of activities being carried out in the body) to:
 • stimulate
 (a) (greatly) the rate of protein anabolism, particularly during growth phases

(b) the rate of protein catabolism.

The *overall effect* is normally an increase in protein anabolism.

In summary, it can be seen that thyroid hormones stimulate the use of carbohydrates and fats for energy production, while sparing proteins to a greater extent for other uses.

Growth Hormone

Growth hormone is produced and secreted from the anterior pituitary gland (adenohypophysis). It has effects on the metabolism of all three food types.

Growth hormone can act in

1. Carbohydrate metabolism to:
- stimulate

(a) glycogenesis
- inhibit

(a) glucose uptake by the cells of the body

(b) glucose utilisation for energy production in most cells of the body

The *overall effect* is to conserve glucose and increase the level of glucose in the plasma.

2. Fat metabolism to:
- stimulate

(a) lipolysis

(b) the use of fatty acids in cells for energy production (gluconeogenesis).

The *overall effect* is an increase in the levels of fatty acids in the plasma and a decrease in the storage of fats.

3. Protein metabolism in a most important way, to:
- stimulate

(a) amino acid transport through cell membranes

(b) protein synthesis in all cells of the body. This is probably its most important role
- inhibit

(a) cell protein catabolism.

The *overall effect* is to increase all aspects of amino acid uptake and protein synthesis while reducing protein breakdown.

In summary, growth hormone increases body protein, decreases fat stores and conserves carbohydrate.

There are some other hormones which have more indirect effects on organic metabolism, such as somastatin, which is secreted by the pancreas. One of the effects of this hormone is to slow down the assimilation of food from the gastrointestinal tract and thus prevent the rapid exhaustion of the absorbed nutrients by tissues.

However, the hormones discussed above are the major ones and have the most specific actions. It is appropriate to point out that these hormones are not all secreted at the maximum rate at the same time, but are secreted to different degrees at various times to cope with different tissue requirements in response to changing body activities.

When the reader has completed the rest of this chapter, the roles of these hormones will become more apparent and a second examination of them will enable the reader to apply them in more specific contexts.

Storage of Energy

Since the production of energy does not necessarily correspond with the body's needs at any given moment, the body uses a storage mechanism for its energy. This is just the same type of arrangement as we have with our water supply. During the night, the supply of water usually exceeds the demand for it, and the reservoir fills. At other times, the demand exceeds the supply and if the reservoir did not exist this demand could not be met. So it is with the energy in our bodies.

The reader is particularly asked to note the distinction between the compound to be discussed below (ATP) and glycogen in terms of energy storage. **ATP** is an 'energy currency', as it were, providing a readily available store of energy. **Glycogen,** on the other hand, is the raw material that is stored in the liver and can be transported (as glucose), when required, to cell 'factories'. These cell factories are able to process glucose to 'extract' the energy from it. Just as ordinary factory products are packed in cartons, bags or other containers, the energy extracted from glucose in cell factories is stored in ATP molecules.

The energy storage mechanism in the body involves a substance called **a**denosine **trip**hosphate (ATP), which is able to release energy when required to form **a**denosine **dip**hosphate (ADP) and an inorganic phosphate group, which is usually represented as 'Pi'. This relationship can be represented thus:

ATP	$\rightarrow$	ADP	+	Pi	+	ENERGY
adenosine		adenosine		phosphate		
triphosphate		diphosphate		group		

Adenosine triphosphate is an organic compound produced in all cells, which can readily liberate its energy, i.e. it is *labile*. It is made up from a five-carbon sugar (a pentose sugar) and a nitrogenous base called adenine (one of the constituents of RNA and DNA.)

It is sometimes represented thus:

$$A - Pi \sim Pi \sim Pi$$

where $\sim$ indicates a 'high-energy' bond. In fact, each mole of

ATP has about 37 kJ (the amount quoted varies somewhat in the literature) of energy available per molecule. Guanosine triphosphate (GTP) is a similar compound that operates in a similar way.

Another important allied compound is CP (creatine phosphate or phosphocreatine) which operates in a similar way to ATP in providing a storage of energy, particularly in muscles. It is this energy store that is called upon by muscles to provide the energy needed for contraction. Unlike ATP, CP cannot release its energy directly to a chemical reaction. Instead it releases it to reform ATP. This compound, or the first part of the name of this compound, should not be confused with the compound creatinine, which is formed as the end product of the metabolism of creatine. Urine tests for creatinine are commonly used, since an elevation of creatinine levels in the urine is indicative of kidney malfunction.

Energy Production, Cellular Respiration and Carbohydrate Metabolism

Cellular respiration is the process by which energy is obtained by the body cells as a result of the oxidation of food material such as glucose. This energy is utilised by the body in two ways:

(i) for our daily activities (e.g. walking, running, writing, respiration, heartbeat and thinking);
(ii) for the maintenance of normal body temperature.

Metabolism is the sum of the physical and chemical processes by which living material is built up and maintained (anabolism) and by which large molecules are broken down into smaller molecules frequently to make energy available to the cells of the body (catabolism).

Let us now take a closer look at cellular respiration. Firstly, a large number of reactions are involved in the overall reaction of the full breakdown of glucose. Secondly, it is an *aerobic* reaction, since oxygen is involved. If the oxygen supply is limited or non-existent, the reaction is described as being *anaerobic*.

The body does not, at any time, function clearly in either an aerobic or anaerobic mode, as indicated in many textbooks. It has been demonstrated by research that some aerobic and some anaerobic activity is always occurring, but the aerobic and anaerobic components vary in extent, depending upon circumstances.

Before embarking into a detailed treatment of this topic, an overall summary should assist students to assimilate this detailed information.

Summary of Aerobic Respiration
Aerobic respiration occurs in four stages – the first stage in the cytoplasm of the cell and the other three in the mitochondrion.

1. The first stage is **glycolysis**, which takes place in the cytoplasm and is anaerobic, in which the 6-carbon glucose molecule is broken down into two 3-carbon pyruvic acid molecules with the production of sufficient energy to recharge *two* molecules of ATP.

2. The second stage is transitional, occurs in the mitochondrion of the cell and is aerobic, and results in the breakdown of pyruvic acid to a 2-carbon acetyl compound with the evolution of carbon dioxide. The acetyl compound attaches itself to a co-enzyme called co-enzyme A to form **acetyl co-enzyme A**.

3. The third stage is once again aerobic and occurs in the mitochondrion of the cell. It is called the **Krebs cycle** or the **citric acid cycle** and results both in the production of heat for the body and the release of 16 atoms of hydrogen, which together with the four atoms released in each of the two previous stages, yields a total of 24 hydrogen atoms.

4. The final stage is once again aerobic and occurs in the mitochondrion of the cell. It is called the **cytochrome chain** or **electron transport chain** and essentially converts the 24 hydrogen atoms mentioned above into useful energy.

Now that the reader is aware of these different stages and the overall pattern of aerobic respiration, we may now proceed to a more detailed study of these processes.

Aerobic Respiration in more Detail

Stage 1. Glycolysis

(a) The overall process of glycolysis can be represented by the summary equation in Fig. 10.6.

For simplicity, the H and O atoms have been omitted from these compounds, so that the representations which we are using here are **not** chemical formulae.

| glucose (a six-carbon compound | → | 2 × pyruvic acid (at least nine steps, each catalysed by its own specific enzyme and needing a total of TWO ATPs for the reaction) | + | sufficient ENERGY to recharge FOUR molecules of ATP |

or, diagrammatically,

| C−C−C−C−C−C glucose | → | 2 × C−C−C pyruvic acid | + | sufficient ENERGY to recharge FOUR molecules of ATP |

Figure 10.6.

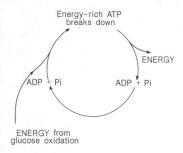

ENERGY from glucose oxidation

Figure 10.7. The energy cycle in respiration. (From Cree & Webb: *Biology Outlines*. Sydney. Pergamon Press. 1984.)

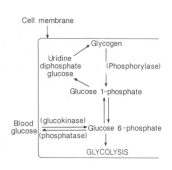

Figure 10.8. Reactions involving glycogen and glucose. (From Guyton: *Textbook of Medical Physiology*. 6th Ed. Philadelphia. W.B. Saunders. 1981.)

It is important to note that the NET gain of ATPs is four minus two = two ATPs. The reaction produces four ATPs, but two ATPs are needed to provide the energy for the reaction to proceed.

(b) The ADP and Pi (phosphate) molecules are able to utilise the energy formed in the reaction above and recharge ATP molecules, i.e. form high-energy phosphate bonds in ATP molecules as already described. When this energy is later put to good use, the ADP and Pi molecules can be recycled, ready to pick up more energy, as shown in Fig. 10.7. Thus:

$$2 \times ADP + 2 \times Pi + energy \text{ [from (a)]} \rightarrow 2 \text{ molecules of ATP}$$

Note: Since no oxygen has been used in Stage 1, the process so far has been anaerobic. Also:

(i) The formation of pyruvic acid from glucose with the release of energy is reversible. This means that the liver can convert pyruvic acid back to glucose and then it can be converted to glycogen for storage.

(ii) The three monosaccharides that are absorbed through the intestine – glucose, fructose and galactose – can all enter cells and provide energy, but the latter two must be converted to compounds that will fit into the glucose catabolism process. Fructose, once phosphorylated (combined with a phosphate radical), is able to move directly into the series of chemical reactions involved in glycolysis in all cells. Galactose, however, has to be converted to glucose before entering this chain of reactions and this conversion can occur only in liver cells.

(iii) The relationship between glucose, glycogen and glycolysis is shown in Fig. 10.8. The names of the enzymes responsible for each reaction are shown in brackets.

(iv) Mention will be made of PGAL (glyceraldehyde-3-phosphate or 3-phosphoglyceraldehyde) from time to time. This is an important compound since it is an intermediate in the assimila- tion of glycerol (from fats) into the glycolysis pathway and in the reverse process.

(v) Finally, it should be noted that the steps of glycolysis between glucose and PGAL (see Fig. 10.9) require a total of two molecules of ATP (i.e. they require energy) before these reactions can occur. However, between the PGAL and the pyruvic acid steps, a total of four molecules of ATP are formed. This means that a total of 4 − 2 = 2 molecules of ATP are gained as a result of glycolysis, as shown in Fig. 10.11 (by crosses through the four ATPs which cancel out).

This represents about 74 kJ of energy, but it should be noted that about 240 kJ of energy is lost as heat, so that the whole process is not particularly efficient (although its efficiency is still better than that of a motor car!).

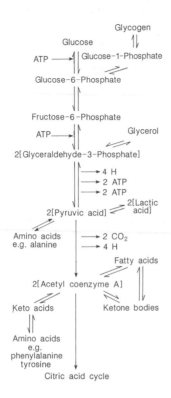

Figure 10.9. Glycolysis and some important interrelationships. Note that this is only a summary, since several of these reactions involve several steps.

(vi) Four hydrogen atoms are also formed in glycolysis, the significance of which will be discussed when we come to stage 4.

Stage 2
This is a *transitional* step that occurs in the mitochondrion of the cell, following facilitated diffusion of the *two* molecules of pyruvic acid formed from each molecule of glucose in the cytoplasm.

The following reactions are *aerobic*, i.e. the breakdown of the two pyruvic acid molecules requires oxygen in this case. Later we will see what happens when oxygen is *not* available.

Before pyruvic acid can be broken down (stage 3), it is converted to a two-carbon compound by losing carbon dioxide, and two hydrogen atoms. So that:

$$\text{C–C–C} \xrightarrow{\text{O}_2} \text{C–C} + 2\text{H} + \text{CO}_2$$

| three-carbon pyruvic acid | a two-carbon acetyl group | hydrogen atoms | carbon dioxide |

Since two pyruvic acid molecules are involved, a total of four H atoms are released. The acetyl group attaches itself to a co-enzyme called co-enzyme A to form **acetyl co-enzyme A**, which then enters the Krebs cycle, which is stage 3. The 2-acetyl co-enzyme A are formed from one glucose. One of the constituents of co-enzyme A is the B vitamins, especially pantothenic acid. The process of formation of acetyl co-enzyme A assists the acetyl group in attaching itself to the matrix of the mitochondria, where stage 3 takes place.

Furthermore, acetyl co-enzyme A forms a link through which keto acids (from amino acids such as phenylalanine and tyrosine) and ketone bodies can enter the pathway leading to stage 3.

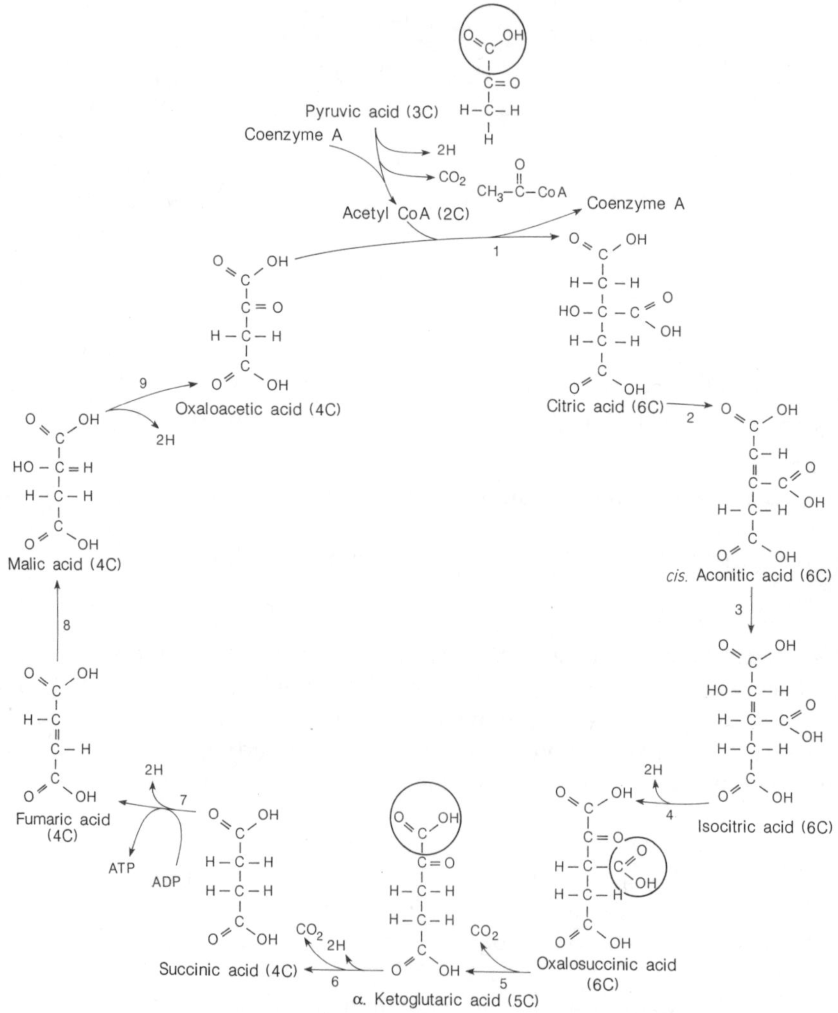

Figure 10.10. As the citric acid cycle turns. (From Solomon & Davis: *Human Anatomy & Physiology.* Philadelphia. Saunders College Publishing. 1983.)

Pyruvic acid (3C)

Coenzyme A

2H

CO_2

$CH_3-\overset{O}{\overset{\|}{C}}-CoA$

Acetyl CoA (2C)

Coenzyme A

1

Oxaloacetic acid (4C)

Citric acid (6C)

2

9

2H

Malic acid (4C)

cis. Aconitic acid (6C)

8

3

Fumaric acid (4C)

Isocitric acid (6C)

2H

2H

7

4

ATP

ADP

Succinic acid (4C)

Oxalosuccinic acid (6C)

CO_2 2H

α. Ketoglutaric acid (5C)

CO_2

6

5

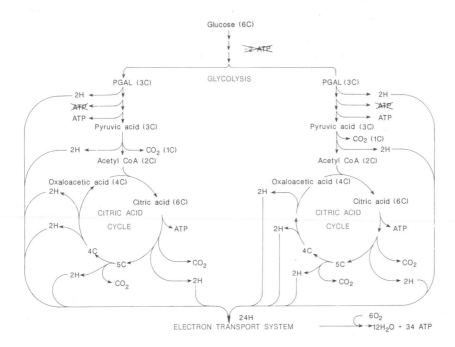

Stage 3. Krebs Cycle or Citric Acid Cycle

This step also occurs in the mitochondrion and involves the following:

(a) Each of the two acetyl co-enzyme A molecules combines with another compound (oxaloacetic acid) and the co-enzyme A is released to combine with more acetyl. The new compound goes through the cycle and releases this oxaloacetic acid to pick up more acetyl co-enzyme A. The fact that oxaloacetic acid is picked up at one stage and later released, only to be picked up again, leads to the description of this stage as a *cycle* (Fig. 10.10).

(b) In the process, oxygen is taken in, carbon dioxide is released and energy is liberated, i.e.

$$\text{accetyl co-enzyme A} + O_2 \rightarrow CO_2 + \text{co-enzyme A} + ENERGY$$

There are eight separate steps in this cycle. Apart from two co-enzyme A and oxaloacetic acid, water, carbon dioxide and *two molecules of ATP are formed* (one from each of the original acetyl groups). In addition, 16 atoms of hydrogen are released at this stage (eight from each acetyl group), following on the four atoms of hydrogen that were released in the glycolysis stage and the four atoms that were released during stage 2, so that a net total of 24 hydrogen atoms are released.

Figure 10.11. Summary of the reactions of cellular respiration. (From Solomon & Davis: *Human Anatomy & Physiology*. Philadelphia. Saunders College Publishing. 1983.) Notes: 1. Multiple arrows indicate that several reactions take place at that point. 2. PGAL (3-phosphoglyceraldehyde) is an intermediate compound formed during stage 1. 3. The electron transport chain (stage 4) yields 34 molecules of ATP. To this must be added the net gain of two molecules of ATP from the glycolysis step (stage 1) and two molecules of ATP from the Krebs cycle (stage 3), as shown in the diagram, to give the aerobic total of 38 molecules of ATP. 4. These 38 molecules of ATP are capable of storing approximately 1270 kJ of the total of approximately 2870 kJ of energy produced by the oxidation (reaction with oxygen) of one mole of glucose. This means that the overall storage efficiency of energy is 44 per cent, the remaining 56 per cent being converted to heat energy. This heat energy is able to maintain body temperature, as discussed in Chapter 2.

Once again, each of the reaction steps requires its own specific enzyme. Also reference has been made to the fact that much of the energy produced in these reactions is released in the form of heat. This provides the heat to maintain normal body temperature. Should this heat be in excess of requirements (such as on a hot day or when exercising vigorously), other homeostatic mechanisms have to operate to dissipate it.

For the benefit of the more advanced or interested reader, the full Krebs cycle is shown in Fig. 10.11. It is emphasised, however, that there is no need for most students to concern themselves with all the detail shown, while at the same time appreciating that these processes are indeed complex.

It is interesting to note that some amino acids can be converted to some of the compounds that are found in the Krebs cycle and thus are able to become direct sources of energy. Examples include aspartic acid (a non-essential amino acid that is widely distributed in proteins), which can be converted to oxaloacetic acid, and glutamine which can be converted to ketoglutaric acid.

Stage 4. The Cytochrome Chain or Electron Transport Chain
Before proceeding further, it is instructive to consider what we have achieved so far in the chemical treatment by the cell of the glucose molecule and its derivatives.

So far we have produced:

- 24 H atoms – for what reason?
- Some waste products – carbon dioxide and water
- Some by-products such as heat to warm our bodies
- Four molecules of ATP – rather inadequate for our energetic bodies!

The next stage of cellular respiration converts the 24 hydrogen atoms into useful energy, in a series of reactions all of which are enzyme catalysed and all of which occur in the mitochondria of the cell. This is called the *cytochrome chain* or the *electron transport chain*. Some institutions of courses will not require students to know this section of cell metabolism in the detail shown, but others may. We have thus given some depth to our treatment for the benefit of students for whom this is required knowledge.

We will take our discussion of the electron transport chain in a number of stages.

Firstly, let us imagine that we want to post an electron overseas (just for fun!). The electron, having reached the post office, will be transported by truck to a central sorting depot, then taken by another truck to be loaded on a ship. (Airmail is too expensive for electrons!) (Fig. 10.12.)

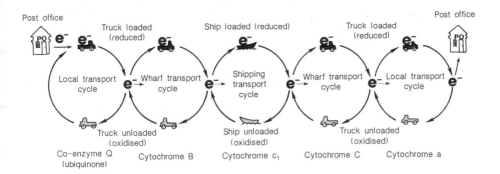

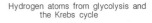

The first truck, having unloaded its electron, will return to the post office to pick up another electron. (This truck and all the other means of transport mentioned specialise in electrons!) The second truck also returns to pick up another electron, as shown in the diagram, and the ship, having transported the electron overseas, does likewise. In the new country, our electron is – transported from the ship by a truck which, having delivered its electron to a central sorting depot, returns to the wharf to pick up another electron. The electron is then transported to the post office to be despatched to its recipient, while the truck returns to the sorting depot to pick up another electron.

Thus we have an imaginary electron transport chain, in which the electron is passed through a series of stages to reach its destination and the electron carrier in each case returns to pick up another electron.

Since reduction has already been described as a *gain* in electrons, we can refer to the truck carrying the electron as the *reduced truck*, and the truck that is no longer carrying the electron as the *oxidised truck*, since oxidation is a loss of electrons. The same applies to our ship. Furthermore, each of the four trucks and the ship are named after compounds in the real transport chain, which are shown under each cycle.

Secondly, our electron has to get to the post office in the first place and be delivered at the other end. We will not take our analogy any further, but hope that the reader will understand the fundamental idea of an electron transport chain, and we will describe what happens at each end.

In Fig. 10.13, we see that before our first truck (co-enzyme Q), there are two other cycles involving two hydrogen carriers called NAD and FAD, which we will discuss in more detail later. These hydrogen carriers take the hydrogen atoms produced in glycolysis and the Krebs cycle and transport them to the rest of the electron transport system that we have described. When the hydrogen atom reaches co-enzyme Q, it breaks up into a hydrogen ion and an electron. The hydrogen ion leaves the chain at this point and rejoins it later as shown, while the electron proceeds along the electron transport chain. For reasons still to

Figure 10.12 Diagram showing an imaginary electron which has been 'posted' passing through various cycles to an overseas destination – as a comparison with the cytochrome (or electron transport) chain

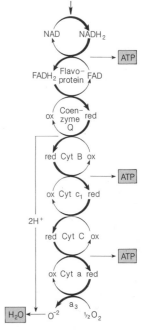

Figure 10.13. Electron transport chain. The successive transfer of hydrogen atoms and electrons results in the formation of ATP at three different places.

be discussed, we consider two hydrogen atoms at once and thus *two* electrons travelling along the electron transport chain.

This takes us to the other end of our transport chain, where the two electrons are given up by **cytochrome a$_3$** (called cytochrome oxidase, because it gives up electrons) and combine with oxygen from the lungs to form O^{2-}, which in turn combines with the two hydrogen ions that are available, to form water.

Note that this is the prime reason for the intake of oxygen into the body for metabolism. Note also that the cytochromes are organic molecules with a central iron atom, similar to haemoglobin. It is the iron which is alternately oxidised and reduced to carry the electron.

Fig. 10.11 reveals that the hydrogen atoms that are released during glycolysis, the intermediate steps and the Krebs cycle are released in pairs. Furthermore, *two* electrons are needed to form the O^{2-} ion. This last ion is then able to combine with the two hydrogen ions formed from the two hydrogen atoms that entered the chain. This is the reason that two hydrogen atoms were considered at once.

The substances NAD and FAD will now be examined in more detail. NAD is *nicotinamide adenine dinucleotide,* which is a derivative of the vitamin niacin, exists as the oxidised form NAD^+ and reacts with two hydrogen atoms to form NADH and H^+:

$$NAD^+ \ + \ H \ + \ H \ \xrightarrow{\text{enzyme}} \ NADH \ + \ H^+$$
oxidised   reduced

form   form

The hydrogen ion is free, although, for convenience, it is not shown separately in Fig. 10.13. FAD (*flavin adenine dinucleotide*) behaves in a similar fashion.

The important result of this is two free hydrogen ions and two electrons, which can be passed on to the electron transport chain for energy generation.

Finally, the most important result of all is that **energy** is produced – three ATPs are recharged for every two out of 20 hydrogen atoms produced by metabolism, the remaining four hydrogen atoms producing only four ATPs. Thus for 20 hydrogen atoms (i.e. 10×2), we have

$$10 \times 3 = 30 \text{ ATPs recharged,}$$

and for four hydrogen atoms we have four ATPs recharged, giving an overall total of 34 ATPs recharged from the 24 hydrogen atoms.

When this 34 is added to the net two ATPs from glycolysis and the two ATPs produced in the Krebs cycle, we have a final total of 38 ATPs being recharged by the energy from each molecule of glucose.

The full energy 'balance sheet' is shown in Table 10.4, which also compares aerobic respiration with anaerobic respiration, which we are about to discuss.

TABLE 10.4   Energy balance sheet—aerobic and anaerobic respiration

ATP profit	Anaerobic	Aerobic
Maximum From glycolysis	2 ATP	2 ATP (oxygen not required)
From the Krebs cycle		2 ATP

From the electron
  transport system
  24 H atoms
		34 ATP

Maximum total	2 ATP	38 ATP
End products	Pyruvic acid Lactic acid in muscle cells	CO_2 and H_2O

Note: The hydrogen input and hydrogen output are not balanced because water provides extra hydrogen atoms, which enter into the reactions. Also note that one ATP produced with each turn of the citric acid cycle is actually produced at the substrate level, not by way of the electron transport system. (Adapted from Solomon & Davis: *Human Anatomy & Physiology*. Philadelphia. Saunders College Publishing. 1983.)

In summary then, this step (consisting of a number of enzyme catalysed reactions) also occurs in the mitochondrion, oxygen is taken in, water is produced and much more energy is released. The overall result is as follows:

One glucose molecule ⟶ enough energy to
recharge 38 molecules of ATP.

Some variations to the quantity of 38 molecules of ATP do exist, but these need not concern us here.

Anaerobic Respiration

Anaerobic respiration tends to occur to a greater extent where the supply of oxygen is deficient. Anaerobic respiration occurs in those circumstances where the supply of oxygen is deficient. It may arise:

1. Locally in some muscles – as a result of vigorous or prolonged exercise.
2. Throughout the body as a result of extensive exercise, lung diseases or severe shock if left untreated.

In local oxygen deficiency, lactic acid builds up:

glucose + 2 ADP + Pi ⟶ 2 lactic acid + 2 ATP

This reaction occurs via the formation of pyruvic acid. The build-up of lactic acid is particularly noticeable in muscles after or during strenuous or prolonged exercise. It causes pain in muscles and results in what is described as muscle fatigue. This is another situation where the body's homeostatic mechanisms come to the fore and buffer this acid. Note that this lactic acid can be converted back to glucose or used directly for energy production as soon as oxygen becomes available. Most of this activity occurs in the liver, but some does occur in other tissues such as the muscles.

This situation – anaerobic respiration – can occur for only very short periods of time, since only *two* molecules of ATP are recharged per molecule of glucose. Compare this to aerobic respiration, in which 38 molecules of ATP are recharged per molecule of glucose. The heart, for example, cannot function if it is not receiving the energy it requires for contraction, and this is what happens under anaerobic conditions. It can be seen that the rate of glucose consumption will rise markedly under anaerobic conditions as the body struggles to produce the energy it requires for cardiac activity, etc., when such a small amount of energy is being produced.

Note: This is a summary treatment only. Some of the steps involved (e.g. in the Krebs cycle and the cytochrome chain) are quite complex. Greater detail will be found in any appropriate physiology or biochemistry textbook. However, Fig. 10.11 gives a summary of the reactions involved in cellular respiration, with the above stages indicated in the diagram.

The Use of ATP

ATP provides the energy necessary for most physiological processes to take place efficiently and completely.

One example of this is the coupling of the reaction in which two simple sugars (monosaccharides) combine to form a complex sugar (a disaccharide). During this reaction, ATP (adenosine triphosphate) breaks down to form ADP (adenosine diphosphate) and a phosphate group, with the release of energy to enable the chemical reaction to take place (Fig. 10.14).

This is a two-step reaction:

1. A molecule of ATP reacts with a molecule of glucose to form ADP and a high energy compound called glucose-l-phosphate; i.e. some of the energy originally contained in the high-energy ATP has been transferred to the compound glucose-1-phosphate and stored in the chemical bonds of that compound.

2. A second reaction occurs in which the energy in the glucose-1-phosphate is transferred to the new compound formed

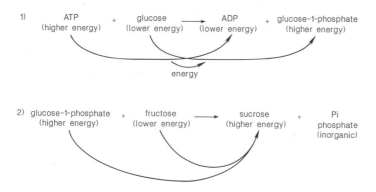

by the reaction with fructose – it is stored in the chemical bonds in the complex sugar molecule that is formed.

Figure 10.14. Acquisition of energy by lower energy glucose to form higher energy sucrose.

Fat Metabolism

It should be noted that the opposite of the reaction, hydrolysis of a fat, is one of the essential reactions in the digestion and metabolism of fats.

Firstly, almost all cells, with the exception of brain tissue, are able to utilise fatty acids interchangeably with glucose for the production of energy. In fact, between periods of food intake, fats are frequently used by many cells for energy, leaving glucose to be used particularly by brain cells, which are completely dependent on glucose supplied by the blood (Fig. 10.15).

Secondly, it follows that fats have to undergo hydrolysis, as indicated above, in order to form fatty acids and glycerol, which can then be utilised for energy production.

Thirdly, the fatty acids thus formed undergo a series of chemical reactions (each of which has its own particular enzyme to help it along) *that break the fatty acids down into acetyl co-enzyme A* (Fig. 10.16). As an example, one molecule of stearic acid yields nine molecules of acetyl co-enzyme A. This process is known as **beta oxidation**.

Fourthly, the acetyl co-enzyme A produced by beta oxidation then enters the citric acid cycle as before, to produce energy in the form of ATP. One molecule of stearic acid, for example, produces 146 molecules of ATP.

Let us now examine some of these reactions more closely. The liver stores no appreciable amount of fat, but is one of the main sites to utilise fats, as is adipose tissue which, as has already been seen, is the main storage site for fats.

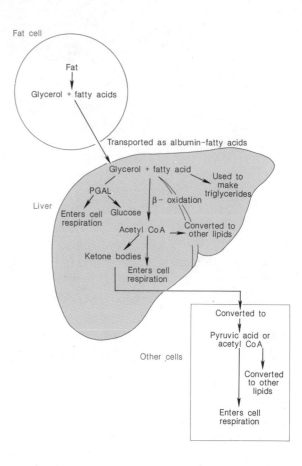

Figure 10.15. Overview of lipid metabolism.

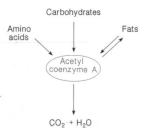

Figure 10.16. Acetyl co-enzyme A is formed from carbohydrates, fats and amino acids. Whatever the source, a large fraction of it is oxidised to CO_2 and H_2O although any excess may be used to form fats for storage. (From McGilvery: *Biochemistry: A Functional Approach.* 3rd Ed. Philadelphia. W.B. Saunders. 1983.)

Fat metabolism occurs in two stages:

1. Mobilisation and breakdown
2. Synthesis and deposit

Mobilisation and Breakdown
The mobilisation and breakdown, or catabolism of fats, is illustrated in Fig. 10.15.

A few points about this diagram warrant comment.

1. Following the initial breakdown of fats in the adipose tissue or fat cells to glycerol and fatty acids, further breakdown may be necessary and this occurs in the liver, since adipose tissue lacks the enzymes necessary to combine glycerol with phosphate, for example. In the phosphated form (PGAL), the original glycerol can then enter into normal cell respiration.

2. The 'ketone bodies' in the diagram are compounds, which may be described as keto acids and acetone, and these may be converted back to acetyl co-enzyme A and used to produce

energy. They may also be excreted in urine, a fact which forms the basis for urine tests for certain disorders, such as diabetes mellitus.

3. The blood concentration of ketone bodies may rise as high as 30 times the normal value if fats are being utilised for energy production, leading to extreme acidosis. This highlights the need for buffers in the blood and also reminds us again that the utilisation of various food types in the body does not consist of a series of independent chemical reactions, but a series of interrelated ones.

Synthesis and Deposit

Synthesis and deposit refers to the manufacture and deposition of fats. The body relies upon dietary intake of fatty acids and glycerol to form fats and other lipids in tissues, but may utilise carbohydrates and their products, e.g. pyruvic acid.

Protein Metabolism

As is the case with carbohydrates and lipids, proteins can be metabolised by the citric acid cycle and the electron transport chain to produce energy. Proteins that are in excess of a cell's requirements can be broken down to amino acids, and stored as fat or used to produce energy. This is achieved by further breakdown to pyruvic acid, acetyl co-enzyme A or to one of the compounds in the citric acid cycle (alpha-ketoglutaric acid) and entry into the pathway as indicated in Figs. 10.17 and 10.18.

In Fig. 10.17, we observe two essential processes occurring:

1. Anabolism – the building of protein molecules from amino acids – protein synthesis.
2. Catabolism – the breaking down of amino acids into other substances – protein breakdown.

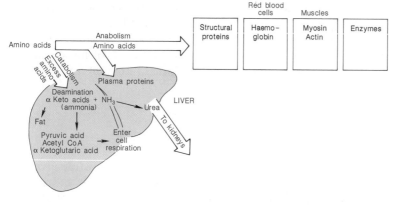

Figure 10.17. Overview of protein metabolism.

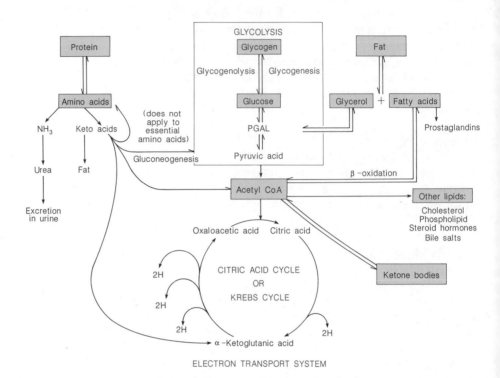

Figure 10.18. Overview of the integrated metabolism of carbohydrates, fats and proteins.

In adulthood, a balance is normally maintained between the two processes of protein breakdown and protein synthesis. An *imbalance* exists, however, in childhood and adolescence, when synthesis exceeds breakdown; in old age when breakdown exceeds synthesis; and in disorders caused by disease, starvation, etc.

Finally, it should be observed that the fact that protein can be used to meet energy requirements means that in some circumstances, cell repair can be secondary to the need to provide energy. This can lead to loss of weight and loss of muscle mass, as in malnutrition and diabetes mellitus. In children it can also lead to failure to grow.

Energy in Foods – Heat of Combustion

The fact that respiration in cells is a form of combustion gives us a means of measuring the energy value of foods. By measuring the heat of combustion of foods, a close approximation of the

TABLE 10.5 Energy values of selected foods (in kilojoules)

Food	kJ/g
Apples, raw	2.68
Beans, navy	14.8
Bread, white	11.1
Butter	33.3
Buttermilk	1.55
Cheese, cheddar	16.5
Chocolate	23.9
Cream 40%	15.9
Egg boiled	6.78
Icecream, plain	8.80
Lard	38.9
Lettuce, leaf	0.84
Meat, lean	1.13
Milk, whole	3.01
Oatmeal, cooked	2.64
Orange juice	1.80
Potatoes, boiled	4.06
Rice, cooked	4.69
Salmon, broiled	7.12
Spinach, cooked	2.43
Sugar, granulated	16.50
Tomato	0.96
Turnip	1.13

From Nave & Nave: *Physics for the Health Sciences.* 3rd Ed. Philadelphia. (W.B. Saunders. 1985.)

energy values of various foods may be found. Values for a number of foods are given in Table 10.5, in kilojoules per gram.

The Role of Oxygen in Cellular Respiration

Most of the oxygen that is consumed by an organism is used for reactions called oxidative phosphorylation in the mitochondria of cells. From our discussion of oxidation reactions above, we realise that:

- oxygen will be consumed,
- energy will be released,
- the oxygen content of the fuel compounds will be increased.

The term phosphorylation refers to the addition of a phosphate group to ADP, which then, with the energy available, forms ATP. We can then represent this as follows:

fuel + O_2 + ADP + Pi $\longrightarrow$ CO_2 + ATP + H_2O
(e.g fat   phosphate
or glucose

It is apparent in this reaction that oxygen is consumed and that lower energy ADP combines with energy from the fuel and a phosphate group to form higher energy ATP.

What then of the relative oxygen content of the compounds formed in this reaction compared to the original fuel? Has it increased as predicted above? Let us examine this question more closely.

If we take as our example of a fat the compound $C_{55}H_{102}O_6$; and glucose ($C_6H_{12}O_6$) as our example of a carbohydrate, we have:

Fat

Number of oxygen atoms: Number of other atoms

$$= 6:(55+102)$$
$$= 6:157$$
$$= \frac{6}{157}$$
$$= 0.04$$

Carbohydrate

Number of oxygen atoms: Number of other atoms

$$= 6:18$$
$$= \frac{6}{18}$$
$$= 0.33$$

Fuel products (CO_2 and H_2O)

Number of oxygen atoms: Number of other atoms

$$= (2+1):(1+2)$$
$$= 3:3$$
$$= 1$$

We are now in a position to compare the oxygen content of the fuel we started with (fat or carbohydrate) to the fuel products (CO_2, and H_2) in terms of oxygen content. The oxygen content ratio of fat is thus 0.04 and of carbohydrate is 0.33, but that of the fuel products is 1. Since 1 is obviously much higher than both 0.04 and 0.33, the oxygen content *has* increased, and we can then describe our reaction as oxidation, i.e. fats and carbohydrates are oxidised in the body. The same applies to protein, of course.

The relationship between oxidative phosphorylation and other metabolic reactions is shown in Fig. 10.18.

Oxygen Usage by the Cells

Under normal circumstances, only a small oxygen pressure is required for chemical reactions taking place in the cell. The reason is that the respiratory enzymes in the cell can function quite satisfactorily at an oxygen pressure as low as 3 to 5 mmHg. This means that there is normally no question of cells being short of oxygen for respiration reactions.

In fact, the factor governing the rate of cellular respiration is *the availability of ADP in the cells*. The reader will recall that when ATP releases energy, it is converted back to ADP. Thus when the rate of energy usage increases, such as during exercise, more ATP will be converted to ADP as energy is released, and the concentration of ADP will increase. This increased concentration will bring about an increase in the rate of cell metabolism and thus in the usage of oxygen to form more ATP.

Therefore, under normal circumstances, *the rate of usage of oxygen by the cells* is controlled by the rate at which *energy is used by the cells* – that is, by the rate at which ADP is formed from ATP – and NOT by the availability of oxygen in the cells.

It may be seen from this that if a patient is at rest, or nearly so, he will be using less energy than he normally does and his oxygen requirements will be less. This principle underlies both treatment and response in a number of diseases, particularly those that alter the capacity of the body to take in oxygen and get rid of carbon dioxide. It also applies to those affecting the efficiency of blood circulation and thus the delivery of necessary nutrients and removal of waste or by-products of energy production.

Basal Metabolic Rate

The basal metabolic rate (BMR) is *the energy expenditure of an individual under basal conditions*. Basal conditions means that the individual is rested, fasted and is not suffering from physical, emotional or environmental stress. It is normally expressed as a rate of heat production per unit time – as kilocalories (dietary calories) per hour in the former system of units, and as kilojoules per hour in the SI system of units.

BMR is essentially a measure of the energy requirements of the body in maintaining its vital functions only, since these energy requirements are being met from chemical energy stores. Clinically, BMR is measured some 12 to 14 hours after the last food intake, usually in the morning after a good night's sleep with the subject awake but resting in a state free of stress. It is noteworthy that this is not the lowest metabolic rate, since that measured when the subject is asleep is usually about 10 per cent lower, probably because of decreased muscle activity.

Nurses are often involved in the preparation of patients for

BMR tests, which are frequently done as part of thyroid function studies. The thyroid gland produces a hormone, thyroxine, which affects metabolism of all three foodstuffs, which in turn alters energy production. When the production of thyroxine is high, the BMR is high, and when the production of thyroxine is low, the BMR is low.

The most important factor in preparing a patient for a BMR test is ensuring that the patient really understands what the test involves, what is required of him or her, and why. This helps to reduce the fear and anxiety that arise whenever people are faced with an unfamiliar or unknown situation. It also gains greater co-operation from the patient when he/she understands the reasoning and expectations behind the test, its preparation and requirements. The need for the patient to rest and relax will certainly not be met unless the nurse fulfils his or her role in helping the patient to do so, since people can find it very difficult to rest and relax even under the best of circumstances.

Factors Affecting Energy Requirements

These may be listed as:

- growth and development
- pregnancy
- age
- exercise, level of activity
- stress – emotional, physical
- disease or illness
- state of alertness – sleep, wakefulness
- climate
- eating

Table 10.6 provides information on protein and energy requirements of patients under varying conditions. It can be seen that disease, trauma and surgical intervention may change energy requirements quite considerably. This should always be taken into account when treating and caring for a patient or client in these circumstances.

Summary

We have come a long way from our baker's slogan at the beginning of this chapter. It is to be hoped that the reader will now have a much better concept of energy in the body and all that this implies for the practising nurse.

TABLE 10.6 Guide to protein and energy requirements

Patient	Protein (g)	Energy kJ	Calories
Medical patient (uncomplicated)	45–75	6300–8400	1500–2000
Surgical patient (uncomplicated)	75–125	8400–14 700	2000–3500
Hypercatabolic state (e.g. major burns)	125–300	14 700–21 000	3500–5000

Source: SHPA, *Pharmacology and Drug Information for Nurses*, 3rd Ed. Sydney, W.B. Saunders/Ballière Tindall 1989.

From our examination of the production of energy and associated factors, it can be seen that the publicity and emphasis which is today being given to diet and exercise is indeed important for health. It should also be noted that the increased awareness of the roles and effects of vitamins and trace minerals in the body is very relevant to the maintenance of health. We are indeed caring for a whole person, not just a small factory on legs that requires energy!

We are dealing with people, not complaints, and an awareness of the diffuse or extensive role of energy will contribute to this holistic approach.

Our treatment of the metabolism of carbohydrates, lipids and proteins has been somewhat simplified. However, the metabolism summary in Fig. 10.18 provides a useful overview of the preceding subject matter. It should be stressed that all of these reactions are often occurring simultaneously, and can be affected by such things as diet, hormones, circulation and cardiac function, functioning of the gastrointestinal tract and lungs, the demands of the body at any one time, the state of general health and state of well-being of the individual. This is an excellent example of homeostasis in action.

REVIEW

1. Give two examples in each case of potential energy and kinetic energy.
2. Of what importance to human beings is —
   (a) the carbon cycle?
   (b) photosynthesis?
   (c) the nitrogen cycle?
3. Distinguish between carbohydrates, fats and proteins, and list the major sources of each.
4. Why are polyunsaturated fats considered to be preferable to saturated fats in the human diet?
5. Discuss the functions of the three classes of lipids in the body.
6. In some areas of the world children are starving to death.
   (a) Which of their tissue types are most likely to be affected by the protein

    deprivation associated with starving?

    (b) Would the lack of sufficient vitamin content have any effect on energy production?

    (c) If so, which vitamins are involved and in what way?

7. (a) Identify the waste products of glucose metabolism.

    (b) In what ways does the body eliminate these waste products?

8. Describe four forms of energy in the body, using examples and possible interconversions.

9. (a) What are amino acids and how are peptide links formed?

    (b) Of what significance are peptide links in the body?

10. Define basal metabolic rate. Under what conditions is it measured? Why, then, is the nurse's role so important?

11

Electricity and magnetism

OBJECTIVES

After studying this chapter, students should be able to:

1. Describe bar magnets and electromagnets and draw the fields associated with the former.
2. Discuss static electricity and the precautions to be taken to avoid any adverse effects arising from this.
3. Define the terms potential difference, electric current and resistance, together with the units for each, and describe the relationship between these in an electrical circuit.
4. Differentiate between insulators and conductors, fuses and earth wires.
5. Discuss electric shock, including the difference between macroshock and microshock.
6. List the safety rules to be observed when using any electrical device.
7. Describe the use of electricity in medical and nursing practice.

INTRODUCTION

If you should poke your finger into a live electrical socket, you would become instantly aware of the effect of electricity on the body. However, since most of us were made aware in our childhood of the extremely dangerous, even fatal, effects of electricity, we would never investigate it in this way. Then, as part of your training in nursing, you see a patient being given a substantial electric shock in an effort to save the patient's life, and you might wonder how lethal electricity can suddenly become a saver of lives.

When you enter today's intensive care units and specialized areas such as coronary care, haemodialysis, and operating rooms, it is sometimes hard to find the patient amongst all the electrical equipment! Sometimes we even become confused as to which requires the most attention – patient or machine. Since electrical devices of all sorts can be useful and, in some instances even life-preserving, we must learn to use them properly and develop priorities when using them.

One major aspect of the nurse's responsibility is *safety*: safety not only of the patient's life, but of the nurse's, and that of other staff and visitors, in the use and presence of electrical equipment. How, in fact, can the necessary protection of people against the hazards of electricity be ensured? All individuals, not just nurses, should be able to answer this question, since electricity plays such a major role in the life of most communities.

Magnetism is also of importance in therapy.

MAGNETISM

Simple permanent magnets such as horseshoe magnets and bar magnets are able to attract metallic objects made of iron, steel and some alloys. One alloy that is superior to iron for most purposes is **alnico**, an alloy of **al**uminium, **ni**ckel and **co**balt.

Such magnets have two poles, a north pole and a south pole. A north pole is simply defined as that part of the magnet pointing north and the south pole is that part of the magnet pointing south. For convenience, only bar magnets will be considered here. The rule governing the behaviour of any two magnets in close proximity to each other is that *like poles repel* and *unlike poles attract*. This means that two north poles will repel each other, as will two south poles. A north pole and a south pole will attract each other.

Associated with any magnet is a **magnetic field**. This is regarded as a region in which a small magnet such as a compass needle would experience an influence. The direction in which the small magnet points is shown by **lines of force** and indicates the direction of the magnetic field (Fig. 11.1). The magnetic lines of force, or field lines, come out of the north pole and go into the south pole, as indicated by the arrows; the lighter end of the small compass needles is the north pole in each case. Also, it should be noted that Fig. 11.1 is a two-dimensional representation of a three-dimensional pattern.

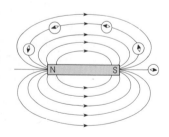

Figure 11.1. A small compass indicating the field pattern around a bar magnet. (From Greenberg: *Physics for Biology & Pre-Med Students*. Philadelphia. W.B. Saunders. 1975.)

The bar magnet in Fig. 11.1 is a **permanent magnet**. Another type of magnet used in medical practice is the electromagnet, which operates on the principle shown in Fig. 11.2(d).

The electric current (I) flowing through the wires gives rise to a magnetic field, by a mechanism which need not concern us here. This magnetic field arises only when the current is flowing and is not present (other than a very slight amount of permanent magnetism that remains) when the current is not flowing. Such electromagnets are used in control valves in the expiratory part of some ventilators to control the flow of gas. These are called solenoid valves, since they operate in a similar way to the solenoid valve shown in Fig. 11.2(d).

When the current (I) is flowing through the many turns of wire wound around the core, the soft iron core becomes magnetic and interacts with the magnetic field around the wire. Note that 'soft' iron is iron that contains little carbon and does not remain permanently magnetised when the current is switched off.

This causes the soft iron core to move, and its movement can be utilised to shut or open a valve. This valve can then be used to control the flow of gas (as in the ventilator), or of liquid in other devices. Furthermore, because the current can be switched on or off at a remote locality such as a control station, this device offers a number of advantages.

An electromagnet is used to extract pieces of material (e.g. iron) with magnetic properties from the eye. The sterilised tip of a small portable electromagnet may be used, or else the tip of a large stationary electromagnet such as the Muller giant eye magnet. The advantage in using an electromagnet is that the strength of the current flowing in the wire, and thus the strength of the magnetism, can be controlled.

It must be remembered that such a situation is a penetrating injury to the eye, that the unsterile object will have created an open pathway to its present position and that its presence does create pressure within the eye. Therefore great care should be exercised, particularly in administering first aid, to ensure that no further pressure is put upon the eye, for example, by the patient bending over or by disturbance of the object. Strict cleanliness and sterility should be enforced where possible and the eye should preferably be covered.

Magnetic-field therapy is a fascinating new development in medical practice which is utilized in the treatment of a wide range of afflictions, including fractures, arthrosis (diseases of joints), sporting injuries. tendonitis, bruising, myositis (inflammation of a voluntary muscle) and neuralgia. It functions by using a very low frequency (1-50 pulses per second) magnetic field, which can either increase or decrease (depending on the frequency used) the blood supply to a particular area.

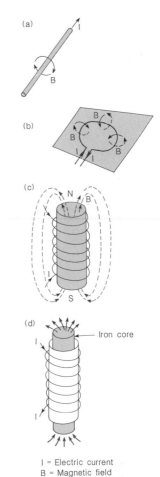

I = Electric current
B = Magnetic field

Figure 11.2. The magnetic fields produced by electric currents. In (a) the current I flowing through the wire produces the circular magnetic field B. In (b) a similar effect is observed. In (c) the current flowing through the wire around the cylinder gives rise to a magnetic field similar to that produced by a bar magnet. This is the principle of the electromagnet. In (d), a similar effect to (c) is observed, but the soft iron core enhances the effect by a factor of thousands. If the core is free to move, it can be used to operate a switch or a valve, in order to control the flow of electric current or liquids and gases (solenoid valves). (From Nave & Nave: *Physics for the Health Sciences*. 3rd Ed. Philadelphia. W.B. Saunders. 1985.)

ELECTRICITY

Why do so many people claim that they do not understand electricity? Is it because it cannot be seen? Perhaps it is because this interesting subject has never been explained properly to them. At least the reader should become sufficiently familiar with the nature of electricity that its fundamental properties will be understood and electricity will be treated with the respect it deserves.

Firstly, it is important to realise that electricity of any kind involves electrons. As we have already seen, electrons are very small entities that carry a negative electrical charge and that can be removed from various elements and compounds with varying degrees of ease.

Secondly, it is appropriate to distinguish between *static* electricity and *dynamic* electricity. Static electricity is electricity that builds up in one place, i.e. it doesn't go anywhere – at least not until circumstances change and it gets the opportunity to discharge (see below). Dynamic electricity is otherwise known as current electricity and involves a *flow of electrons*.

Static Electricity

Just a few things need to be said about static electricity. Firstly, it is generated by means of rubbing or friction. If we take a comb and rub it on almost any piece of fabric, we find that it acquires a small electric charge. If this comb is placed near some small pieces of paper (say 1–2 cm wide) we find that the pieces of paper are attracted to the comb. This is because the comb has become charged by the transfer of electrons to or from the comb.

If electrons are transferred *to* the comb from the fabric, the comb will become *negatively* charged. If electrons are transferred *away* from the comb to the fabric, the comb will become *positively* charged.

Some other everyday examples are:

- Combing your hair when both the hair and the atmosphere are dry (transfer of electrons in this way is much more probable in dry air since they are likely to be absorbed by the moisture in humid air). Under these conditions, you can often hear a crackling sound and sparks are sometimes observed in the dark (the sparks being caused by the movement of electrons). Note that these effects are much more pronounced in dry air than in humid conditions.
- Some types of clothing, particularly if made from synthetic

materials such as nylon and terylene, tend to cling to your skin while you undress, since these fabrics either gain or lose electrons very readily.

- Motor vehicles can sometimes build up a considerable charge because of friction with the atmosphere. For this reason, petrol tankers used to trail chains along to conduct any static electricity to the earth. Similarly, the toll collectors on the Sydney Harbour Bridge used to be protected from electrostatic shocks by small pieces of flexible wire protruding up out of the road. These caused electrons to flow to or from the motor vehicle to remove the static electric charge. Alternative methods are now used. Such electric shocks are relatively harmless (as we shall see), but rather distressing.

- Lightning is the discharge (or passage of electrons from clouds to the earth) of static electricity, which builds up in clouds under certain conditions. Whereas normal *static* electric shocks do not harm an individual, lightning can be fatal, essentially because of the extremely large number of electrons involved.

But what of the nurse who is not combing his/her hair, undressing, driving over a bridge or even, hopefully, not being struck by lightning?

The first encounter the new nurse may have with static electricity may be in the process of making a bed (Fig. 11.3). The friction generated here may give the unfortunate nurse something of a lift in life! This is one reason why cotton blankets are preferred to woollen ones, because wool easily builds up static electricity. While static electricity will not harm the patient or the nurse, it does cause unnecessary discomfort for both.

The second encounter may be with the precautions taken to prevent any sparking due to electrostatic charges in operating theatres, e.g. the type of clothing to be worn by personnel and the fabrics used. Thus cotton fabrics and loose-fitting clothing is preferred for nurses, and women are asked not to wear nylon slips. This used to be much more significant when anaesthetics such as ether and other highly flammable gases were in more common use and the very real danger of an explosion or fire existed, particularly if oxygen was present. In addition, operating rooms and equipment are now designed with special floors and equipment to reduce static build-up, and anaesthetic machines are designed to prevent gas leakages.

Some people seem to think that oxygen is flammable also and that this is consequently a hazard. As we saw in Chapter 7, oxygen is *not flammable* but *does support combustion*. This means that in the event of fire, oxygen would assist the combustion of ether or any other flammable material.

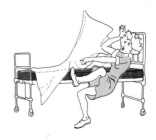

Figure 11.3. The effect that static electricity can have on a nurse making a bed.

Dynamic Electricity

As was mentioned above, this consists of a flow of electrons. Why do electrons flow anyway? Why don't they just stay where they are? The answer is that electrons normally do stay where they are and don't go wandering about unless there is a reason. Before proceeding let us look at some of the terms used in connection with dynamic electricity, and we will do this by comparing the flow of electricity with the more familiar flow of water, which should assist understanding. Various terms will be explained, for the time being considering direct current only.

Voltage or Electrical Pressure

For water to flow in a pipe, pressure is needed. As we have already seen, the greater the difference in height between the water reservoir and the tap, the greater will be the pressure of the water. Water supply authorities normally achieve this by siting reservoirs at the highest point available. It follows that the water pressure in houses up near the reservoir will not be as great as the pressure for the houses in the valley below. We say that the *gravitational potential energy difference* is greater for the valley dwellers.

The same principle applies to electricity. In this case, however, height is not involved. The potential energy difference in electrical situations arises by virtue of the *state of charge* of the two points between which the electric current flows. Thus if one point has a higher concentration of electrons than another, the electrons will tend to flow 'downhill' from the point of high concentration to the point of low concentration. The greater this difference in electron concentration, the greater will be the potential difference between the two points, or the greater will be the electrical pressure between the two points (Fig. 11.4).

The difference in energy in the example (Fig. 11.4) using water results from gravity, but in the electrical example the difference in energy arises from the battery or whatever other source of electrical energy is used. In a battery, for example, a difference in electrical potential exists between the two terminals of a battery, since there is a much greater concentration of electrons on the negative terminal compared to the positive terminal. This is the reason why electrons flow when given the chance – a source of energy such as a battery provides the electrical pressure or electromotive force. If the two points A and B are joined by a wire, electrons will then flow from A to B as shown.

It is important to note that our forefathers *guessed* the direction of flow of electric current and had a 50 per cent chance

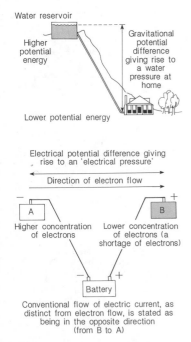

Figure 11.4. Comparison between water and electricity to show the generation of an 'electrical pressure' or voltage.

of being correct. They weren't! This has left us with the unfortunate situation whereby we say that electric current flows from *positive to negative* while all the time the little electrons are doing their own thing and going from *negative to positive*. The reader should make sure, then, that the difference between the direction of conventional current flow and electron flow is appreciated.

The **volt** is the unit of measurement for electrical potential difference or electrical pressure. This is defined as follows:

If the work done in moving a charge of one coulomb between two points is one joule, the potential difference between those two points is one volt.

In this definition:

- A 'charge of one coulomb' means an object carrying an electric charge – it has an excess or shortage of electrons. The unit coulomb is used because it is of a more practical size than the charge on an electron, for example. This should be apparent from the fact that the coulomb is 6.25×10^{15} times as large as the charge on an electron!
- The joule is simply a measure of energy (as we have seen previously when considering energy in the body), or of work done, as in this case. This means, in fact, that work and energy are measured using the same unit. This is not unreasonable when it is remembered that energy is the capacity to do work and that energy is consumed when work is done.

Current or Rate of Flow
Returning to our water pipe, let us look at the effect on the rate of flow of using different water pressures. If we use a very low pressure, the flow rate will be low, as shown in Fig. 11.5(a). If we use a higher pressure, however, the flow rate will look more like Fig. 11.5(b).

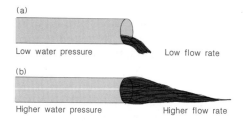

(a)

Low water pressure   Low flow rate

(b)

Higher water pressure   Higher flow rate

Figure 11.5. Effect of water pressure on flow rate.

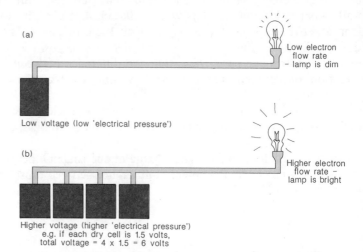

(a)

Low electron
flow rate
– lamp is dim

Low voltage (low 'electrical pressure')

(b)

Higher electron
flow rate –
lamp is bright

Higher voltage (higher 'electrical pressure')
e.g. if each dry cell is 1.5 volts,
total voltage = 4 x 1.5 = 6 volts

Figure 11.6. Effect of 'electrical pressure' on electron flow rate.

The rate of flow of water could be measured in litres per second. If an electrical example is now considered, it can be seen in Fig. 11.6 that we have two wires of the same diameter and made from the same metal. In Fig. 11.6(a), the voltage (or electrical pressure) is low, so the rate of flow of electrons will be low, and the lamp will be dim. With the higher voltage in Fig. 11.6(b), the rate of flow of electrons will be much higher and the lamp will glow brighter.

The rate of flow of electrons is measured in *coulombs per second* (compare litres per second for water), the coulomb per second being called the *ampere* or *amp*. Thus we now have a unit for rate of flow of electrons or electric current.

Resistance

If a pipe of small diameter is used for a particular task, we know that it will not be able to deliver as much water as one with a large diameter. It is just as well that firemen don't have to put out fires with garden hoses!

In just the same way, in electrical applications a fine wire is used to carry a small current and a thicker wire to carry a larger current. In a car, for example, the wire used to run the car radio will be very much finer than the wire used to carry current to the starter motor, because the latter has to carry a much larger current.

This assumes that in both cases the wire is made of the same metal, because some metals are better conductors than others, i.e. they offer less resistance to electron flow than other metals and other materials. Copper, silver and aluminium are all good for this purpose, that is they are good conductors. Solids are normally better conductors than liquids, which are better conductors than gases. Other factors can affect conduction, such as:

- **Temperature**. Higher temperatures mean that electrons tend to collide with vibrating atoms more frequently, and thus conduction is impeded. Low temperatures mean that electrons are less impeded, so that conduction is increased.
- **Length of wire**. The longer the wire through which the current has to travel, the greater will be the resistance.
- **Purity of the metal**. Impurities in the metal tend to impede current flow.

Poor conductors, or insulators, are discussed below, but water warrants special mention. Pure water is a very poor conductor indeed, but water is very rarely pure. The presence of some electrolytes (and there are usually some present in town water) turns water from a very poor conductor into quite a good conductor. It is for this reason that the presence of water near any electrical appliance increases the danger to the user.

Any energy loss occurring as a result of poor conduction is dissipated as heat and light. By designing an appliance using appropriate metals and thickness of wire, we can deliberately produce heat, as in the following examples:

- Heaters, such as electric radiators.
- Heat lamps, which are used in treatments to promote drying, healing and comfort, and to promote circulation in an area.
- Electrocautery irons, which are often used in surgery to seal small blood vessels. They may also be used to seal fallopian tubes: adhesions are created, tubes are blocked and sterilisation results.

The unit of resistance is the **ohm**, which is defined by the following relationship, known as Ohm's law:

$$I \text{ (amperes)} = \frac{V \text{ (volts)}}{R \text{ (ohms)}}$$

where I is current, V is voltage or potential difference and R is resistance.

This means that *if a voltage of one volt drives a current of one ampere through a resistance, the resistance will be one ohm.*

In the body, skin, bone and oil (produced by the sebaceous glands) all present resistance to the flow of an electric current. If the skin is dry, it presents the greatest resistance of all – about 100 000 ohms. If the skin is wet, the resistance is much lower. The resistance of a current path from one extremity of the body

to the other on intact moist skin is about 1,000 ohms. Special jellies are used to lower skin resistance for the electrodes used in
electrocardiographs (ECGs) and electroencephalographs (EEGs).

It should be noted that a *voltage drop* is said to occur over a
resistance. Just as a pressure drop occurs in a water reticulation
system such as a domestic water supply when it has done its work
of spurting from a tap, so a drop in voltage occurs when works
is done on an electrical resistance such as the heating element of
an electric jug, i.e. the electrical energy is dissipated in the form
of heat.

These ideas are summarised in Fig. 11.7.

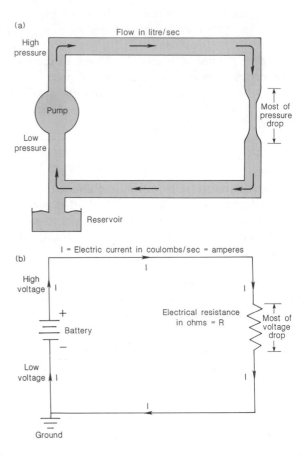

Figure 11.7 Analogy between an electric
and hydraulic circuit. (a) Hydraulic circuit.
(b) Direct current electric circuit.

Insulators and Conductors

We have just described a good **conductor** as a material that offers little resistance to the flow of electrons. This is because it is largely free from impurities and because its electrons are able to flow readily. What happens when a current flows is that an electron can be thought of as 'hopping' onto the end of a wire, which displaces another electron, which displaces the electron next to it, and so on. The effect is rather like pushing over a line of dominoes that have been stood on end and spaced about two-thirds of a domino length apart. When the end domino is pushed over, the impulse passes very rapidly along the line as each domino fells its neighbour.

An **insulator** is a material that offers very high resistance to the flow of electrons. This normally means that an electric current will not flow through that material. However, it must be remembered that there is no such thing as a perfect insulator – if the voltage is high enough even the best of insulators will break down. Typically good insulators are rubber, plastics, glass and ceramics.

In the body, one notable insulator is the myelin sheath separating one nerve cell, or neurone, from another in a nerve, and separating the nerve from fluids and body tissue. This is a comparable structure to a telephone cable, which consists of a number of insulated wires all forming part of the cable, which is then insulated from other cables. Myelin is a lipid substance that acts as an insulator and prevents any form of electrical connection between nerve fibres and their surroundings. This will be discussed in more detail in Chapter 13.

As with insulators, there is no such thing as a perfect conductor. Even copper wires that are very pure offer some resistance to the flow of electric current. If a perfect conductor did exist, a relatively fine wire would be able to carry an extremely large current.

Fuses

These are pieces of resistance wire that are put into electrical circuits to act as 'safety valves'. They are designed in such a way that they are just thick enough to carry the required current. If a larger current is sent through them as a result of some kind of malfunction, they overheat and burn through, thus effectively cutting off the electricity supply. However, the current necessary to blow a fuse is usually lethal, even in a domestic supply, and thus may cause a fatality, particularly if the fuse does not blow quickly.

Other devices such as circuit breakers are designed to perform the same function.

Earth Wire

An electric current will usually take the path of least resistance. Therefore, if a current is flowing around a circuit, insulation is required around the conductor to prevent electrons from travelling into surrounding materials with lower resistance and thus from taking an uncontrolled or undesired pathway – called a 'short circuit'.

Typical power cords have three wires, as we shall see, but the green (or green and yellow) wire is the 'earth' or 'ground' wire. An **earth wire** is one which, as its name suggests, is connected (from the appliance, through the power point) to a piece of water pipe or a water service, which has direct contact with the ground. Electrical appliances usually have earth wires (and, with the exception of 'double insulated' devices *should* have earth wires), which serve to conduct electric current away from the appliance straight to the ground in the event of a fault. This means that, if an appliance is faulty, the electric current will take the line of least resistance and travel through the earth wire to the ground, rather than through the body of someone in contact with the appliance, which has greater resistance than the copper earth wire.

Various types of faults occur in electrical equipment, but one of the most common is the one we have called a short circuit. This arises because of the breakdown of electrical insulation, meaning that the electric current is then able to flow through any metal parts of a ventilator or cardiac monitor, for example, which come into or form a contact with the live conducting path. The equipment may then become 'live', i.e. it will be carrying a current. Note that this does not normally happen with a double insulated piece of equipment.

If no earth wire is present and a nurse touches the metal, the current will flow through the nurse's body, since this is a convenient pathway to an area of lower potential – the earth (Fig. 11.8).

If all is as it should be and an earth wire is present, the electric current (i.e. electrons), will flow through the earth wire as a path of least resistance. The fuse will then blow (because of the large current passing through it and the wires), and the machine can then be repaired. If, however, the wiring is not as it should be, anyone touching the machine will probably be electrocuted. Outer casings made of materials such as plastic, rather than metal, give the user extra protection.

Circuit

Electricity requires a circuit in order to flow. A complete circuit will, as a very minimum, consist of a source of electrical energy,

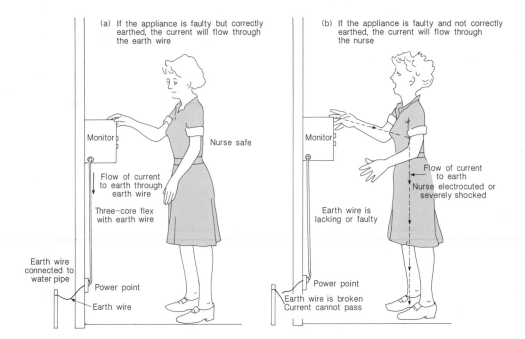

(a) If the appliance is faulty but correctly earthed, the current will flow through the earth wire

Monitor

Nurse safe

Flow of current to earth through earth wire

Three-core flex with earth wire

Earth wire connected to water pipe

Power point

Earth wire

(b) If the appliance is faulty and not correctly earthed, the current will flow through the nurse

Monitor

Flow of current to earth

Nurse electrocuted or severely shocked

Earth wire is lacking or faulty

Power point

Earth wire is broken Current cannot pass

Figure 11.8. The importance of the earth wire.

a 'load' and wires to connect these together to enable current to flow from high potential to low potential. Note that electrons will flow only if the circuit is complete.

The source of electrical energy may be a dry cell such as a torch battery, a wet battery such as a car battery or a power supply such as a typical hospital, domestic or industrial supply. The load may be a simple light bulb or a highly sophisticated piece of equipment that uses up the electrical energy. More complex circuits will incorporate switches, fuses or circuit breakers and other components.

Wiring

A conventional three-pin plug that we typically use as a means of access to our domestic or hospital electricity supply, has three wires attached to it, which are colour-coded as follows:

- The **active** wire, which is the *live* wire and carries the current from the supply. This is either *red* or *brown*.
- The **neutral** wire, which forms the completed circuit back to the supply, is either *black* or *light blue*, and *is not active* - **if, and only if, the wiring is correct**. This does **not** mean that this wire is safe to touch – always regard **all** wires as dangerous.

- The **earth** wire, which has already been mentioned, is normally coloured *green* or *green-yellow* and connects the appliance through an earthing circuit to the ground.

The red/black/green coding has been used in Australia for many years, but many suppliers are changing to the internationally recognized brown/blue/green-yellow system, which has been adopted as an Australian standard to avoid problems with red/green colour blindness.

It should also be noted that much of the imported equipment used in hospitals may have colour coding different to either of the above.

Power

This is a measure of the electrical energy consumed in a given time. It is equal to a joule per second (energy per unit time) and is calculated by multiplying the voltage by the current.

$$\text{power} = \text{voltage} \times \text{current}$$
$$\text{(watts)} \quad \text{(volts)} \quad \text{(amps)}$$

For example, if the domestic supply is operating on 240 volts and the maximum permissible current that can be consumed by one appliance operating from a power point is 10 amperes:

$$\text{power} = \text{volts} \times \text{amps}$$
$$= 240 \times 10$$
$$\text{Therefore power} = 2400 \text{ watts.}$$

This is why so many electric room heaters are rated at 2400 watts.

Table 11.1 summarises these quantities.

TABLE 11.1

Electrical unit	Definition	Physical quantity measured	qUsual symbol for physical quantity
volt (V)	joule/coulomb	potential difference – electrical pressure	V
ampere (A)	coulomb/sec	electric current	I
ohm (Ω)	volt/amp	resistance to current flow	R
watt (W)	joule/sec	power	P

Direct and Alternating Current

Much of our discussion so far has involved direct current mainly because it is somewhat easier to comprehend, but it is now time to consider both types of current.

Direct current (DC) is current that travels in *one direction only*. As we have already seen, it is a convention to regard current as travelling from positive to negative (even though the electrons travel the other way).

Alternating current (AC) is current that travels backwards and forwards, usually at a frequency of 50 hertz or 50 cycles per second. This means that the current travels one way for a short time and then in the reverse direction for the same short time. This whole operation is called a cycle, so that 50 of these occur in each second.

Domestic supplies usually utilise alternating current because it offers a number of advantages, which we will not discuss here. However, one of the most important of these is that *we can use transformers with alternating current, but not with direct current.* Transformers offer the advantage of being able to change a voltage to suit our purposes, as we shall see when electric blankets are discussed.

Electricity and the Body

To understand the effects of electricity on the body, we should first be aware of the most important – *electrocution*. This first occurs when the body becomes part of an electric circuit and the passage of current through the body results in death. Current medical opinion regards the probable cause of death as ventricular fibrillation. This condition is one in which the heart engages in random chaotic activity rather than the regular, co-ordinated activity necessary to pump blood. This reflects the electrical nature of the signals sent throughout the heart by the natural pacemakers, which cause the heart to contract.

Fig. 11.9 shows the normal pattern of electrical stimulation in the heart, which produces the PQRST curve seen on an electrocardiograph (ECG). This pattern is completely overridden by lethal currents and disrupted.

The danger of electrocution occurring depends upon several factors:

1. The *duration* of the current, i.e. a *sustained* current of anything greater than 100 milliamperes can lead to cardiac arrest.
2. The *location* of the contact point, since this will determine

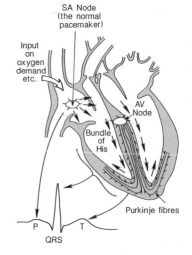

Figure 11.9. The electrical conduction process which controls the heart's pumping cycle. (From Nave & Nave: *Physics for the Health Sciences.* 3rd Ed. Philadelphia, W.B. Saunders 1985.)

the amount of resistance presented to the current on its way towards the heart, through legs, arms, skin or bone.

3. The *amount of current*. This factor is very significant, as the above discussion indicates. Sustained currents of anywhere between 30 and 200 milliamperes and above (depending on the individual and other circumstances mentioned) may bring about fibrillation.

4. The *voltage*. This is not as significant as most people expect, because provided the voltage is high enough to drive a lethal current through the body, the voltage is unimportant. Obviously, this will vary from one individual to another, but about 30 volts may well be sufficient. Many warning signs attest to the voltage available (e.g. DANGER – 33 000 VOLTS) but the important point here is *the current that such a voltage can drive through the body*. Thus, a shock from the sparkplug of a car (about 12 000 volts) or an electrostatic shock (as previously discussed) will not normally hurt an individual, because *the current is low*. The normal hospital and domestic supply is 240 volts, although some parts of most hospitals have a 415-volt supply to service certain types of equipment.

5. *Frequency*. A frequency of 50 hertz (cycles per second) can be lethal, depending on the current. In some medical applications such as cautery and electrosurgery, very high frequencies (of the order of two million hertz) are used, which tend to produce heat and thus result in burns rather than muscle contraction or ventricular fibrillation.

6. *Resistance*. The electrical resistance of the body can vary from over 1 000 000 ohms for very dry skin to less than 1 000 ohms for wet skin. Skin resistance is increased by thicker skin, the presence of bone and oil from sebaceous glands. Skin resistance is lowered by water on the skin, perspiration, the presence of electrolytes and conduction gels.

What happens when an electric current enters the body? We will now examine some of the effects:

1. The body tissues are heated, leading to burns - which can range from trivial burns to complete charring, depending on the factors discussed above.

2. Active cell functioning is disrupted, the effects of which may range from unconsciousness to paralysis of the respiratory centre and/or fibrillation of the heart.

A nurse may have to deal with two types of shock arising from contact with an electric current.

1. **Macroshock**. This occurs through an electrical contact with the skin surface. The current passes through the body tissues

to the heart and passes out to an area of lower potential such as the floor, the earth, etc. In this case, no direct contact occurs between the source of the current and the heart, and this constitutes the most common form of electrocution. The current necessary to produce severe abnormalities of heart rhythm is of the order 30–200 milliamperes, as previously indicated.

2. **Microshock**. This occurs when current flows directly to the heart muscle. The current does not need to flow through other body tissues, which provide resistance, to reach the heart. This type of situation occurs most frequently in hospitals where patients are undergoing treatments or being monitored for severe problems, such as heart disorders. Direct pathways to the heart may be created by the following:

Transvenous pacemaker wires, which are insulated metal wires inserted through a vein to the heart to allow an external electrical device to be connected. The device will be used to initiate heartbeat when the heart's own pacemaker is damaged and unable to perform effectively.

Monitoring devices, such as normal saline-filled catheters (0.9 per cent sodium chloride solution), which are used to monitor or check venous pressures. These are placed just outside the right atrium (upper chamber) of the heart and provide a solution through which current can travel directly to the heart. Similar devices are used to check arterial pressures.

Drainage catheters (urinary), which carry an electrolytic (i.e. current-conducting) solution in the form of urine.

Two important differences exist with microshock, associated with the direct pathway:

Only a very small current (of the order of 0.06 milliamperes or 60 microamperes) is needed to cause ventricular fibrillation, since the current does not meet with any significant resistance in the direct pathway and a high current density at the heart results from the fact that no current dispersion occurs.

Since a current of less than one milliampere is not perceived by the body, it follows that such a current may be transmitted through another person without that person realising it, even though it might be lethal to a patient in the circumstances described (Fig. 11.10).

In a defibrillator (i.e. a machine used to deliver an electric shock to the body in an attempt to restore normal heartbeat) as a comparison, a large current of the order of several amps is used, driven by a voltage pulse of up to 10 000 volts.

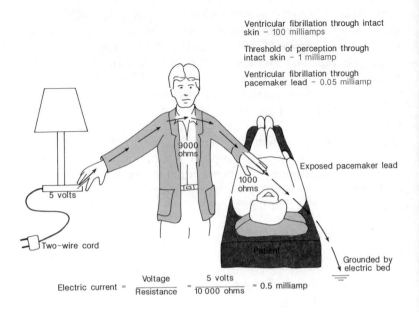

Ventricular fibrillation through intact
skin – 100 milliamps

Threshold of perception through
intact skin – 1 milliamp

Ventricular fibrillation through
pacemaker lead – 0.05 milliamp

9000
ohms

Exposed pacemaker lead

1000
ohms

5 volts

Two–wire cord

Patient

Grounded by
electric bed

$$\text{Electric current} = \frac{\text{Voltage}}{\text{Resistance}} = \frac{5 \text{ volts}}{10\ 000 \text{ ohms}} = 0.5 \text{ milliamp}$$

Figure 11.10. An example of a microshock hazard. From Nave & Nave: *Physics for the Health Sciences.* 3rd Ed. Philadelphia. W.B. Saunders. 1985.)

In electric shock therapy, currents of the order of one amp are used over a period of about one-tenth of a second. With this very large current the necessity for restricting the current flow to the temple area between the electrodes cannot be overstressed.

SOME SAFETY RULES WITH ELECTRICITY

Nurses in particular are involved with the use of electricity. In the course of a day's work, whether in a hospital or in community nursing, a nurse might be involved with the use of a defibrillator or in making a decision on whether it is safe to leave an incontinent patient on an electric blanket. In the case of an elderly patient, the visiting nurse may be one of the few contacts that person has with the outside world, and anything that may endanger the life or well-being of the patient, electrical or otherwise, is very much that nurse's concern.

The following rules should always be observed:

1. Never take short cuts of any sort with electricity or with any of the rules that follow.

2. Always seek the services of a licensed electrician in repairing faulty appliances and frayed cords, whether in a hospital, at home or in someone else's home. There are many people around who are good at fixing things, but there are others who only think they are, and some of their victims are now dead

as a result. Furthermore, the law has some definite things to say on such matters.

All electrical equipment, especially when used in institutions, should be checked and labelled as having been checked on a regular basis. For example, an earth wire could become loose or damaged without the user being aware of it, causing metal parts on the equipment to become live. Remember that it is still possible for current to flow or leak, even with the apparatus turned off and a cardiac monitor carries a potentially lethal charge inside the back of the unit (on the tube) even when the current is switched off.

3. If a fuse blows, call an electrician to replace it – the cause may be serious. As previously mentioned, a fuse may not protect a human life, because the damage may be done before the fuse blows. In the case of those who are susceptible to microshock, this is even more important. The lesson is clear: rely on good safety awareness, not fuses, to save lives.

4. Three-pin plugs are a constant problem. If they are broken or damaged, or if any wires are showing other than the outside covering of three-core flex, they *must* be repaired. No electrical device (not even a bedlamp) should **ever** be used if it is not connected to an approved (by the local electricity supply authority) three-pin plug by a **three**-core flex. Two-core flex is an absolute 'no-no', unless the particular appliance is clearly marked '*double insulated*', to which might be added '*do not earth*'. Such appliances have a double provision of electrical insulation, so do not require earthing – and should not be earthed.

Never disconnect appliances by pulling on the cord. This practice can cause the earth wire to come loose. Pull out the plug itself. Note also that the power *must* be switched off before a plug is inserted or pulled out.

Also, avoid the use of extension cords – these can be a real problem. Because they may not always be wired correctly, considerable voltage drop may occur and earthing problems can arise (see below). In addition, there is the hazard of an extra link in the circuit at some distance from the power source, which means the circuit is not always checked for full connection before power is turned on.

5. Equipment such as defibrillators must always be handled with the greatest respect. These are normally used only in emergencies, and in such stressful situations it is so easy to forget safety. However, remember the potential consequences of such oversights. See below for special precautions in the use of defibrillators.

6. Always be particularly conscious of the extra hazards involved in using any kind of electrical equipment or appliance on wet surfaces. Pure water is in fact not a conductor, but the

water obtained from most domestic supplies is *not* pure, and of course it becomes even less pure on a laundry floor, for example. Under such circumstances, the danger of electrocution is considerably increased.

7. Always ensure that the patient cannot become part of an electric circuit, i.e. the patient should be isolated from the ground by avoiding contact with a metal bed frame whenever electrical devices are connected to him or her. Remember that even a catheter can conduct current.

8. Any electrical equipment with bare metal casing must be kept out of the patient's reach. Even though all electrical equipment should be earthed, a leak can occur. This makes it particularly important to avoid touching any two pieces of electrical equipment at the same time.

9. Where the potential for microshock exists, extra precautions should be taken. Do not handle bare pacemaker wires or the conducting part of a catheter while in contact with any metal object. In fact, a nurse should not adjust equipment while in contact with a patient or a bed. Any exposed wires should be covered and taped.

10. *All electrical equipment associated with one patient should be connected to the one panel.* In intensive care units and modern hospitals, multiple power outlet panels are provided on a one-per-bed basis. If a patient is linked to different pieces of equipment that are connected to different power outlets, the potential of the outlets may not be the same. If one piece of equipment is connected to a power outlet by means of an extension lead, for example, and a fault develops in that circuit (which may not be the same as the circuit feeding the outlet near the patient's bed), a significant potential difference may exist between the two earth wires of two pieces of equipment. It then follows that a significant potential difference may exist between two metal casings on pieces of equipment. While this may not be dangerous for an individual where contacts are made to intact skin, it may well be fatal if one of the contacts to the equipment is attached to a catheter.

11. In any situation where it is possible to remove an electrical cause of a problem, such as an electrical fire, SWITCH OFF THE CURRENT.

12. Should an oxygen tent be in use at any time, electrical equipment must be kept away, as discussed in Chapter 7. Oxygen does not burn but supports combustion and thus increases the possibility of fire. Also, since electric drills and saws tend to spark, all drills and saws used in operating theatres are driven by compressed nitrogen (an inert, non-flammable gas).

13. It must be remembered that a nurse is responsible for the safety of the patient at all times, so that he or she also has a

responsibility to ensure that all visitors and non-medical personnel are aware of safety precautions.

Finally, all these safety rules are provided to enable us to use electricity safely and wisely.

MEDICAL USES OF ELECTRICITY

If treated with the respect it deserves, electricity is a most useful servant – an essential component of our modern lifestyles, in fact. Even more importantly, it offers numerous advantages in medical practice in the constant endeavour to save lives, of which the following are but a sample.

Diagnosis

Electricity is widely used today to aid the physician and, in some circumstances, the nurse. It can be used in identifying the presence, location and nature of a problem that a patient may have. For example, an electrocardiograph records variation in electrical activity of the heart muscle, just as an electroencephalograph records electrical activity of the brain. Other examples include the **electrocystoscope**, which uses an electric light to see inside the bladder, and an **ophthalmoscope**, which uses an electric light to see inside the eye.

Monitoring

A wide range of electrical and electronic devices are available that will constantly check and record – visually, audibly or graphically – particular aspects of the functioning of the body. They provide instant access to information in many situations, without disturbing the patient. They may also reduce the need to inflict further discomfort on the patient every time information is required. For example, heart activity, blood pressure, pulse and temperature can all be monitored by various devices, requiring the nurse simply to read a screen or push a button to obtain readings (Fig. 11.11). Of course, the nurse should be aware of the particular problems associated with these devices in caring for the patient who is connected to them.

Treatment

The following are examples of applications of electricity in treatment:

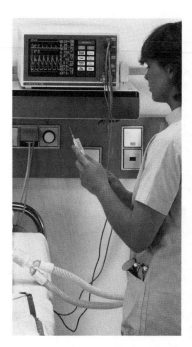

Figure 11.11. This photograph shows a modern sophisticated monitor which provides the nurse or doctor with comprehensive physiological data. (Courtesy of Medical Applications P/L.)

- Blood vessels can be sealed off by electrocautery.
- Some types of excisions can be done electrically.
- Relief from pain can be obtained in some cases by using low intensity electric currents in the technique called electro-therapy.
- Electrotherapy can also be used in the electrical stimulation of damaged muscles.
- *Electric shock therapy.* This form of treatment is used in psychiatry, but not to the same extent as it used to be. It involves passing an electric current, of a particular frequency and strength and for a specified period of time, through the brain, usually to treat certain types of psychoses. It induces convulsive seizures in an attempt to alter the electrical activity of the brain. As previously indicated, currents used are of the order of one ampere over a period of about one-tenth of a second. The necessity for restricting the current flow between electrodes to the temple area cannot be over-stressed.
- *Defibrillation.* This is an emergency procedure in which an electric current is delivered to the heart to terminate an abnormal heart rhythm that is life-threatening, usually ven-tricular fibrillation. A specific large current is used, driven by a voltage pulse of up to 10 000 volts. The objective is to stop the abnormality and allow the heart to return to a more uniform (and thus more effective) contracting pattern (Fig. 11.12).

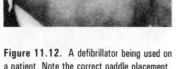

Figure 11.12. A defibrillator being used on a patient. Note the correct paddle placement. (Courtesy of Medical Applications P/L.)

An important responsibility of the nurse and all others concerned is to ensure that everyone *stands clear* of the patient's bed and that no one actually touches the patient while the shock is being delivered, for obvious reasons.

Electric Blankets

It is appropriate to discuss these briefly, since they are used not only in creating general warmth, but in the treatment of hypothermia, discussed in Chapter 2.

Two types exist: high-voltage and low-voltage.

High-voltage electric blankets are safe under normal circum-stances, which include:

1. The simple annual precaution of sending the blanket back to the manufacturer or his agent for a thorough check. Remem-ber that if the insulation breaks down, the possibility of electric shock is very real.

TABLE 11.2 The physiological effects of 50 Hz AC current through intact skin into the body trunk

Current (1 second contact)	Physiological effect	Voltage required to produce the current with assumed body resistance	
		10 000 ohms	1000 ohms
1 milliampere	Threshold of feeling	10 V	1 V
5 milliamperes	Accepted as maximum harmless current	50 V	5 V
10–20 milliamperes	Beginning of sustained muscular contraction ('can't let go' current)	100–200 V	10–20 V
50 milliamperes	Pain, possible fainting and exhaustion. Heart and respiratory functions continue	500 V	50 V
100–300 milliamperes	Ventricular fibrillation, fatal if continued. Respiratory function continues	1000–3000 V	100–300 V
6 amperes	Sustained ventricular contraction followed by normal heart rhythm (defibrillator). Temporary respiratory paralysis and possibly burns	60 000 V	6000 V

(From Nave & Nave: *Physics of the Health Sciences*. 3rd Ed. Philadelphia. W.B. Saunders. 1985.)

2. The assumption that the user is not incontinent or a bed-wetter for emotional or other reasons. Urine contains a number of electrolytes and is thus a very good conductor of electricity. This, coupled with a wet skin, is a recipe for potential disaster.

Low voltage electric blankets are less popular with many people because they are much more expensive. The reason for this expense is the transformer (a large heavy object, with its controls, compared to the light and simple control unit on a high-voltage blanket). The transformer changes the voltage down to about 17 volts, which is not normally enough to drive a current of any significant magnitude through the body. Thus, even if the electrical insulation breaks down, the low-voltage electric blanket is *normally* not lethal.

However, points 1 and 2 made above for high-voltage blankets still apply.

In summary then, low-voltage electric blankets are very much safer than high-voltage ones, but the same precautions must be faithfully observed for both types, together with those points covered in the general discussion on safety. Table 11.2 summarises the physiological effects of 50 Hz AC current on the body.

In conclusion, electricity is a marvellous servant of humanity. We should not be frightened of it, but should always treat it with the respect it deserves.

REVIEW

1. Give an example of the use of an electromagnet in medicine.
2. (a) Give an example of the need to avoid static electricity.
   (b) How is this related to oxygen and why are precautions against the effects of static electricity so important when oxygen is being used?
3. What is the relationship between voltage and electric current?
4. Why are gels used under electrodes when taking ECGs?
5. Why are fuses included in electric circuits?
6. How does an earth wire function as a safety device?
7. Discuss the safety rules to be observed when using electricity.
8. What are the safety advantages of low-voltage electric blankets?
9. It is sometimes claimed that medical and surgical treatments create more problems for the patient. Discuss this statement in relation to microshock.
10. An electric shock does not always result in electrocution. Which factors might determine whether electrocution occurs?
11. There are situations in which the delivery of a predetermined level of electric current to the body is considered to be beneficial. Identify some of these.
12. The flow of an electric current along a wire is dependent on mobile electrons. Is this the case in the body? Why?

12

Light and sound

OBJECTIVES

After studying this chapter students should be able to:

1. Differentiate between longitudinal and transverse progressive waves and define the terms wavelength, amplitude and frequency.
2. Describe properties of light such as reflection, refraction, dispersion, colour and polarisation.
3. Outline the function of each of the major structures of the eye through which light passes and is received. Discuss the use of lenses to correct defects of vision.
4. Describe the electromagnetic spectrum and the relevance of each type of radiation in terms of (a) possible effects on the body and (b) the application of these in medical and nursing practice.
5. Define terms such as transmission, reception, frequency, pitch and loudness of sound waves.
6. Outline some other modern imaging techniques such as MRI (magnetic resonance imaging) and the use of lasers and optical fibres in medical practice.
7. Distinguish between the two types of deafness.

INTRODUCTION

It has been stated that energy is of vital importance to the human being. Following this, chemical energy in the body and electrical energy were discussed, but two other forms of energy also have great impact on the functioning of the human being – light energy and sound energy. These two forms will be discussed in this chapter since they are both associated with wave formation and the senses.

LIGHT

Light is normally emitted at the same time as heat and results from the energy given out by electrons as they move back to their respective energy levels in the atom after having risen to higher levels. This explanation oversimplifies a complex process, but we will not need to pursue this aspect any further, as sufficient understanding of light itself and its value to us can be gained without it.

Light is far more important to us than most of us realise. To get some idea of the dramatic role light plays in your life, it would be instructive to try blindfolding yourself and see what you discover. Certainly, you would bump into things because you wouldn't be able to see them. However, the effect on your sense of balance, your orientation and your perception of the surrounding world and the people in it may come as a great surprise.

The ability to see, which depends not only on the nervous system but also on the presence of light, is a fantastic achievement when we think about it. Unfortunately, space does not permit the complete exploration of the idea of vision here. We can only take a brief look at the subject of light energy.

To do this we must first discuss the subject of waves, because light travels in the form of waves.

Waves

We will be concerned with two different types of waves in this chapter.

- **Transverse progressive waves**, such as light waves, X-rays, gamma-rays, infra-red and ultra-violet waves.
- **Longitudinal progressive waves**, such as sound waves.

Longitudinal progressive waves will be dealt with in more detail in the next section: suffice it to say at this time that these waves are formed by a vibration or an oscillation (a to-and-fro motion).

In transverse progressive waves, the direction of vibration or oscillation is *at right angles* to the direction in which the wave is moving – hence the term 'transverse'.

In longitudinal progressive waves, the direction of vibration or oscillation is in the *same* direction as the direction in which the wave is moving, i.e. the direction of propagation.

This is illustrated in Fig. 12.1.

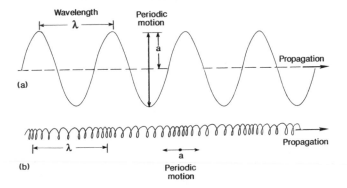

Figure 12.1. Transverse (a) and longitudinal (b) (compression) waves. In each case 'a' is the amplitude. In (b), the regions where the spring coils are close together are called 'compressions' and the regions where they are further apart are called 'rarefactions' or 'expansions'. (From Nave & Nave: *Physics for the Health Sciences.* 2nd Ed. Philadelphia. W.B. Saunders. 1980.)

Transverse Progressive Waves

It is important to note that in treating light as a wave motion, we are oversimplifying a complex concept, in that light has some of the properties of waves, but also some of the properties of particles. For example, light rays are stopped by dense materials and they can be made to do mechanical work – both these facts show that light rays can be regarded as particles.

Of course, this is difficult for us to visualise, but one cannot deny the facts. However, having made that comment we will now treat light as a wave motion only, as a matter of convenience.

Visible light or white light makes up a very small portion of the electromagnetic spectrum, which is described later in this chapter. White light consists of a mixture of the colours red, orange, yellow, green, blue and violet. Note that in some books (especially old ones) indigo (a dark blue) is included.

In Fig. 12.1 we see that two factors associated with waves are indicated:

1. **Wavelength** This is the distance between any two successive crests or any two successive troughs in a transverse wave. In a longitudinal wave it is given by the distance between two successive compressions or rarefactions.

2. **Amplitude** This is the maximum displacement of a point from a mean, or average, position.

Also, the **frequency** of a wave is equal to the number of complete waves that pass a given point per second. The frequency thus depends on the source and not the medium through which the wave is passing.

The speed or velocity at which waves are propagated normally depends upon the medium in which the wave is travelling, whether it is travelling through air or water or steel, and not upon the frequency or amplitude of the wave. Thus, when we speak of the velocity of sound, for example, this usually has meaning only if the medium is specified. If this is not specified, it is understood to mean through air (or, more correctly speaking, through a vacuum). As we will see shortly, the 'speed through a vacuum' has no meaning for sound since sound does not travel through a vacuum.

The following relationship is useful:

$$v = f\lambda$$

where v = velocity of propagation
f = frequency
and λ = wavelength

The velocity of propagation is constant for a particular type of wave motion (under a given set of conditions), such as light travelling through air. In this case, the velocity is 3×10^8 m/s. Light travels about a million times faster than sound.

Since the velocity is constant, it follows that a higher frequency will result in a shorter wavelength and a lower frequency will result in a longer wavelength.

Properties of Light

It should be noted that substances that transmit light are described as being *transparent* (e.g. air, glass and clean water), those that do not transmit light are described as being *opaque* (bricks, concrete, timber, steel) and those that transmit some light in a diffuse way, so that objects may not be clearly distinguished, as *translucent* (frosted glass).

Reflection
Reflection is the bending or 'bouncing back' of a light ray or wave at a *surface*. If the surface forms part of an opaque medium, the light is not able to pass into that medium and so is bent back into the original medium (or absorbed). If the surface forms part of a completely transparent medium, less reflection will occur and the light will pass into the medium.

Furthermore, if the surface of an opaque medium is not smooth, the light will be reflected (bent back) at a variety of angles, i.e., it will be *scattered*. Scattering explains why the sky is blue (blue light is scattered more than red light and so the sky appears blue), gives rise to polarisation (which is discussed later in this chapter) and is important in vision when considering focusing of the eye, perception, etc.

A line drawn on a diagram perpendicular to the surface, at the point where the light ray impinges on that surface, is called a **normal.** When a light ray strikes a reflecting surface, the angle formed with the normal is called the **angle of incidence**, and it is found that this is equal to the **angle of reflection**, which is the angle that the reflected ray makes with the normal, as shown in Fig. 12.2.

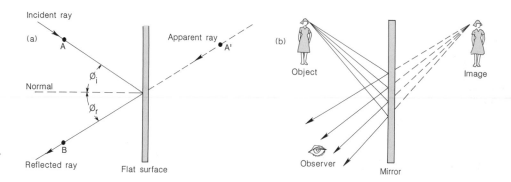

Refraction

The word refraction simply means 'bending'. The reason light bends is that it passes from one medium to another, and its velocity in the second medium is different from its velocity in the first. For example, if light passes from air into glass, it slows down to a velocity about two-thirds of its velocity in air. In passing from air into water, its velocity is about three-quarters of its velocity in air.

Figure 12.2.(a) A light ray undergoing reflection. The angle of reflection ϕ_r is equal to the angle of incidence ϕ_i. (b) The reflected image appears to the observer to be behind the mirror.

This bending effect resulting from different velocities is illustrated in Fig. 12.3. The diagram illustrates a succession of waves passing from, say, air into glass. As each wave front reaches the boundary, it is checked, or slowed down, by the denser material, the glass in our example. Thus, the lower portion of the wave front B is not able to travel as fast as the upper portion (for the instant illustrated) and so it is bent.

For a light ray or wave travelling from a less dense medium to a more dense medium, the bending is *towards* the normal.

For a light ray or wave travelling from a more dense medium to a less dense medium, the bending is *away from* the normal.

This is illustrated in Fig. 12.4, together with the fact that, at any interface, some reflection and some refraction will usually occur.

This bending effect is used in lenses, as illustrated in Fig. 12.5. *Convex* lenses cause light to converge (they are sometimes called converging lenses for this reason), and *concave* lenses

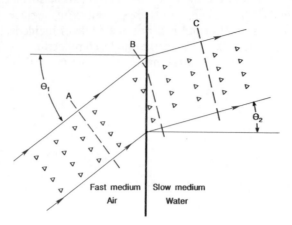

Figure 12.3. Refraction of light waves on passing from a less dense medium into a much denser medium. The resulting change in the velocity of the wave causes the wave to bend at the interface.

Figure 12.4. In (a), showing light passing from air into glass, the refracted ray is bent *towards* the normal, and $\phi > \theta$. In (b), showing light passing from glass into air, the refracted ray is bent away from the normal, and $\phi < \theta$.

cause light to diverge (and thus the term diverging lenses is used). 'Converge' means 'to come together' and 'diverge' means 'to move apart'.

A **lens** may be defined for our purposes as a transparent object with curved faces that causes a beam of rays to converge or diverge. As a result of this, images may be created.

Within the context of this general science text, it is sufficient simply to describe what happens with lenses and not be too concerned about *why* such things happen, while assuring the

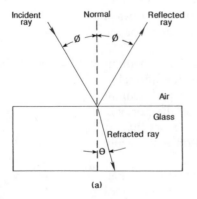

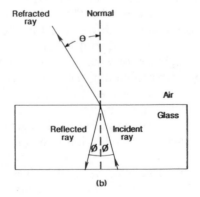

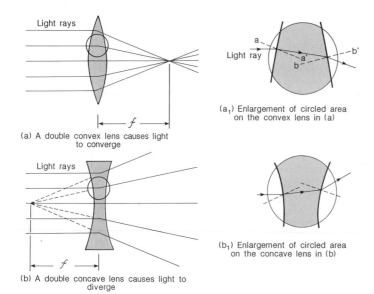

Light rays

(a₁) Enlargement of circled area
on the convex lens in (a)

(a) A double convex lens causes light
to converge

Light rays

(b₁) Enlargement of circled area
on the concave lens in (b)

(b) A double concave lens causes light to
diverge

Figure 12.5. Refraction in lenses.

student that the light paths indicated in Fig. 12.5 may easily be demonstrated. In the case of compound lenses (those that are made up of several individual lenses) and of multiple lens systems, the optics of lenses can become very complex indeed and require an in-depth study of the field of optics. The eye is a two-lens system.

The letter f is used to designate the **focal length** of the lens, which is the distance from the centre of the lens to the focal point. The focal point is the point at which parallel rays converge after passing through a convex lens, or at which they converge after being projected backwards from a concave lens, as shown in Fig. 12.5.

The focal length, f, of a lens can be used to calculate the 'strength' or focusing ability, S, of that lens, using the formula:

$$S = \frac{1}{f}$$

where f is in metres and S is in a unit called the **dioptre**. Determining the strength of a lens is very important in the prescription of spectacles, in assessing the properties of the lens of the eye and in manufacturing lenses for microscopes, etc.

For example, a lens that focuses parallel light rays at a point 25 cm beyond the lens has a strength given by:

$$S = \frac{1}{0.25} = 4 \text{ dioptres}$$

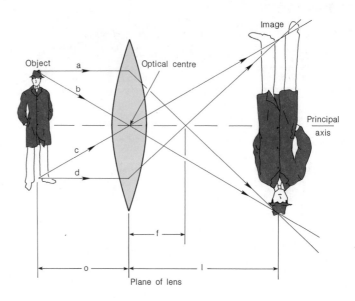

Figure 12.6. The formation of a real, inverted, magnified image by a convex lens. O = object distance, I = image distance, f = focal length.

Parallel rays of light are normally obtained only from very distant sources of light such as the sun. Since the sun is so far away, for all practical purposes light from the sun can be regarded as being parallel when it arrives at the earth. For all the normal applications of this work in nursing, 'point sources' of light will be considered. The concept of a point source makes description and understanding easier, but it should be remembered that any source of light is finite in size and cannot, strictly speaking, be regarded as a point source.

In Fig. 12.6, note the following points:

1. The lenses with which we are concerned normally have at least one plane of curvature in the vertical plane, as shown in the diagram, and at least one other in the horizontal plane, which cannot be shown in the diagram.

2. An imaginary line, called the **principal axis**, is drawn through the optical centre of the lens at right angles to the plane of the lens. Other rays that show the formation of an image may then be described in relation to the principal axis and the optical centre.

3. Some of the basic rules by which optics are determined are illustrated here:

- Rays such as b and c that pass through the optical centre continue in a straight path.
- Rays such as a and d that travel parallel to the principal axis are refracted (bent) through the focus.

- Where rays intersect, images are formed. If rays do not intersect, no image will be formed.
- In some cases, such as where the rays are diverging, rays have to be projected backwards before they will intersect.

4. The images formed may be of several types:

(a) *They may be magnified or diminished.* Most of the images that are to be formed on the eye need to be diminished so that the image can form in the space available. If the image has already been magnified (as in a simple magnifier), the eye's own lens system needs to compensate for this. The images formed by both converging and diverging lenses for *distant* objects are *diminished.*

(b) *They may be real* (i.e. they may be projected on to a screen) or *they may be virtual* (they may not be projected on to a screen but may be seen, as in the image in a mirror or a simple magnifier). If rays are projected backwards, as described above, the image formed will be virtual. Note that all images formed by a *converging* lens are *real,* unless the object is between the lens and the focus, i.e. very close to the lens, and all the images formed by a *diverging* lens are *virtual.*

However, diverging lenses are used in spectacles. How can they form a real image? The answer is that the diverging lens forms only part of the system – it supplements what the eye's own lens system is doing.

(c) *They may be erect or inverted.* The images formed on the retina are inverted, but the brain turns the image back up the correct way.

The image in Fig. 12.6 is magnified, real and inverted. However, the nature of the image formed at any time depends upon the type of lens, the position of the object in relation to the focus, etc.

5. The refractive index (the ability of a material such as glass to refract light rays) will be a significant factor in all the above, since this will determine the extent of refraction of any light ray.

6. It is almost impossible to manufacture a perfect lens. Any flaws in materials or faults in curvature cause distortion of the image formed, even if very slight. For this reason, true double convex or double concave shapes are not used where high clarity of images is required, i.e. in spectacles, microscopes, etc. In these cases, lenses with complex shapes (a mixture of concave and convex or a shape that is more cylindrical) together with a mixture of plastics, glass and other materials, are used to overcome such problems. However, all such lenses are a compromise and some distortions still occur on the outer edges. For this reason, only the centre portion of the lens is normally used – this is just as true for the lens in the eye as for a camera lens.

(a) CONSTRUCTIVE INTERFERENCE. If the two waves (i) and (ii) are combined by adding the amplitudes at each point, the result is wave (iii). Note that crests and troughs coincide. This is constructive interference.

(i)

(ii)

(i) + (ii) = (iii)

(b) DESTRUCTIVE INTERFERENCE. If the same two waves are combined but with the crests and troughs in opposition, the result is (iii). This is destructive interference.

(i)

(ii)

(i) + (ii) = (iii)

Figure 12.7. Results of interference in sound waves.

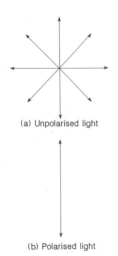

(a) Unpolarised light

(b) Polarised light

Figure 12.8. Planes of vibration of unpolarised and polarised light.

Interference

When any two waves meet, they may *interfere* with each other, and the final wave form produced will be the sum of the two individual wave forms. If two crests (or two troughs) coincide, *constructive interference* occurs and the amplitude of the result-ant crest is the sum of the amplitude of the two waves at that point, as shown in Fig. 12.7(a), i.e. the light is brighter.

If a trough and a crest coincide, *destructive interference* occurs and the amplitude of the resultant crest or trough is the sum of the amplitude of the two waves at that point, as shown in Fig. 12.7(b), i.e. the light is dimmer.

The colours we see in an oil slick on the road or in a soap bubble are produced by interterence of the colours which make up white light. Interference phenomena are very useful in detecting flaws and optical irregularities in lenses.

Polarisation

In transverse waves, the plane of vibration may be oriented randomly or it may be restricted to a single plane, as shown in Fig. 12.8. In Fig. 12.8(a), the vibration is shown as occurring in a number of different planes, but in Fig. 12.8(b) only one plane of vibration occurs. The light in Fig. 12.8(b) is said to be *plane polarised*.

If light is passed through material such as polaroid, which

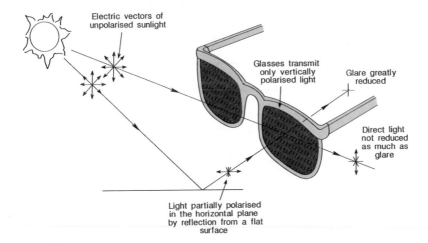

Electric vectors of
unpolarised sunlight

Glasses transmit
only vertically
polarised light

Glare greatly
reduced

Direct light
not reduced
as much as
glare

Light partially polarised
in the horizontal plane
by reflection from a flat
surface

has the capacity to polarise light, the light which formerly had unlimited modes of vibration can now vibrate in one direction only. In Fig. 12.9, the sunglasses have their polaroid lenses arranged so that only the light vibrating in the vertical plane can pass through them. This achieves two things:

1. *It reduces ordinary direct light* by one-half. To understand the reason for this, it is really necessary to consider vectors. However, suffice it to say that any mode of vibration can be resolved so that it has a vertical component and a horizontal component, When all these components are added together, one half of the light can be regarded as vibrating vertically and the other half horizontally.

2. Light reflected from a horizontal surface, such as a road surface, beach or water, tends to be *partially polarised* so that it is vibrating horizontally. Such horizontal vibrations are not able to pass through polaroid lenses, so that this light, and thus 'glare' is considerably reduced, as shown.

Colour

We have already made reference to the fact that white light is composed of a number of colours, which we try to describe by naming some of them.

These colours are easily produced by passing a ray of white light through a prism, as shown in Fig. 12.10.

In fact, no object is coloured. In a perfectly dark room, everything is black. Furthermore, a pure red object would look black when illuminated by blue or yellow light. What so-called 'coloured' objects can do is to absorb some colours and reflect others and it is these reflected colours that we see: this is called a 'subtractive' effect. To understand this, it must first be said that

Figure 12.9. The reduction of glare by polaroid sunglasses demonstrates the wave nature of light. (From Nave & Nave: *Physics for the Health Sciences.* 3rd Ed. Philadelphia. W.B. Saunders. 1985.)

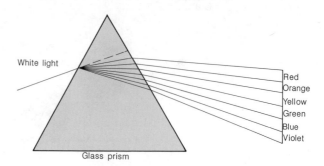

White light

Red
Orange
Yellow
Green
Blue
Violet

Glass prism

Figure 12.10. When white light passes through a prism, it is broken up (dispersed) into the colours of the spectrum. It is seen that red light is refracted least and violet light the most.

three primary colours of subtraction exist – *red, yellow* and *blue*. These are the three primary colours that artists use, and must be pure – they must have no colour other than the primary colour itself. This means that these colours will reflect light only from a narrow band of frequencies (or wavelengths).

If pure red light then falls on a jumper, the pigments of which can reflect red light only, the jumper will look red. If pure blue light falls on the jumper, it will look black, however, since the blue light will be absorbed and no red light is available to be re- flected. The same would occur if the jumper were illuminated by yellow light.

In practice, most objects show a colour that is a mixture. A 'red' jumper, for example, may have some yellow present, in which case it looks more orange than a 'red' jumper with blue present, which looks more violet. Note that it doesn't look violet, but it looks more violet than does the jumper with some yellow present. Many readers will be familiar with the fact that this happens only when the source of illumination has these colours present, such as white light. The colour of a jumper is observed to 'change' if illuminated by yellow light, for example.

Remember that it is the pigments used to dye the jumper that cause it to look 'red', a red that may have some yellow or some blue as well, or perhaps both. The *secondary* colours of subtraction are then:

- orange (red plus yellow),
- purple or violet (red plus blue)
- green (yellow plus blue)

The primary colours of *addition* are *red, blue* and *green*, and apply to spotlights in a theatre and to television receivers. The *secondary* colours of addition are:

- magenta (red and blue)
- yellow (red and green)
- cyan or blue-green (blue and green)

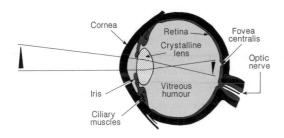

Figure 12.11. Image formation by the eye. (From Nave & Nave: *Physics for the Health Sciences*. 3rd Ed. Philadelphia. W.B. Saunders. 1985.)

All three added together (i.e. red, blue and green) give white. In addition, we are normally starting with pure colours and the light reflected simply adds together to give the colours indicated.

Some people are colour-blind – some eight per cent of men and about one to two per cent of women. Most are able to see only two of the three primary colours (usually yellows and blues) satisfactorily, but a small percentage sees everything in black and white only.

The cells that make up the retina of the eye (see Fig. 12.11, the retina is the light-sensitive lining of the back of the eye) are either rods or cones, the cones being the cells that make colour perception possible. The **cones** tend to be most concentrated around the central area of the retina, the fovea centralis, so that colour vision is at its best when one is looking directly at an object and almost non-existent in the far peripheral vision.

On the other hand, **rods** are much more effective in the dark, because they are more sensitive at low light levels. Animals, for example, have no cones in the retinas of their eyes and thus all cells in their retinas are rods. Animals therefore have excellent night vision, but having no cones, they are colour-blind. That much-maligned creature, the bull, responds to red rags no more than to rags of any other colour, since he is colour-blind!

The eye is able to adjust its sensitivity to light by a factor as great as 1 million. When light strikes the eye an image is formed on the retina, the nerve endings in the rods and cones transmitting electrical impulses along the optic nerve to the brain.

The Eye

Light from the sun or some other source travels to various objects, where it undergoes reflection. This reflected light can then travel towards the eye, where it passes through the cornea, the aqueous humour, the crystalline lens and the transparent vitreous humour before forming an image on the retina of the eye, as shown in Fig. 12.11. Nerve endings in the retina transmit electrical impulses along the optic nerve to the brain, which also turns the image the right way up.

The cornea of the eye is probably the most important refractive medium in terms of gross refraction. When we consider all the light rays striking the eye from many different sources at any one time, indeed not only from different sources but of different strengths, some rationalisation becomes necessary. Furthermore, the cornea, like the lens, is curved both in the vertical and the horizontal plane but is rarely perfectly curved, thus adding to the problem. The cornea has to do all the 'coarse tuning' and adjustment before the light rays enter the lens. The lens then does the 'fine tuning', adjusting for distance and increasing the sharpness and clarity of images, assisted by the gel-like humours.

The eye is also able to adjust for brighter or dimmer light by adjusting the size of the iris, and thus the size of the apperture or opening, which we call the pupil. When the pupil is large, more light can enter (e.g. in a dimly lit room), and when the pupil is small, less light enters (e.g. on a bright sunny day at the beach).

The other function the iris performs is to concentrate light rays to a greater degree after they emerge from the cornea. This serves to eliminate peripheral, disorganised and weaker rays, which only cause confusion and tend to prevent clear focusing.

The **ciliary muscles** surround the lens and are able to adjust the thickness of the lens by relaxing and contracting, so that it can be used to focus on very close objects or those in the far distance, as shown in Fig. 12.12. In the case of distant objects, the eye is able to focus by relaxation of the ciliary muscles, which enables the suspensory ligaments to contract, and the lens thus becomes thinner and less powerful. The focal length is lengthened in the process so that the focal point falls on the retina and the image is thus formed on the retina. This gives the lens of the eye an effective focal length of about 2.2 cm and a strength of about 45 dioptres. The thinner lens is all that is needed to focus the light rays on to the retina in this case, but in the case of a close object, the rays are more divergent and have to be 'pulled in', as it were, to focus on the retina.

If closer objects are being viewed, the ciliary muscles contract, thus allowing the suspensory ligaments to relax, and the lens becomes more rounded and more powerful. This has the effect of shortening the focal length of the lens, so that the focal point occurs on the retina. The formation of an image is illustrated in Fig 12.11.

As light passes through the four stages before forming an image, it undergoes refraction to some extent in all stages, but the

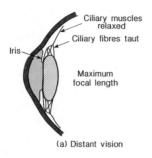

Ciliary muscles relaxed
Ciliary fibres taut
Iris
Maximum focal length

(a) Distant vision

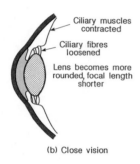

Ciliary muscles contracted
Ciliary fibres loosened
Lens becomes more rounded, focal length shorter

(b) Close vision

Figure 12.12. Accommodation of focus. (From Nave & Nave: *Physics for the Health Sciences*. 3rd Ed. Philadelphia. W.B. Saunders. 1985.)

major refraction occurs in the cornea and the lens. The cornea has a fixed focal length, whereas the lens is able to alter its focal length. It does this by changing the normally relaxed, almost spherical shape of the lens to a much thinner shape (with a shorter focal length), by contraction of the ciliary muscle. Thus the refractive power of the lens, i.e. the accommodation, is altered. In young children, the accommodation can be increased from about 15 dioptres to about 29 dioptres – a range of 14 dioptres. This decreases to about two dioptres in many people in the 45–50 age group. It is significant, however, that the eye retains some refraction, and thus some vision, even if the lens is removed. This is one reason why blindness occurs in varying degrees.

Convergence of the eyes

We are fortunate in having been designed with two eyes. One of the immediate benefits of such a system is that we enjoy **depth perception**. This is the facility that enables us to be able to estimate distances, as we commonly have to do when driving a car, for example. The situation is analogous to the spotlights in an auditorium, which can be manipulated to come together on a particular subject, but which require constant adjustment to maintain this situation when the subject moves. Our brain is able to interpret and co-ordinate the messages it receives from both eyes to enable us to estimate distance. This is not possible with one eye only.

It is important that the two eyes function together as 'partners', moving together and producing clear, sharp images that co-ordinate the two images into a single *clear*, final image.

Artificial lenses and the eye

The ideal optical condition of an eye, in which parallel rays focus precisely on the retina, is described by the term *emmetropia*. If parallel rays fail to come to a focus on the retina, a condition known as *ametropia* is present. This term includes myopia, hyperopia and astigmatism, each of which is subsequently described.

In some defects of vision, the light rays do not focus properly on the retina, resulting in various effects such as blurring, distortion or shadowing of the images. This may occur because of abnormalities in the lens system or in the shape of the eyeball. The effects of **myopia** or 'short-sightedness' and **hypermetropia** (hyperopia) or 'far-sightedness' in focusing in front of and behind the retina, respectively, are shown in Fig. 12.13, together with the lenses that are used to correct such defects.

In Fig. 12.13(a), it may be seen that the rays from a distant object have converged in front of the retina. In this case the

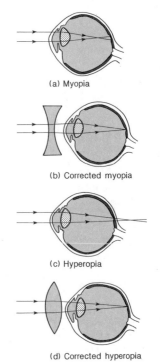

(a) Myopia

(b) Corrected myopia

(c) Hyperopia

(d) Corrected hyperopia

Figure 12.13. The use of lenses to correct common eye defects.

eyeball is usually too long, or the lens system may be too strong, giving rise to a focal length that is too short to be able to focus on the retina. This means that even when the ciliary muscles are completely relaxed, the lens is still not 'weak' enough to allow distant objects to be focused. However, as the object is brought closer to the eye, a point is reached at which the image will focus on the retina, assisted by the accommodation of the eye as the object moves nearer.

It is thus necessary to *diverge* these rays more, so that they now converge at the retina. This myopia (short-sightedness) is corrected as indicated in Fig. 12.13(b), enabling the owner of the eye to focus distant objects more clearly.

In Fig. 12.13(c), the two light rays have not converged on the retina, but rather at a theoretical point behind the retina, because the eyeball is too short or the lens system is too weak when the ciliary muscle is completely relaxed. In this situation, distant objects can be focused on the retina by the accommodation powers of the eye, i.e. the ciliary muscles contract. However, the capacity of these muscles to contract is limited, so that the accommodation of the eye may be insufficient to enable it to focus on objects brought closer to it.

This hyperopia (long-sightedness) is corrected by a converging lens, which causes the light rays to converge and form an image on the retina, thus assisting the focusing of near objects.

With the onset of middle and old age, some changes in the lens occur, for example, a loss of elasticity or **presbyopia** often giving rise to long-sightedness as part of the ageing process.

Very commonly, the lens of the eye has different focal lengths in different planes, so that an object such as a window appears to be out of shape. This arises from defects in the curvature of the cornea. These defects may be on any axis – that is vertical, horizontal or diagonal. This is a problem that often goes unrecognised in children, frequently until well into their school years, when they experience problems reading a book or the board.

Figure 12.14. (a) Astigmatism. It may be seen that the focal length of the horizontal plane (f^1) is not the same as the focal length of the vertical plane (f). This means that the image formed on the retina is distorted. (b) Fan chart (see text).

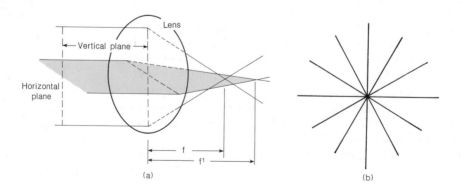

(a)   (b)

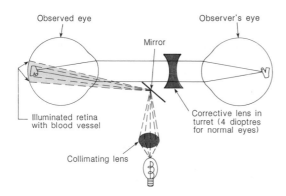

Figure 12.15. The optical system of the ophthalmoscope. (From Guyton: *Textbook of Medical Physiology.* 6th Ed. Philadelphia. W.B. Saunders 1981.)

This defect is known as **astigmatism** and can be detected by means of a fan chart, such as that shown in Fig. 12.14. To a person with normal vision, the lines of the chart appear equally dark, but to a person with astigmatism, some of the lines appear darker than others. Astigmatism is corrected by using a cylindrical lens – a special lens formed like a cylinder with the curvature adjusted to compensate for the corneal defects.

Apart from the correction of defects of vision, lenses can be used to assist the eye. Instruments such as the simple magnifier, the microscope and the ophthalmoscope (used for detailed examination of the eye – see Fig. 12.15) all use lenses to achieve their object, i.e. to provide a magnified image.

Light and lenses are used extensively in many medical instruments and have proved invaluable in the examination of internal tracts and cavities of the body. These instruments have the general name **endoscopes** and include:

- Bronchoscopes, which are used to examine the lungs and bronchi.
- Gastroscopes, which are used to examine the gastrointestinal tract.
- Cystoscopes, which are used to examine the bladder.

An endoscope is essentially a fairly long, rigid, metal tube with an optical system (utilising light and lenses) which, when inserted down or up a passage, allows the area of concern of be viewed and specimens to be obtained. Instruments which utilise optical fibres are now in use.

The Electromagnetic Spectrum

Visible light, X-rays, radar, radio waves, microwaves, infra-red and ultra-violet rays all form part of what is called the

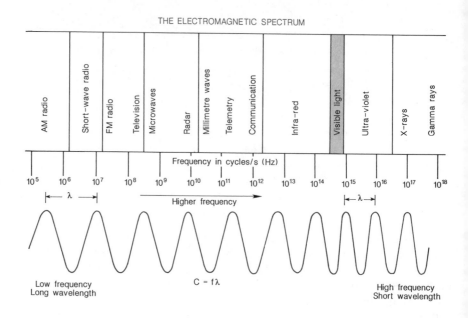

THE ELECTROMAGNETIC SPECTRUM

Figure 12.16. Types of electromagnetic waves.

electromagnetic spectrum, and these different types of radiation are called **electromagnetic waves**. All these waves:

- Have frequencies, wavelength and amplitude, as shown in Fig. 12.16.
- Do not require a 'material medium' for their propagation, i.e. they are able to travel through a vacuum (at the same speed, 3×10^8 m/s).

The electromagnetic spectrum is shown in Fig. 12.16.

We will now look at some of these types of radiation and discuss their relevance and application to the human body and clinical work.

Infra-red radiation

This term covers a wide range of frequencies (very much wider than visible light, for example), as may be seen in Fig. 12.16. The portion of the infra-red section of the electromagnetic spectrum that is used in most medical applications is the 'near' end – the portion closest to visible light and having wavelengths from 750 to 3000 nanometres (a nanometre is 10^{-9} m).

The heat emitted from any hot object is essentially infra-red radiation. Infra-red lamps are sometimes used for heat therapy, especially on patients with musculoskeletal disorders, but the rays do not penetrate very deeply, so that these lamps are not suitable where warming of deep tissues is desired. However, since infra-red light penetrates the skin, veins and other structures that are invisible to the eye can be photographed using infra-red photography. This technique has also been used in diagnostic studies of the eye and for studying healing patterns under certain scabs.

Another technique known as **infra-red thermography** relies on the fact that the body gives off heat, and that temperature variations shows up as varying amounts of radiation. This enables early detection of breast cancer, for example, since the temperature of a tumour will often be one to two degrees Celsius higher than that of normal tissue and can be as much as five degrees higher. This then shows up in a pictorial representation of the infra-red radiation given out by the body, which is normally displayed on a cathode-ray oscilloscope screen, as used in heart monitors. This same technique can also be used for the examination of burns and frostbite, for checking on the vitality of skin grafts and for checking the blood flow to particular areas such as the limbs when vascular disorders are in question or after surgery for such.

Ultra-violet radiation
In this case also, the radiation in which we are essentially interested is at the 'near' end of the spectrum – from 250 to 400 nanometres. The sun is a strong source of ultra-violet radiation, but fortunately most of this radiation of wavelengths below 300 nanometres is screened out by atmospheric gases and the ozone layer. In passing, it should be noted that any depletion of the ozone layer by aerosols or high-flying jet aircraft may have very serious consequences.

Since these shorter wavelengths are injurious to tissue, it is just as well that this absorption does occur, and it should be noted that those rays which are not absorbed are responsible for sunburn. Some of the higher frequency rays are thought to be implicated as a cause of skin cancer.

Sun-blocking agents have chemicals such as zinc or titanium oxides present, which prevent the penetration of ultra-violet radiation and thus prevent sunburn. The extent to which people are burned by ultra-violet radiation depends on the amount of a pigment called **melanin** in the skin – those with a high melanin content being much less susceptible to sunburn than those with a low melanin content. Albinos are particularly susceptible because of the lack of melanin in their skin.

Ultra-violet radiation does not have high penetration and thus can be used therapeutically in the treatment of such skin conditions as psoriasis and acne. Since this radiation is also effective in killing fungi and bacteria, it has been used to kill these organisms on the skin and in the sterilisation of instruments and operating theatres.

The part of the body most susceptible to damage from ultra-violet radiation is the eye. 'Snow-blindness' and the acute inflammatory conditions caused by looking at the electric arc produced in electric welding both result from the effects of ultra-violet radiation.

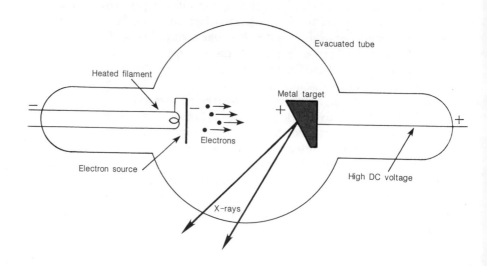

Figure 12.17. X-ray production. (From Nave & Nave: *Physics for the Health Sciences.* 3rd Ed. Philadelphia. W.B. Saunders. 1985.)

X-ray radiation

This form of radiation has wavelengths falling in the range 10 to 10^{-2} nanometres. It is produced by accelerating electrons through high voltages and directing them towards a metal target, as shown in Fig. 12.17. The formation of a picture depends upon the fact that various tissues are penetrated to different extents by X-rays, bones being the most resistant to penetration. Substances such as barium sulfate strongly resist the penetration of X-rays and thus find considerable use in providing contrast in the stomach and gastrointestinal tract, for example in the form of barium meal.

It should also be mentioned that X-rays have a cauterising (destruction of tissue) effect.

It is important for the reader to appreciate, that while the benefits of X-rays for diagnostic purposes generally far outweigh the risks, risks *do* exist.

These *risks are greater with the X-ray fluoroscope* (an instrument that permits visual observation of the form and motion of the deep tissues), since the patient is exposed to X-rays for a greater length of time than with a photograph. However, this device is very useful in observing the motion of internal parts of the body.

A more sophisticated approach is provided by the **CT scan**, or computed tomography scan. If used in an axial plane (normally a 'slice' about one centimetre thick through the patient's body), this is then called a computed axial tomography scan, or CAT scan (Fig. 12.18). The basic principle is that a very large number of thin X-ray beams are passed through the body from many different directions in the plane of the 'slice' to a particular point at which they all meet, and a similarly large number of detectors pass information for storage into the memory of a computer, some thousands of points being examined within a few seconds of expo-

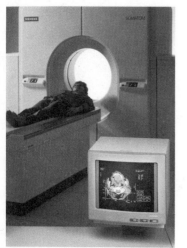

Figure 12.18. A CAT scanner. (Courtesy of Medical Applications P/L)

sure time. The computer is then able to iron out distortions and produce a display on a television monitor or a photograph. This technique is very much more sensitive and produces a better picture than standard X-ray methods.

Much progress has been made recently, however, in the use of other techniques that do not expose the patient to ionising radiation and its hazards (which are discussed later). These include ultrasonic scans and NMR (nuclear magnetic resonance) techniques, although the latter is more often called MRI (magnetic resonance imaging), since the word 'nuclear' has other connotations.

The great promise that MRI offers concerns its demonstrated greater sensitivity in detecting malignancies, ischaemic regions (regions where the blood supply is deficient) and other functional changes in the tissue of an organ before they have progressed so far that gross anatomical changes have been produced. Note that, as a comparison, CAT scans are effective only in these later stages, since it is necessary for gross anatomical changes to have occurred before detection is possible with a CAT scan.

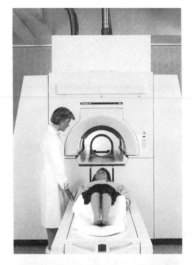

Furthermore, the contrast between grey and white matter in the brain is much distinct with MRI, while the image is almost unaffected by bone, and thus by the skull (Fig. 12.19). This applies equally well to the spine, where even a vertical sagittal (front-to-back) image can be produced. Computer technology can then be combined with the detailed imaging data to produce a cross-sectional image in almost any plane, or a sequence of these to give a 'slice' effect. From this a clinician can calculate the exact size of a tumour, for example. Further advances will no doubt arise as research progresses.

Lasers
This is an acronym for Light Amplification by Stimulated Emission of Radiation. The medical importance of lasers arises from the fact that these light rays can be concentrated into a very narrow, parallel beam of light. It is also possible to focus the beam even further to an almost microscopic point, with an extraordinary concentration of energy at that point.

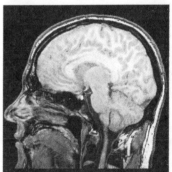

One of the most significant applications of laser technology has been in ophthalmology, in the treatment of haemorrhages of the retina, retinal detachments and tears, and some other retinal conditions. If the haemorrhage occurs in the fovea centralis, where many of the colour receptors (cones) are located, the advantages of the capacity of the laser to be focused on an area with a diameter of only 50 micrometres is obvious, since this area is only about 1000 micrometres in diameter. Earlier xenon technology was able to focus to only 500–1000 micrometres. (A micrometre is 10^{-6} or one-millionth of a metre.) The other outstanding feature of the laser is that the pulses are less than a millisecond in length and thus many more doses can be administered in each treatment session.

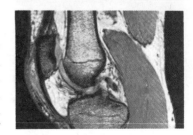

Figure 12.19 (a) (top) An MRI scanner. **(b and c).** Examples of MRI images. (Courtesy of Medical Applications P/L.)

The laser beam has a cauterising effect and this, together with the very accurate focusing possible with this beam, means that bloodless surgery is possible, at least in some specific applications. The removal of birthmarks and tattoos has been achieved with lasers. The laser can induce coagulation and clotting, and thus is most useful in the control of haemorrhage and also has a photocoagulation effect, i.e. it alters protein in tissues. Ordinary light rays can be utilised for this purpose, but not as effectively, in the treatment of a detached retina. The laser incites a thermal inflammatory response in the specific area, leading to localised adhesions between the retinal and the underlying coat, along with other responses.

Various types of lasers have been developed, and research will no doubt eventually result in many other clinical applications of this fascinating technology.

One other application of laser technology should be mentioned – holography. This is a technique whereby a three-dimensional image of an object is produced (and may be recorded), in such a way that the object can be viewed from any direction in the horizontal plane. Furthermore, magnification can be achieved.

Fibre optics

This technology offers a considerable advance on the bronchoscopes, cystoscopes and similar instruments developed for viewing internal tracts of the body. A **'light pipe'** is used, consisting of a bundle of light fibres, each of which is able to transmit its own small piece of information (Fig. 12.20). When the small pieces of information from each of a large number of light fibres are added together, an image is formed, in the same

Figure 12.20. A bundle of very thin fibres, each acting like a light pipe, will transmit an image if the arrangement of the fibres is the same at both ends. (From Greenberg: *Physics for Biology & Pre-Med Students*. Philadelphia. W.B Saunders. 1975.)

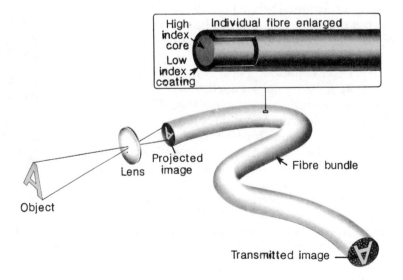

High index core
Low index coating
Individual fibre enlarged

Object
Lens
Projected image
Fibre bundle
Transmitted image

way that a photograph in a newspaper is produced from a large number of dots. A lens system is used at each end, and the light pipe can be considered to consist of a large number of flexible, parallel glass rods that conduct the light from one end to the other. These instruments are very useful when doing biopsies or minor surgical procedures in deep internal tracts or areas, e.g. in some sterilisation procedures in women.

One of the outstanding advantages of the light pipe is its flexibility, enabling it to follow the change of direction of an internal tract of the body. Together with the fact that these pipes are available in lengths in excess of three metres, they offer tremendous advantages in the applications described.

SOUND

Stress is a word at the forefront of today's societies. It is sometimes seen as a 'disease' of our fast-paced, highly competitive society and a reflection of living in crowded cities with large urban sprawls.

One of the factors that has been found to contribute to stress is **sound**, particularly in the form of noise. Noise can be difficult to define, since one person's music can be another's noise, and a crying baby can elicit love from one person and physical abuse from another. One of our tasks in this chapter is to examine the properties of sound, some of which will help us to define noise in general, including an awareness of an individual's perception of what constitutes noise.

Although sound can have such negative effects, it is a major contributor to our survival, to the progress of civilisation and to the aesthetic aspects of life that give us pleasure and help us to develop into fuller, more complex, human beings.

One wonders where we would be without this particular form of communication. It could be assumed that we would be in relative isolation, living in a silent world without the benefit of the spoken word, music, birds and so on. Yet many in today's society abuse sound in such a way that such isolation may seem a relief – isolation from excessively loud stereos, noisy vehicles and motor mowers, etc.

This chapter should assist the reader to develop an understanding of sound, its uses in medicine and some of its abuses which have led to hearing problems. Many opportunities exist in nursing, particularly for the community and industrial nurse, to participate in the promotion of hearing conservation, to assist in the detection of hearing disabilities and to intervene in hazardous situations in this area.

We have made reference to longitudinal progressive waves as the means by which sound is propagated. (Refer to Fig. 12.1) In the case of sound waves, the following properties are observed:

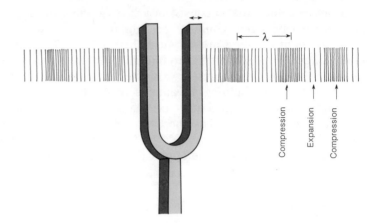

Figure 12.21. The vibration of an elastic object produces sound waves.

1. Sound is transmitted by particles that vibrate backwards and forwards in the direction of propagation, i.e. in the direction in which the wave is travelling. These can be regarded as pressure waves.

2. It follows as a consequence of (1) that a *material medium* must be present, that is a substance (solid, liquid or gas) which can provide the particles, which can then vibrate. It also follows that a sound wave cannot travel through a vacuum.

Properties of Sound

Production
Sound is produced by a *vibration*. Fig 12.21 illustrates the production of sound by the vibrating prongs of a tuning fork.

In this case the prongs of the tuning fork vibrate backwards and forwards, as shown by the arrows. Each outward movement of a prong causes the air to be compressed in its path, giving rise to a **compression**, whereas each inward (return) movement causes the pressure of the air behind the prong to be lowered, giving rise to a **rarefaction** (expansion). This process continues, forming a series of compressions and rarefactions (expansions) and thus a longitudinal progressive wave. This wave carries **energy.**

In the above example, the vibrations occur in the prongs of the tuning fork but they may be produced in strings, where the vibrations are fairly easily observed, as with the guitar, violin or piano; or in a column of air as with the trumpet, organ or clarinet; and in a complete object such as the triangle. In the two latter cases the vibrations are not so easily observed. In the body, sound (i.e. voice) is produced by the vibration of vocal cords in the larynx.

The larynx is a cartilaginous structure in which the vocal ligaments or vocal cords are controlled by an extensive system of muscles. The vocal cords are actually folds along the walls of the larynx and produce sounds of varying pitch, depending upon the tension of the cords and the shape and mass of the vocal cord edges.

Transmission

This will depend upon the medium through which the sound is travelling: in air (at 0°C) sound travels at 331 m/s, but in iron it travels at about 4900 m/s, and in sea water at 1540 m/s. It will be noted that in air the speed is temperature-dependent, the speed increasing by about 0.6 m/s for every degree Celsius above 0°C. However, the frequency and amplitude do not affect speed.

Reception

Our sound receptors are, of course, the ears. We are provided with two of these for a good reason: just as the two sources of a stereo sound system not only enable us to hear sound, but give us the impression that sound is coming from different parts of the room, so our ears give us stereo hearing and enable us to detect the *direction* of the source of a sound.

The direction from which a sound has come is determined by two main mechanisms:

1. By the time lag involved between the reception of the sound in one ear and the reception of the sound in the other ear. If a sound comes from the right, for example, the right ear hears the sound before the left ear and the brain then collates this information and relays it back so that we recognise the direction of the source of the sound. If the sound comes from in front, for example, both ears hear the sound together.

2. By the difference in intensity of the sounds that are heard by the two ears.

The exact location of the sound, especially in the presence of other sounds, may require turning of the head.

The ear is illustrated in Fig. 12.22. It consists of a collecting system (the pinna and auditory canal), an amplifier (some of the structures of the inner ear), a processing system (the cochlea) and a transmitting channel (the auditory nerve). The human ear is normally able to detect sounds having a frequency range of 20 to 20 000 Hz, with the greatest sensitivity in the range 2000 to 5500 Hz. It has a remarkable sensitivity, sometimes being able to detect changes of frequency as low as 1 Hz, and it is also very sensitive to the 'quality' of a sound or musical note.

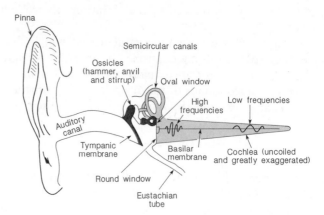

Figure 12.22. Sketch of a human ear with cochlea uncoiled. (From Nave & Nave: *Physics for the Health Sciences*. 3rd Ed. Philadelphia. W.B. Saunders. 1985.)

Resonance

Any object has its own natural frequency of vibration. While it will vibrate at other frequencies, it will vibrate most vigorously at its own frequency. Thus, if a note is played that has the same frequency the object will also start vibrating, sometimes to such an extent that the results can be serious. On one occasion, the gusts of wind in a storm happened to occur at just the same rate as the natural frequency of a bridge and the bridge collapsed. Soldiers are always given a command to break step when crossing a bridge for this reason – if the frequency of their marching is the same as the natural frequency of the bridge, the results could be disastrous for both the bridge and the soldiers!

These are all examples of **resonance** – *the tendency of one object to vibrate 'in sympathy' with another* – an effect that is most marked at the natural frequency of the object. The famous opera singer Caruso was able to shatter wine glasses by singing a note of the same natural frequency as the glass, causing it to resonate and then shatter.

Musical instruments often use a sounding board or a sounding chamber to produce resonance and thus improve the quality of the sound of the instrument. In a similar way the larynx uses the mouth, nose, the associated nasal sinuses, the pharynx and sometimes even the chest cavity as resonators.

The basilar membrane (see Fig. 12.22) has a number of fibres associated with it which vary in their degree of stiffness, which means that different fibres can resonate to different frequencies. The mass of the fluid in the cochlea also varies in different localities and so responds to different frequencies, in this way assisting the generation of resonance. Thus the higher frequencies of the basilar membrane resonate near the base of the cochlea and the lower frequencies resonate near the apex of the cochlea, as shown in the diagram. Intermediate frequencies resonate between these two extremes.

Pitch
Pitch, for most purposes, is related to the frequency of a note. However, there is a subjective element involved, in that pitch tends to depend on the individual's perception of that note as being 'high' or 'low'. Furthermore, following our discussion above, the major method used by the nervous system to detect different pitches is by determining the position along the basilar membrane that is stimulated the most, or that resonates the most. This is called the 'place principle'.

The pitch of a sound emitted by the vocal cords can be changed in two different ways:

1. By stretching or relaxing the vocal cords. A high note is achieved by stretched vocal cords and a low note by relaxed vocal cords.
2. By changing the shape and mass of the vocal cord edges. They become sharp and thin to emit high frequency sounds but thicken and increase their mass to emit low frequency sounds.

Pitch is therefore dependent on frequency and the following general principles apply to objects that produce sound (including the vocal cords):

1. The *higher* the frequency, the *higher* is the pitch of the note produced, and vice versa.
2. The *higher* the tension in a body that is stretched (such as a string), the *higher* the pitch (all other things being equal).
3. The *higher* the mass of a given length of string, the *lower* is the note produced (all other things being equal).
4. The *shorter* the vibrating medium (such as a length of string), the *higher* is the note produced (once again, all other factors being equal, since these factors all depend on each other and all determine the pitch of the note produced).

Loudness or volume
The auditory system determines loudness in at least three different ways:

1. As the sound becomes louder, the amplitude of vibration of the basilar membrane and hair cells also increases, so that the hair cells excite the nerve endings at an increased rate.
2. As the amplitude of vibration increases, it causes more and more of the hair cells on the fringes of the vibrating part of

the basilar membrane to become stimulated, resulting in transmission of impulses through a larger number of nerve fibres.

3. Some of the hair cells do not become stimulated until the vibration of the basilar membrane reaches a relatively high intensity, once again reflecting the fact that the sound is loud.

Measurement of sound intensity or loudness utilises the decibel scale.

The decibel scale

This scale enables a *quantitative comparison* to be made *between 'loud' and 'soft' sounds*. Because of the enormous range of intensity of sound that the human ear can detect (the loudest sounds are more than 10^{12} times the intensity of the softest sounds that can be heard), a logarithmic scale is used. This means that a sound level of 100 decibels is not 20 times greater than a sound level of 80 decibels, but 10^2 or 100 times as great. This may be seen in Table 12.1.

Table 12.1 Typical decibel levels for normal sounds

Decibel level at 1000 Hz		Multiple of threshold intensity
160	Bursting of eardrum	10^{16}
140	Severe pain	10^{14}
120	Pain threshold	10^{12}
100	Damage to hearing after prolonged exposure; average factory, loudest passages of orchestra for close observer (*fff*)	10^{10}
80	Class lecture, loud radio	10^8
60	Conversational speech	10^6
40	Very soft music (*ppp*) typical living room	10^4
20	Very quiet room	10^2
0	Threshold of hearing	1

From Nave & Nave: *Physics for the Health Sciences.* 3rd Ed. Philadelphia. W.B. Saunders. 1985.

Noise or music?

As previously stated, this distinction is inclined to be very subjective. However, a working definition may be stated as follows:

Noise does not have definite pitch or steadiness and its nature tends to change, but musical notes are identified by definite pitch, regularity and smoothness.

Reflection

When a sound wave arrives at a barrier between two different media such as air and water, air and concrete or air and human tissue, part of the sound wave is reflected and part is usually absorbed and/or transmitted by the new surface. Some surfaces reflect a considerable amount of the incident sound, giving rise to *echoes*.

Refraction

When a sound wave passes from one medium to another, as described above, its direction of travel changes because its velocity in the new medium is different from that in the old medium.

Interference

Just as interference occurs with light waves, similar effects are observed with sound waves, and both constructive and destructive interference may occur. With *constructive* interference, the sound becomes *louder*, and with *destructive* interference, the sound becomes *softer*.

Furthermore, if the frequencies of two sound waves are very similar but not quite the same, *beats* may be heard. This is a waxing and waning effect produced by the addition of the two sound waves that musicians utilise in tuning their instruments.

The Doppler Effect

The speed of sound in air is quite rapid, but slow enough to be affected by any relative motion between the source and the observer. If a train that is sounding its hooter sweeps by, a distinct change in the pitch of the note is heard by a stationary observer as the train passes. A similar effect can often be noticed with ambulance and police sirens, even though the pitch is already changing as a result of the siren itself.

If the observer is moving, again there is a similar effect. For example, a passenger on a train notices a drop in pitch of the sound produced by a railway bell that is clanging at a level crossing.

This effect is illustrated in Fig. 12.23. In case (a), the sound emitted by the stationary source has a frequency of 330 Hz. Sound has a velocity in air of 330 m/s and the sound reaches the observer at a velocity of 330 m/s. The distance between successive compressions (represented by shadings) is the wavelength of the sound wave and is equal to 1.0 m.

In case (b), the source is emitting sound of the same frequency, but is moving towards the observer at a velocity equal to half the speed of sound. This means that the compressions are reaching the observer more rapidly than before, and with a greater frequency than before – because of the combined effect of

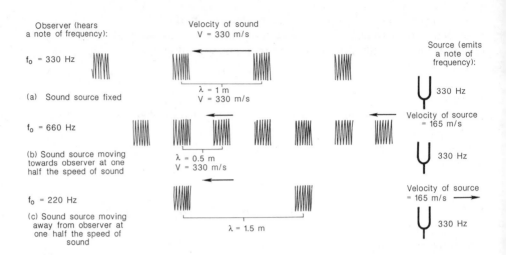

Observer (hears a note of frequency):

f_o = 330 Hz

(a) Sound source fixed

f_o = 660 Hz

(b) Sound source moving towards observer at one half the speed of sound

f_o = 220 Hz

(c) Sound source moving away from observer at one half the speed of sound

Velocity of sound V = 330 m/s

λ = 1 m
V = 330 m/s

λ = 0.5 m
V = 330 m/s

λ = 1.5 m

Source (emits a note of frequency):

330 Hz

Velocity of source = 165 m/s

330 Hz

Velocity of source = 165 m/s

330 Hz

Figure 12.23. The Doppler effect. The frequency heard by the observer depends on the relative motion of the sound source with respect to the observer. Thus a note of frequency 330 Hz is heard as a frequency of 330 Hz in case (a), 660 Hz in case (b) and 220 Hz in case (c). Note the entities shown above are meant to represent the 'crests' of waves, which each form part of an *extended wave*.

the velocity of sound and of the observer, both moving towards the observer. The observer then hears a note of *higher* frequency, i.e. 660 Hz.

In case (c), the source is emitting sound of the same frequency, but is moving *away from* the observer at a velocity equal to half the speed of sound. This means that the compressions are reaching the observer less rapidly, and with a lower frequency than before – because of the combined effect of the velocity of sound towards the observer and the velocity of the source away from the observer. The observer then hears a note of *lower* frequency, i.e. 220 Hz.

In medicine, the Doppler effect can be utilised to assist the diagnosis of the thromboses. The instrument determines the velocity of blood flow by measuring the apparent difference in frequency between an emitted signal and a received signal after reflection from a moving red blood cell. If a blood clot is present, blood flow is restricted in the vessel, the red blood cell slows down and this registers on the instrument. This new reading may indicate the position of a clot or thrombus.

Sound in Medicine

Ultrasonics

Brief reference has already been made to ultrasonics. Frequencies above the range of normal hearing are utilised, and use is made of echoes in a similar way to the use of sonar for locating schools of fish and submarines. Sonar is just a sound wave that is reflected from the fish or submarine and indicates the presence of same. In a similar way, some body tissues reflect these waves more than others.

The pattern of reflections produces a 'picture' of internal body structures. This technique is particularly useful in obstetrics and shares none of the dangers of X-rays (Fig. 12.24). A 'picture' of the fetus is thus gained, enabling a determination of its size, location, position and sometimes even physical abnormalities (Fig. 12.25). This provides useful information for the doctor and patient in making decisions regarding the progress of the pregnancy, preparation for delivery or labour, and potential problems.

It is also used to locate tumours, cardiovascular disorders and eye defects. Ultrasonic scanners employing the Doppler effect are used to study heart motion and function, the passage of blood through major arteries and fetal heart sounds.

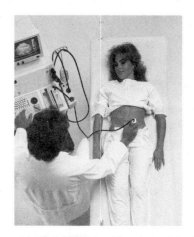

Figure 12.24. An ultrasound scanner being used in an obstetrics applications. The scan may be seen on the monitor. (Courtesy of Medical Applications P/L.)

Ultrasonic Lithotripsy

This technique has the great advantage of being non-invasive and thus much less traumatic than the surgery which it can replace in some 90–95 per cent of all renal pelvis and upper ureter stones.

The principle of this technique depends on the generation of a shock wave which is concentrated in the region of the location of the stone. This wave is transmitted through a fluid in a specially designed bath or, with newer machines, a fluid cushion or a belt and is then transmitted through tissues with a high water content. On reaching the stone, however, release of energy from the shock wave causes the stone to gradually disintegrate. However, since 500 to 1500 shock wave impulses could be required, anaesthesia may be necessary.

A great deal of work is being done overseas utilising this technique with gallstones, so that it may be expected that this application will also increase in this country.

Stethoscopes

These are really very simple instruments in which the 'bell' acts as a small sound detector that amplifies the sound of a heart beating or the passage of air in and out of the lungs. The amplified sound is passed through the tubes to both ears in the same way that sound is passed through air, and the vibrations are then registered by the user's ears.

Hearing aids and deafness

Deafness may be classified into several types:

1. **Sensorineural** or **nerve deafness** is caused by a malfunction of neural structures in the inner ear, the auditory nerve to the brain or in the brain itself. Apart from other causes, this may result from a cerebrovascular accident (or 'stroke').

2. **Conduction, canal** or **transmission deafness** results from

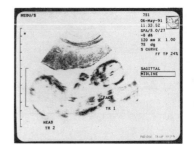

Figure 12.25. The outline of triplets is visible in this ultrasonic scan. (Courtesy of Diasonics P/L.)

impairment of the outer and/or middle ear mechanism so that sound is not transmitted into the cochlea.

A common cause of conduction deafness in young children is chronic middle ear infections.

3. **Mixed deafness** results from disturbances to both the conductive and the nerve mechanisms.

4. **Functional deafness** has an emotional or psychological origin. In this case there is no organic lesion evident.

Hearing aids often produce good results with conduction deafness, since the bone can act as a conductor to take sounds (which the hearing aid amplifies) through to the auditory nerve, which is still functioning satisfactorily in this type of deafness. The **bone conduction test**, whereby the stem of a vibrating tuning fork is placed on the mastoid process behind the ear, is used to help determine whether deafness is of the conduction or the nerve type and thus whether a hearing aid or surgery is required. The audiometer, an instrument capable of emitting pure tones of varying frequencies, is used to determine more exactly the nature of the disability.

This is important to help decide the nature of possible treatment, as prostheses (artificial substitutes) are available to replace parts of the middle ear, as well as various types of hearing aids.

Sensorineural deafness, which results from disturbances of the inner-ear neural structures or nerve pathways leading to the brain, has been particularly common in industry and some types of business due to the level and/or consistency of noise. This type of deafness often leads to loss of the higher frequencies of speech (2–4 kHz) so that most consonants are not heard – the sufferer hears only muffled vowel sounds. A hearing aid is usually of no help in this type of deafness.

Preventive programmes in the field of industrial or occupational health have reduced the occurrence of these types of hearing injuries. Various methods have been used to lower noise levels such as the use of sound-absorbing materials, isolating high level noisy machines as much as possible, utilising sound insulation on machines, or parts of machines, and keeping machines in good working order by oiling, repairing, etc., as required.

People working in such environments should be directly protected by the use of ear plugs or special ear muffs designed to reduce sound entry, and even by placing large shields over the entire head, as in jet-engine factories, mining (where explosives are employed) and in gunnery in the armed forces. This is very much the concern of the industrial and occupational health nurse. Such a nurse to also responsible for periodic hearing checks, which are essential in high noise conditions.

Injury to hearing that occurs in teenagers as a result of electric amplification of modern music – 'disco deafness' – is also common among people who work in clubs etc. It is also found that problems are occurring with the use of earphones operated from radios and stereo systems. These are especially dangerous where young people go about wearing them for long periods. The sound is always completely directed into the ears and is not dispersed throughout a room, and as a result hearing deficiencies may follow. This provides opportunities for health teaching since many parents are not aware of these facts.

Sounds can also be irritating at low levels, often because they are consistent, periodic and regular. These can cause problems, to which people respond by becoming irritable and stressed. Illness, for example, can reduce the capacity of the individual to cope with the stress induced by noise – from the sound of trolleys, floor polishers, voices, footsteps and even dripping taps at night, together with constant background noise from cars, trains, buses, trucks, loud music in shops, road works and crying babies.

Nurses are also very involved in screening for hearing problems in schools, baby health centres, etc.

In conclusion, it can be seen that a knowledge of the properties of light and sound is most important for the practising nurse to work effectively, particularly in relation to the prevention of sight and hearing disabilities.

REVIEW

1. Select those properties of light which have some relationship to vision and discuss these relationships in terms of the structure of the eye.
2. A friend informs you that the school nurse thinks that her son may be myopic and asks for an explanation. What would you say?
3. Some types of electromagnetic waves are being used to benefit humans in the course of diagnosis and treatment of various disorders. Discuss these in terms of their positive uses and negative effects.
4. In your role as a community health nurse, you have been asked to give a talk to parents on the causes and prevention of sight and hearing losses. Outline some of the points you would make.
5. Many advertisements are being run which recommend the use of chemical sun-blocking agents and other sun-blocking measures. (a) Why it is considered important to reduce exposure to the sun? (b) How do chemical sun-blocking agents function?
6. A patient who is to receive laser treatment for a partial retinal detachment asks for an explanation of what a laser is and what it will achieve for him. How would you answer?
7. How is the Doppler effect used in medicine?

13

Electrical activity in nerve and muscle cells

OBJECTIVES

After studying this chapter students should be able to:

1. Draw a diagram of a resting nerve cell, showing the distribution of charge in terms of the concentration of Na^+, K^+ and negative ions on either side of the membrane.
2. Fully describe the generation of an action potential and the stages called depolarisation and repolarisation.
3. State the 'all-or-nothing' principle, and define the terms 'threshold' and 'refractory period', indicating both portions of the latter.
4. Draw diagrams to illustrate the passage of an action potential along both myelinated and unmyelinated neurons, and contrast the speed of transmission of an impulse in each.

INTRODUCTION

A child reaches out, touches a hotplate on a stove, immediately withdraws his hand, begins to cry and, clutching the injured hand, runs away from the stove to his parent. Later a blister forms in the burnt area.

What was involved in this situation? How did the body detect the heat, determine that it was of an intensity to be dangerous or damaging, decide what actions to take, initiate an immediate response, and a later response to seek further safety and comfort? Although the situation appears simple and straight-forward, it is indeed complex, involving many responses – physiological, physical, emotional and psychological, some responses having been learned, others being automatic.

However, a major factor here is the involvement of the body's extensive communication system which picks up or senses the changes at the skin surface and carries this information to the spinal cord and brain. This system is also responsible for carrying the response demands to other areas or systems, such as the musculoskeletal system, voice box, tear ducts, etc. We have discussed electricity, which involves the flow of electrons along wires to create changes – producing heat, light and movement. Now we will see that this concept underlies an understanding of the communication of information and its comprehension in and by the body.

The communication system we are thinking of is the 'nervous system' and the passage of information throughout the nervous system is based on electrical changes and movement. You will find that major differences exist between electric current flowing to a light bulb in a home and electric current in the body flowing to the brain. The conducting medium is also very different: a solid inanimate, metallic wire, compared to fluids and live cells. What is flowing is likewise different – electrons compared to charged ions. However, in each case, electrical potential is created in order for flow and change to occur, and this is the subject of this chapter.

It is not the function of this book to deal with the complete physiology of nerves, which is quite complex, but very satisfactorily treated in many physiology textbooks.

However, it *is* the function of this book to deal with those aspects of the operation of nerves that involve an appreciation of the importance of such things as:

- Ions and the result of the movement of these.
- The potentials which occur in cells.
- The application of our knowledge of electricity to cell situations, both in the resting cell and the activated nerve.

We have already described an electric current as a flow of electrons. Thus when a current is flowing along a wire, the movement of electrons constitutes an electric current. In solution (and thus in the body), the *movement of charges* also constitutes an electric current. However, in the body or in a solution, the moving charges are *ions*, which may be positively or negatively charged and can be of different types, e.g. Na^+, K^+, Ca^{2+}, Cl^- and HCO_3^-. The ions will not move of their own accord, but require an electrical potential or some other influence (such as a *concentration gradient*) to drive them. From Chapter 11 it will be recalled that an electrical potential exists between two points when there is a difference in the state of charge of those points and this difference can cause a current to flow. This means that an electric current can flow in body cells by virtue of the *movement of ions*. Remember that pure water does not conduct electricity, but becomes a conductor when ions are present. Being aware of these facts, we can proceed to study electrical activity in the human body cell and its purpose. Before doing so, however, a brief examination of chemical cells will assist further understanding of electrical activity in the human cell.

CHEMICAL CELLS AND ELECTRICITY

To understand what happens in living cells, we need first to consider non-living chemical cells.

An arrangement such as that shown in Fig. 13.1 shows the use of chemical cells (or galvanic cells) to produce electricity from a chemical reaction. The arrangement consists of a piece of zinc rod dipping into a solution of Zn^{2+} [zinc (11)] ions and SO_4^{2+} [sulfate] ions and a copper rod dipping into a solution of Cu^{2+} [copper (11)] ions and (SO_4^{2-}) ions.

The two rods are connected by wires to a voltmeter as shown. To complete the electric circuit, the arrangement includes a 'salt bridge', which simply contains an electrolyte and is separated from the beakers by cotton plugs. The latter permit the slow migration of positive and negative ions.

Figure 13.1. A typical electrolytic cell based on the reaction Zn(solid) + Cu^{2+} (aq) → Zn^{2+} (aq) + Cu(solid).

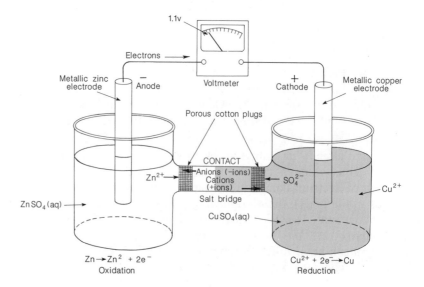

The zinc rod tends to dissolve slowly, so that zinc passes into the solution, giving up electrons to the zinc rod in the process, i.e.

$$Zn \longrightarrow Zn^{2+} + 2e^-$$
(a *loss* of electrons – oxidation)

This means that the zinc rod now has a *surplus* of electrons and is *negatively charged*.

At the same time, in the other beaker, copper ions from the solution are being deposited on the copper rod, taking electrons from the copper rod in the process, i.e.

$$Cu^{2+} + 2e^- \longrightarrow Cu$$
(a *gain* in electrons – reduction)

This means that the copper rod now has a *shortage* of electrons and is *positively* charged.

We have then set up a potential difference, which causes electrons to flow as shown, thus constituting an electric current.

The movement of the positive and negative ions in solution through the salt bridge completes the electric circuit to enable this to happen. In this sense, we can regard these ions as charge carriers, forming part of the electric current in the circuit. If these ions did not move, the electrons would *not* be able to flow and no current would flow.

The rods used are called **electrodes**. The negative electrode is called the **cathode** and the positive electrode is called the **anode**.

Negative ions move towards the anode and are called **anions**.

Positive ions move towards the cathode and are called **cations**.

The cotton plugs that have been used should be noted. In living cells, a membrane acts in the same way, with the important difference that the cell membrane is able to *change* its permeability to the movement of ions, i.e. it is able to inhibit or enhance the movement of ions by changing pore sizes, as was discussed in Chapter 6. This will be most important in the discussion of nerve cells.

THE RESTING CELL IN THE BODY

Electrical Activity in the Cell

If an electrode is inserted into any resting cell (as distinct from a cell engaged in the transmission of a nerve impulse, for example) and if another electrode is inserted into the surrounding intracellular fluid, and these electrodes are then connected to

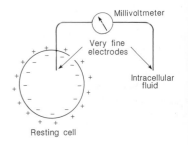

Figure 13.2. A voltage is observed between a resting cell and the intracellular (or extracellular) fluid.

a millivoltmeter, a reading is obtained (Fig. 13.2). The actual value of the reading may range between about 5 and 100 mV, depending on the particular chemical environment of the cell and the type of cell.

The reading obtained, which represents the difference in electrical potential between the inside and outside of the cell, i.e. between the inside and outside of the cell membrane, is called the **resting membrane potential** (RMP).

Development of an electric potential across a cell membrane

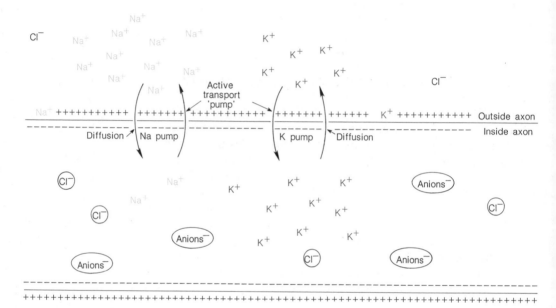

Figure 13.3. Diagram of part of a cell. We see that the active transport mechanisms which were described in Chapter 6 as 'pumps' maintain a higher concentration of $Na^+_{(aq)}$ ions outside the cell than inside and a lower concentration of $K^+_{(aq)}$ ions outside than inside. The 'pumps' have to work to maintain these concentrations since the ions tend to move (as shown) to restore the balance, by diffusion. The particular anions shown are produced within the cell by catabolism and consist of large molecules such as proteins which cannot get out because of their large size. (From Solomon & Davis: *Human Anatomy & Physiology*. Philadelphia. Saunders College Publishing. 1983.)

The situation in a resting nerve cell is illustrated in Fig. 13.3.

The following factors are involved in the development and maintenance of an electrical potential:

1. All of the ions shown are aquated, i.e. since the ions carry a charge, they attract water molecules (probably four), and these four molecules of water 'cling' to the ion so that the whole thing moves around as a single entity. These are represented as $Na^+_{(aq)}$, $K^+_{(aq)}$, $Cl^-_{(aq)}$, etc, where 'aq' means 'aquated'. The reason for this attraction is that water develops a slightly negative end and a slightly positive end. The slightly negative end arises because oxygen 'loves' electrons, so that the electrons tend to move towards the oxygen end, leaving the hydrogen end slightly short of electrons, as shown in Fig. 13.4(a).

Thus water becomes a **dipole** (having two poles – one negative and the other positive). Positively charged ions will then form a chemical bond with the negative end, as in Fig. 13.4(b).

Negatively charged ions will then form a chemical bond with the positive end, as in Fig. 13.4(c).

In Figs 13.1 and 13.3, therefore, the ions shown should be represented as being aquated. (This is omitted for convenience.) One noteworthy point is the fact that $K^+_{(aq)}$ is *smaller* than $Na^+_{(aq)}$. This should be borne in mind when considering diffusion through membranes, e.g. in the caption to Fig. 13.3.

2. The concentration of $Na^+_{(aq)}$ ions *outside* the cell (i.e. in extracellular fluid) is *greater* than that inside the cell in the normal cell. The situation is maintained by the sodium 'pump':

(a) Thus, since sodium ions will tend to move down the concentration gradient, they will tend to move *into* the cell, if given the opportunity.

(b) In Fig. 13.3, we see that a larger concentration of *negative* ions exists inside the cell, compared to the outside, in which a larger concentration of *positive* ions existed compared to the inside. This difference in ion concentration gives rise to an *electrical potential* or an *electrical gradient*. Since an electric gradient also exists, the $Na^+_{(aq)}$ ions will tend to move down the electric gradient. Once again, this means that $Na^+_{(aq)}$ ions will tend to move *into* the cell, given the opportunity.

Some $Na^+_{(aq)}$ ions do, in fact, diffuse in, as shown, but these are removed by the sodium pump, that is by active transport.

3. The concentration of $K^+_{(aq)}$ ions inside the cell is greater than the concentration of these ions outside the cell.

(a) Since the potassium ions tend to move *down* a concentration gradient, they will tend to move *out of* the cell, given the opportunity.

(b) Since an electrical gradient also exists, the $K^+_{(aq)}$ ions will tend to move down the electrical gradient. This means that $K^+_{(aq)}$ ions will tend to move *into* the cell, given the opportunity.

Thus we have a situation where a concentration gradient is trying to drive $K^+_{(aq)}$ ions *out of* the cell, while the electrical gradient is trying to push $K^+_{(aq)}$ ions *into* the cell. These two factors tend to operate quite independently of one another – so it appears that the strongest will win.

Potassium ($K^+_{(aq)}$) ions also do have the opportunity to move into or out of the cell, since they are small and can fit through pore spaces in the membrane. Their smaller size means that they are able to move more freely than $Na^+_{(aq)}$ ions.

The electrical driving force tending to move $K^+_{(aq)}$ ions *into* the cell is not as strong as the concentration gradient or driving force tending to move $K^+_{(aq)}$ ions *out of* the cell, so that $K^+_{(aq)}$ ions tend to diffuse *out of* the cell (see Fig. 13.5).

However, the $K^+_{(aq)}$ pump simply accounts for this by pumping the same number of $K^+_{(aq)}$ ions back *into* the cell to maintain the initial concentrations of $K^+_{(aq)}$ inside and outside the cell. That is the sodium and potassium pumps remove two

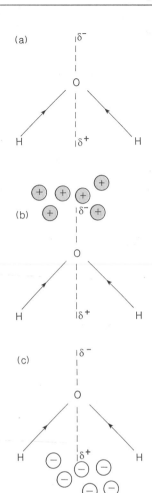

Figure 13.4. The dipole nature of water. (a) A water molecule. The arrows indicate the direction in which electrons tend to move, causing the oxygen end of the molecule to become slightly negative (δ^-) and the hydrogen end to become slightly positive (δ^+). This means that the molecule functions as a DIPOLE (having two poles) – a negative pole (δ^-) and a positive pole (δ^+). (b) Positively charged particles (ions) are attracted to the negative end of the dipole water molecule. (c) Negatively charged particles (ions) are attracted to the positive end of the dipole water molecule.

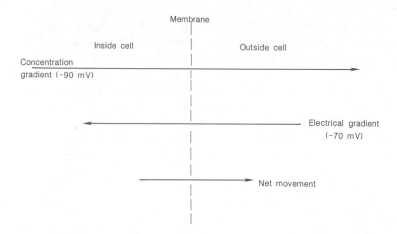

Figure 13.5. Movement of potassium ions into and out of a cell, showing the opposing influences of the concentration gradient and the electrical gradient. Since the former has a 20 mV greater electrical potential, the net movement of ions is in the direction shown.

sodium ions for every potassium ion that is pumped back, which maintains a high concentration of sodium ions outside the cell and a low concentration of sodium ions inside the cell.

This helps to maintain the normal resting membrane potential of the cell, that is the state of affairs whereby *the inside of the cell is negatively charged and the outside is positively charged.*

4. The negative ions involved are as follows:

- chloride ions;
- large non-diffusible anions such as proteins and phosphate ions; and
- hydrogen carbonate (bicarbonate) ions.

The concentration of chloride ions ($Cl^-_{(aq)}$) outside the cell is very much larger than the concentration of these ions inside the cell, but no chloride pump exists. This means that the migration of $Cl^-_{(aq)}$ ions in and out of the cell is passive and in equilibrium, i.e. the rate of movement of $Cl^-_{(aq)}$ ions into the cell is equal to the rate of movement of $Cl^-_{(aq)}$ ions out of the cell so that the overall concentration of $Cl^-_{(aq)}$ ions inside and outside the cell remains constant. The different concentrations arise partly because of the repulsion of $Cl^-_{(aq)}$ ions by other negative ions inside the cell.

5. The remaining ions in the cell are simply shown as anions and consist mainly of proteins and phosphate ions, together with hydrogen carbonate ions. The protein and phosphate ions are large ions, which are not normally able to pass through the membrane. They are formed by cellular activity in sufficient numbers to outnumber the positive ions within the cell and thus

make the inside of the cell negative with respect to the outside (the extracellular fluid).

The hydrogen carbonate ion $HCO_3^-{}_{(aq)}$ is able to pass through the membrane but is not significant in the maintenance of the resting membrane potential or the transmission of signals along nerve fibres. In other situations, for example the red blood cell in plasma, $HCO_3^-{}_{(aq)}$, is very significant indeed.

6. In conclusion, we see that a difference in potential exists between the inside and the outside of the cell of about *70 mV*. Since the inside of the cell is negative this is expressed as -70 mV.

This difference in potential means that the ions involved (e.g. $K^+{}_{(aq)}$, $Na^+{}_{(aq)}$) possess potential energy, since they are influenced by the electric potential to try to move into or out of the cell.

Remember that, because $K^+{}_{(aq)}$ ions are smaller, they tend to move much more freely than $Na^+{}_{(aq)}$ ions.

Should this situation change, however, i.e. should the permeability of the cell membrane to $Na^+{}_{(aq)}$ ions increase, the $Na^+{}_{(aq)}$ ions would be able to move in and *decrease* the potential difference. The potential energy of these ions would then be changed to kinetic energy (energy of movement).

Furthermore, the previously *polarised* cell (having a potential difference) would then be *depolarised* (having lost this potential difference).

Development of an Action Potential

1. Depolarisation
If the resting cell membrane is disturbed in some way, changes occur in the permeability of the membrane, resulting in the creation of an electrical signal. A stimulus in a receptor (the cones of the retina, for example) will cause such a disturbance and thus give rise to an electrical signal. This signal or pulse is called an **action potential** and is initiated when pores in the disturbed region of the nerve cell membrane – called *sodium channels* – allow sodium ions to pass into the cell. In fact, the permeability of the membrane to sodium ions is considered to be increased 5000-fold. Thus we have the first stage of our theory or model of the generation of an action potential. This stage is called **depolarisation** and arises by virtue of the *rush of sodium ions into the cell*. The sudden influx of positive charges neutralises the negative charges inside the cell and **removes the resting membrane potential**.

However, the rush of sodium ions does not stop immediately depolarisation (i.e. neutralisation of the negative charge) is achieved. In fact, an 'overshoot' occurs and the inside of the cell becomes more positive than the outside. This accounts for the change in the electrical polarity or electrical state of the cell, from negative to positive.

Another change then occurs in the *permeability* of the membrane. It now becomes almost impermeable to sodium ions, but much more permeable to potassium ions. This means that the cell is in a state of depolarisation and cannot accept another impulse or action potential.

2. *Repolarisation*

Since the permeability of the membrane to potassium ions has now increased, potassium ions move to the outside because:

(a) The higher concentration of potassium ions and the greater number of positive charges now inside the cell, compared to the outside, means that potassium ions flow down a *concentration* gradient.

(b) The fact that the outside of the cell is now negative means that the potassium ions can now also flow down an *electrical* gradient.

As the potassium ions begin to flow out, **repolarisation** occurs. This represents the *changing of the electric potential of the cell from positive back to negative*. This change results from the loss of potassium ions from inside the cell, making the inside of the cell once more negative compared to the outside of the cell (Figs 13.6 and 13.7).

3. *Restoration of ion concentrations to normal state*

The final step in the restoration of the cell to its former state is to restore the balance of sodium and potassium ions. While the cell has now regained its electrical condition (the resting membrane potential), the concentration of sodium ions inside the cell is higher than normal, as is the concentration of potassium ions outside the cell.

The restoration occurs by means of the sodium-potassium pump, which moves two sodium ions out for every potassium ion that it moves in.

4. *The normal state*

The cell remains in this normal resting state until the next disturbance or stimulus is received. Three other points should be made:

(a) The changes we have described occur initially in the region of the disturbance. From that point, the changes then affect adjacent regions on both sides, so that the disturbance is rapidly transmitted to other parts of the nerve cell membrane.

(b) The number of sodium ions and potassium ions involved in these processes compared to the total number of ions in the locality is very slight indeed. It should be remembered that when

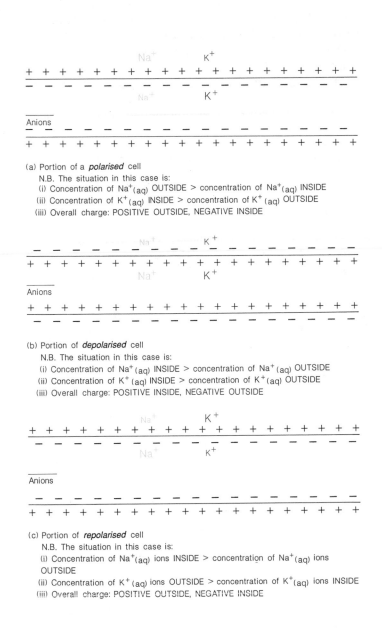

Figure 13.6. Portions of (a) a polarised cell (b) a depolarised cell and (c) a repolarised cell, showing the electrical state of the cell membrane in each case, as a result of ion concentrations.

(a) Portion of a *polarised* cell
   N.B. The situation in this case is:
   (i) Concentration of $Na^+_{(aq)}$ OUTSIDE > concentration of $Na^+_{(aq)}$ INSIDE
   (ii) Concentration of $K^+_{(aq)}$ INSIDE > concentration of $K^+_{(aq)}$ OUTSIDE
   (iii) Overall charge: POSITIVE OUTSIDE, NEGATIVE INSIDE

(b) Portion of *depolarised* cell
   N.B. The situation in this case is:
   (i) Concentration of $Na^+_{(aq)}$ INSIDE > concentration of $Na^+_{(aq)}$ OUTSIDE
   (ii) Concentration of $K^+_{(aq)}$ INSIDE > concentration of $K^+_{(aq)}$ OUTSIDE
   (iii) Overall charge: POSITIVE INSIDE, NEGATIVE OUTSIDE

(c) Portion of *repolarised* cell
   N.B. The situation in this case is:
   (i) Concentration of $Na^+_{(aq)}$ ions INSIDE > concentration of $Na^+_{(aq)}$ ions OUTSIDE
   (ii) Concentration of $K^+_{(aq)}$ ions OUTSIDE > concentration of $K^+_{(aq)}$ ions INSIDE
   (iii) Overall charge: POSITIVE OUTSIDE, NEGATIVE INSIDE

(d) The *repolarised* cell is then restored to the situation in (a) by means of the sodium–potassium 'pump'

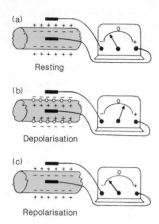

we speak of large concentration changes, we are speaking of large *relative* concentration changes: that is, concentration changes that are important in terms of the *balance* of charge and concentration, but not in terms of the *total* number of ions present.

(c) The mechanisms of these processes are not well understood. However, it is also known that calcium ions are involved in some of the changes of membrane potential, particularly in cardiac conducting cells.

Figure 13.8 illustrates the appearance of an action potential on an oscilloscope, when the electrodes of that instrument are inserted into a nerve:

- The point A shows the normal resting membrane potential of about −70 mV.
- The section of the curve labelled AB illustrates *depolarisation*.
- The section of the curve labelled BC represents the overshoot.
- The section of the curve labelled CD represents the *repolarisation* phase.

Physiology of the Nerve Cell

Before proceeding further, we will digress to consider some definitions and to briefly examine the structure of a nerve cell.

Figure 13.7. Sequential events during the passage of an action potential. A, the normal resting potential, which is negative. B, the development of a positive potential during depolarisation and C, the restored normal resting membrane potential after repolarisation. (From Guyton: *Textbook of Medical Physiology.* 6th Ed. Philadelphia. W.B. Saunders. 1981.)

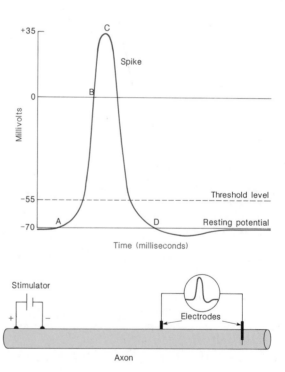

Figure 13.8. An action potential recorded with one electrode inside the cell and one just outside the membrane. When the axon depolarises to about −55 mV, an action potential is generated. (From Solomon & Davis: *Human Anatomy & Physiology.* Philadelphia. Saunders College Publishing. 1983.)

A **nerve cell** or **neuron(e)** is the basic unit of neural tissue and consists of an axon, a cell body and dendrites (see Fig. 13.9).

An **axon** or **nerve fibre** is the process along which impulses travel away *from* the cell body. It is usually considerably longer than the dendrites.

A **dendrite** is a branched process that carries impulses *to* the cell body.

The **cell body** is the central structure of a neuron and contains a nucleus and many other organelles. It performs all the functions that keep the nerve cell alive and operative.

A **nerve** is a collection of nerve fibres (axons and/or dendrites) held together by connective tissue. It conveys impulses between the central nervous system (brain and spinal cord) and another part of the body.

Myelin is a lipid substance which forms a sheath around the axons of the same nerve fibres and acts as an electrical insulator. These axons are then described as being *myelinated*. Gaps in the myelin sheath around axons are called **nodes of Ranvier**. As we will see, they are important when the transmission of nerve impulses is considered.

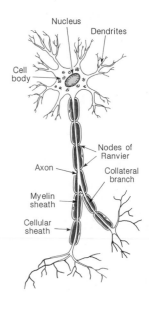

Figure 13.9. Structure of a multipolar peripheral neuron.

Special Characteristics of Nerve Cells

Excitability

A **stimulus** is a physical or chemical change in the environment which may cause an individual or nerve cell to respond in some way. It may be electrical, mechanical, thermal, chemical, or caused by light or sound.

The special ability of nerve cells to respond to stimuli and effectively convert these into nerve impulses (i.e. electric signals) is called **excitability**.

Any substance, such as acids, bases or strong salt solutions, that causes sodium ions to begin to diffuse through the membrane by increasing the permeability of that membrane will generate an electrical signal. This is **chemical stimulation**.

It will be seen during a study of physiology that some substances, called neurotransmitters, have the property of being able to change the chemical environment, and thus the permeability of cell membranes, at the junction of two nerves – called a synapse. The same applies at the junction of a nerve and a muscle – called a neuromuscular junction or myoneural junction. Acetylcholine is such a substance.

If we crush, pinch, prick or even (in some cases) exert slight pressure on some nerve fibres, an influx of sodium ions into the cell will occur. This is **mechanical stimulation** and an electrical signal will be generated.

Electrical stimulation will also give rise to an electrical signal, since a flow of sodium ions into the cell *may* occur. As an example, if we touch the spark plug of a car or motor mower while the engine is running, an electric current is transmitted into the body causing electrical disturbances to nerve membranes.

Thermal stimulation once again gives rise to an inward flow of sodium ions into the cell, as a result of the influence of heat on some nerve cell membranes. Remember the child touching a hotplate on a stove in our introduction?

The same concepts apply to the other types of stimuli. The reader may like to take note of the important fact that, like all animals (including the simplest), we consist of a mass of cells. However, in the human being these cells are usually specialised in function. Nerve cells are highly specialised to respond to the stimuli discussed. In fact, there is further specialisation within the response to stimuli, so that some nerve cells have one kind of receptor (mechanical) and others have other kinds (pain, light, etc), and this helps the brain to differentiate between stimuli. Other cells in the body are specialised to perform other functions, e.g. skeletal muscle cells to move bones, and so on.

All-or-nothing principle

We have spoken above of the types of stimuli that lead to the generation of an electrical signal. However, some stimuli are so weak or faint that we are not able to detect them. Why is this?

It is a direct consequence of the all-or-nothing principle, which simply says that a neuron fires or it doesn't. There are no half measures. The stimulus must be strong enough to cause the cell membrane's permeability to $Na^+_{(aq)}$ ions to increase sufficiently so that they flow through the membrane and cause depolarisation. It is simply not possible for the stimulus to generate a weak or partial electrical signal in a neuron. Note, however, that it is possible to have some neurons (nerve cells) stimulated (and thus firing) and others not stimulated (and thus not firing). It is also possible to have a series of signals passing through single neurons, subject to the restrictions imposed by the refractory period.

Refractory Period

After the passage of an impulse (electrical signal) through a nerve fibre, the nerve fibre is *inactivated* and unable to conduct another signal for the period of time that the cell takes to 'recover'. This period of time is called the **refractory period** and is covered by the portion of the curve CD in Fig. 13.8.

The refractory period has two components:

1. The *absolute* refractory period is a period of time during which no conduction is possible, no matter how strong the stimulus. In the human body, it lasts for or about one millisecond

(0.001 s) but ranges between about 0.5-15 milliseconds. This is the period of time during which the nerve cell membrane is *depolarised*.

2. The *relative* refractory period is a further period of time during which conduction is possible, but it requires a much stronger stimulus than would normally be required. This usually lasts about one to two milliseconds and is the period of time during which the nerve cell membrane is *repolarising*.

Threshold

The weakest stimulus that will still cause a nerve cell to fire is described as being at the **threshold level**. Any stimulus *above* this level will cause the permeability of the cell membrane to $Na^+_{(aq)}$ ions to increase and cause depolarisation. Any stimulus *below* this threshold level will not cause the permeability change in the cell membrane required to permit $Na^+_{(aq)}$ ions to flow and thus will *not* cause depolarisation.

During the relative refractory period, then, the threshold value or level is much higher than normal and a much stronger stimulus will be necessary to cause the permeability change in the cell membrane that allows the $Na^+_{(aq)}$ ions to flow.

The normal threshold level is about -55 mV, as shown in Fig. 13.8. This means that depolarisation will occur if the stimulus is sufficiently strong to generate an electrical potential of about 55 mV. Below this value, a slight local disturbance of the cell membrane will occur, but full depolarisation will *not*.

Transmission of an Action Potential

Unmyelinated Neurons

Firstly, we will consider a length of the axon of a neuron that is in its normal resting state (Fig. 13.10). If the axon then receives a stimulus in the middle of the section shown, transfer of ions will occur as indicated by the arrows, causing depolarisation to occur outwards in *both* directions. The portion of the area first stimulated is in its refractory period, as is each portion of the axon which is behind the 'wave' of depolarisation in each direction. Thus the signal (i.e. the action potential) is transmitted each way as a wave of depolarisation which cannot change direction – it cannot go backwards.

This illustrates an important point, that the *direction of flow of an action potential is away from the site of stimulation*.

Normally, however, action potentials are generated by stimulus at one end of the nerve cell and travel towards the other end.

A typical case is represented in Fig. 13.11, and explained in the caption, the direction of action potential travel being indicated by the arrows.

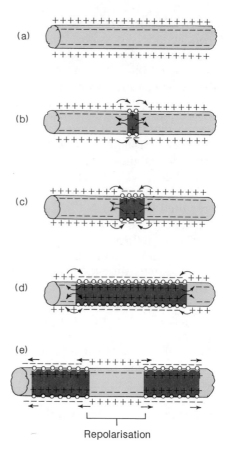

(a)

(b)

(c)

(d)

(e)

Figure 13.10 A, B, C & D – propagation of action potentials in both directions along a conductive fibre. E – propagation of repolarisation in both directions along a conductive fibre. (From Guyton: *Textbook of Medical Physiology*. 6th Ed. Philadelphia. W.B. Saunders. 1981.)

Repolarisation

Myelinated Neurons

The same general principles apply for myelinated nerve fibres, with the important difference that depolarisation can occur only at the nodes of Ranvier. Since myelin is adipose (fatty) tissue, it is an electrical insulator, so that depolarisation cannot occur in any portion of the axon that is covered by a myelin sheath. At the nodes of Ranvier, however, no myelin exists and depolarisation can occur. Transmission of the action potential then occurs in a similar way, but the electrical charges have to 'jump' across the myelinated section between the nodes, as indicated by the curved arrows in Fig. 13.12.

This type of jumping transmission is called **saltatory transmission** or conduction. Two advantages of this means of conduction of an action potential are:

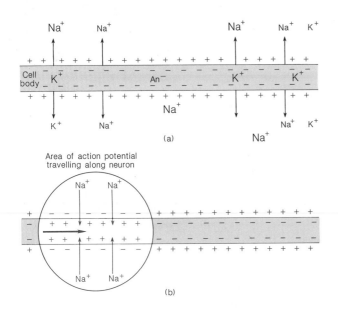

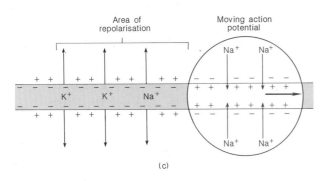

Figure 13.11. Transmission of an impulse along an axon. (a) The dendrites (or cell body) of a neuron are sufficiently stimulated to depolarise the membrane to firing level. The axon in (a) is shown still in the resting state. (b) and (c) An impulse is conducted as a wave of depolarisation that travels down the axon. At the region of depolarisation, sodium ions diffuse into the cell. As the impulse passes along from one region to another, polarity is quickly re-established. Potassium ions flow outward until the resting potential is restored. Sodium is slowly pumped back out of the axon so that resting conditions are re-established.

1. That much less energy is used by the cell in restoring resting conditions once the impulse has passed.

2. The speed of transmission is increased (see below).

If the myelin sheath is damaged and/or destroyed, severe problems occur with nerve impulse transmission, which may be slowed or stopped. Of the disorders that primarily affect the myelin sheath, **multiple sclerosis** is one of the commonest.

The cause of multiple sclerosis is unknown, but it has been attributed to autoimmune mechanisms (destruction or damage being done by the body's own defence systems), infection by a slow virus, toxic agents (metallic poisons), trauma, metabolic elements (myelin-splitting factor[s] in the blood) and vascular

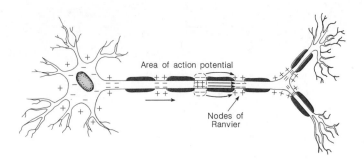

Area of action potential

Nodes of
Ranvier

Figure 13.12 Saltatory conduction. In a
myelinated axon the impulse leaps along from
one node of Ranvier to the next.

lesions resulting from abnormal blood clotting mechanisms.

This disease is characterised by disseminated (scattered)
patches of demyelination in the brain and spinal cord. The
degeneration of the myelin results in hardening of the tissues
(sclerosis).

The resulting problems are variable, develop slowly and
progressively, and are characterised by periods of remission
(lessening or abatement of symptoms) and exacerbations (increase or aggravation of symptoms). The symptoms of the
disease include such problems as weakness of the extremities or
even total paralysis, spasticity, mental changes such as apathy
and poor attention span, loss of co-ordination, visual disturbances (e.g. double vision, nystagmus – involuntary, rapid rhyth-
mic movements of the eyeball), impairment of bladder control
and many others, depending on the nerves affected.

Speed of transmission
The speed of transmission of an action potential in an unmyelinated fibre is of the order 1 m/s and can be as low as 0.5 m/s. On
the other hand, the speed of propagation in a myelinated fibre is
of the order 100 m/s, and can be as high as 130 m/s, which is
equivalent to about 470 km/h!

Apart from whether or not the axon is myelinated, factors
affecting the speed of transmission include:

1. The diameters of axons. Axons with large diameters
normally conduct faster than those with smaller diameters.
2. The degree of myelination – the greater the myelination,
the faster the action potential is transmitted.
3. The distance between the nodes of Ranvier – the further
they are apart, the faster is the transmission.

Note: Our discussion so far has centred upon transmission of
action potentials in axons. It should be noted that the dendrites
of some neurons, notably sensory neurons, have sections between

the cell and the dendrite end that are identical to axons and may be myelinated in just the same way.

REVIEW

1. Discuss the importance of the following characteristics of nerve cells to daily living: (a) excitability (b) the all-or-nothing principle (c) absolute and relative refractory periods.
2. In what way(s) do $Na^+_{(aq)}$, $K^+_{(aq)}$ and protein ions contribute to the transmission of a nerve impulse?
3. If a myelinated nerve lost all or much of its myelin sheath, what effects would this have on the transmission of an action potential in that nerve?
4. Describe the generation of an action potential in terms of:
   (a) depolarisation (b) repolarisation (c) restoration of the resting membrane potential.
   Draw a diagram of an action potential, labeling each section in terms of (a), (b) and (c).
5. Water is a most important compound in the body. Many of its properties depend upon hydrogen bonding. Explain what this is and how it arises. .

14

Radiation – therapy and diagnosis

OBJECTIVES

After studying this chapter students should be able to:

1. Describe radioactivity and ionising radiation.
2. Compare and contrast the properties of alpha particles, beta particles and gamma radiation.
3. Describe the changes that occur in an atom of an element as it undergoes each of these types of decay.
4. Define radioisotopes and describe their diagnostic and therapeutic applications.
5. Outline the factors that determine tissue susceptibility to radiation.
6. Define half-life and discuss the implications of this in medical treatments.
7. List and detail the safety precautions that must be observed whenever radioactive materials are being used.

INTRODUCTION

Whenever the word 'radiation' is mentioned, people tend to associate the term with nuclear war, nuclear weapons, disposal of nuclear waste, horrendous devastation and sickness. These are all highly emotional and controversial issues that seem to be arousing people all around the world. Certainly the question of the use of radiation in relation to its possible, devastating effects is something about which all individuals and communities ought to be concerned.

However, there is also no doubt that materials that produce certain types of radiation are very effective in various specific roles in the field of medicine, e.g. cancer treatment and diagnosis. Many people owe their lives to it.

A problem that many health personnel, including nurses, may face is fear concerning their own safety and that of others when they first come into contact with the use of radiation. Quite often the individual has been exposed more to the negative aspects of radiation than to its exact nature, its many positive uses and the well-established controls and policies concerning its use in medicine. Frequent questions arise not only in the mind of the nurse, but also in that of visitors and patients. For example:

— If my patient is receiving radiation for treatment or diagnosis will I be in danger of exposure or contamination?

— Is it safe to touch or go near the patient?

— Will the patient's belongings and room become radioactive from the patient?

— Can it be passed on from one person to another?

— Will I be radioactive after my treatment? (patient)

— Will I be able to have visitors? (patient)

Unfortunately, unnecessary fears and accidents may arise from a lack of sufficient knowledge and understanding, the results of which can be destructive, damaging or stressful for both nurse and patient. The patient may not receive the quality and level of care to which he or she is entitled, he or she may be left very much alone, specimens might be collected incorrectly or not collected at all, extra stress may be added by a nurse's fears, and so on. The nurse may fail to follow instructions regarding the care of the patient and disposal of the patient's wastes, the care of therapy sites or the procedure for radioactive inserts.

The specific nursing care related to the individual patient and treatment plus individual hospital policies concerning the handling and disposal of radioactive materials will vary, but the basic scientific principles will be the same. It is our role here to examine these principles in terms of the nature of radiation, the forms used in medicine and the general implications of its usage in these areas. Specific care and policies or procedures will be found in hospital manuals and nursing or specialised texts.

Revise those sections of Chapter 4 that dealt with the structure of the atom, atomic number, mass number, etc., and the discussion of electromagnetic radiation in Chapter 12, before proceeding further.

It is important for the reader to remember that we have discussed much of the chemistry of elements and have emphasised that this is dependent upon the *arrangement of electrons* in an atom. Electrons can now be ignored, because we are going to be looking at nuclear reactions, in which the structure of the nucleus is important; that is we are essentially interested in both the absolute and the relative numbers of protons and neutrons in the nucleus.

THE NATURE OF RADIATION

Radioactivity may be defined as the spontaneous emission of particles and electromagnetic radiation. This happens spontaneously because the nuclei of the isotopes of some elements are unstable (they break up) and *decay* (in a radioactive sense). **Isotopes** have been defined as atoms which have the same number of protons but different numbers of neutrons in their nuclei.

Isotopes that are radioactive are called **radioisotopes**. A limited number occur naturally, such as uranium-235 and uranium-238, while the majority with which we will be concerned are produced artificially in a nuclear reactor by bombarding a stable isotope with neutrons. As an example, a stable isotope of cobalt is bombarded with neutrons to produce radioactive cobalt-60, an unstable isotope.

Types of Radioactive Decay

Three important types of radioactive decay exist: alpha, beta and gamma.

Alpha (α) Decay
Alpha particles are helium nuclei ($^4_2$He), i.e. helium atoms that have lost their electrons, leaving a nucleus consisting of two protons and two neutrons. The first example of an alpha-emitter is uranium-238. This isotope spontaneously emits α particles:

$$^{238}_{92}U \longrightarrow ^{234}_{90}Th + ^4_2He$$

This equation represents the radioactive decay of uranium-238, to leave thorium-234, with the emission of an alpha particle ($^4_2$He). If we look at the atomic masses, we have:

$$238 \longrightarrow 234 + 4 = 238$$

Thus the overall sum of the atomic masses of the products is 238. If we look at the atomic numbers, we have:

$$92 \longrightarrow 90 + 2 = 92$$

Similarly, the overall sum of the atomic numbers of the products is 92.

Thus we see that the sum of the atomic masses of the products of the radioactive decay (called the daughter nuclei) is the same as the atomic mass of uranium-238. The same applies to the atomic numbers.

This is a most important general principle which must apply in *all* nuclear reactions. Also, it should be noted that the radioactive decay of an atom is independent of its state of chemical combination. Thus the uranium-238 above will decay in this manner (and at the same rate) whether it exists in the free state (that is, as separate atoms) or as a compound. Furthermore, it should be emphasised that since the uranium atom has now lost two protons and thus its atomic number has decreased by two, it can no longer be considered to be a uranium atom. Its identity will be determined by the number of protons present – 90 – so that the atom remaining after this decay is now thorium.

This isotope of thorium, however, is unstable (as happens in the decay of many isotopes) and it will proceed to decay in the same manner in turn, becoming a different element each time it undergoes alpha decay (and, as we shall soon see, in the same manner each time it undergoes beta decay, although by a different kind of transformation). Uranium goes through many of these stages before it eventually becomes an isotope of lead – a process which takes many years overall.

When we speak of *alpha rays*, we are describing a stream of alpha particles, i.e. a stream of helium nuclei. Since the two electrons of each of the neutral helium atoms have been lost, it follows that the helium nuclei left will have a charge of $+2$. By convention, however (and possibly to add to the student's confusion), it is customary to represent the alpha particle as the Greek letter α, or as ^4_2He, rather than as He^{2+} or $^4_2\text{He}^{2+}$.

Note: The matter of ionisation will be discussed a little later in the chapter.

The positively charged particles have very low penetrating power (see Table 14.1 and Fig. 14.1) compared to the others we are going to discuss. Because of their very short range and penetration, these particles are not used for therapy. They are relatively harmless (once again because of their low penetrating power), unless the source is swallowed or inhaled (uranium dust in mines, for example), or leaked from sealed implants in the body.

One further example of alpha decay is:

$$^{222}_{86}\text{Rn} \longrightarrow {}^{218}_{84}\text{Po} + {}^4_2\text{He}$$
$$\text{radon} \qquad \text{polonium} \qquad \alpha \text{ particle}$$

The reader should check that our rules for atomic masses and atomic numbers holds true in this instance.

TABLE 14.1

Type of radiation	Nature	Charge	Mass	Penetration
α-particle	helium nuclei ($^{4}_{2}$He)	+2	4	very low
β-particle	electron	−1	approx. 0	low
γ-ray	electromagnetic radiation	0	0	very high

Beta (β) Decay

To understand this decay we should first look more closely at the neutron. This uncharged particle has a mass of one unit. Under some circumstances, the neutron is able to break up into a proton and an electron.

$$^{1}_{0}n \longrightarrow {}^{1}_{1}p + {}^{0}_{-1}e$$

neutron   proton   electron

It will be seen that the rule for atomic mass $(1 \rightarrow 1 + 0 = 1)$ still holds, as does the rule for atomic number $[0 \rightarrow 1 + (-1) = 1 - 1 = 0]$. But what do all these symbols mean?

- $^{1}_{0}n$ is a means of representing the fact that a neutron has a mass of one unit but makes no contribution to the atomic number.
- $^{1}_{1}p$ represents a proton, which has a mass of one unit and makes a contribution of +1 to the atomic number.
- $^{0}_{-1}e$ represents an electron, which has a mass of 0 and makes a contribution of −1 to the atomic number.

While the mass of the electron is given as 0, this is only an approximation, the actual mass being 1/1837 of a unit. Also, the idea of the electron making a contribution of −1 to the atomic number may seem a little confusing. However this can be explained as follows.

In a neutral atom, we know that the electric charge is balanced, because the number of protons equals the number of electrons. The neutron is not involved in these considerations because it carries no charge, but since, as explained above, it can be regarded as consisting of an electron and a proton, the emission of an electron (as a particle) from the neutron leaves an extra proton in the nucleus. This means that the atomic number has increased by 1, as in the example below. The allocation of −1 to the electron then compensates for the increase of +1 in the atomic number and our equation remains balanced.

Returning now to beta emission. A beta (β) particle is an

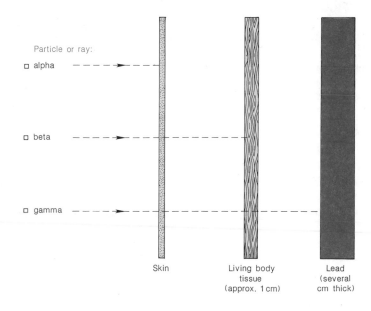

Particle or ray:

□ alpha

□ beta

□ gamma

Skin   Living body tissue (approx. 1 cm)   Lead (several cm thick)

Figure 14.1. Relative penetration of particles and rays resulting from radioactive decay.

electron and is thought to arise in the manner described above, i.e. by the breaking up of a neutron into a proton and an electron.

$$^{131}_{53}I \longrightarrow {}^{131}_{54}Xe + {}^{0}_{-1}e$$

Once again, both the atomic mass rule ($131 \rightarrow 131 + 0 = 131$) and the atomic number rule [$53 \rightarrow 54 + (-1) = 54 - 1 = 53$] holds. Notice that the atomic number (Z) has *increased* in this reaction, and that iodine (Z = 53) has been transformed to xenon (Z = 54).

Beta rays consist of a stream of electrons. Similarly:

$$^{234}_{90}Th \longrightarrow {}^{234}_{91}Pa + {}^{0}_{-1}e$$

As before, the rule for atomic mass ($234 \rightarrow 234 + 0$) and for atomic number [$90 \rightarrow 91 + (-1) = 91 - 1 = 90$] holds, and the atomic number has increased as thorium (Z = 90) is changed into protactinium (Z = 91).

Table 14.1 and Fig. 14.1 contain data on the properties of beta rays. These and γ-rays are the only particle emissions that will be discussed at any length. Other particulate radiations include neutrons, protons and deuterons. Of these, neutrons have been tried in limited therapy in Great Britain with some encouraging results. However, their use has been limited by the lack of appropriate equipment and radiation techniques to adapt them to effective therapy.

Gamma (γ) decay

During the radioactive decay of some isotopes, the nucleus can attain an unstable energy state, which it solves by emitting gamma (γ) rays, thereby giving up its excess energy in the form of electromagnetic radiation.

At this stage, it should be pointed out that the essential difference between gamma radiation and X-rays is that *gamma radiation is emitted as a result of nuclear energy changes but X-rays are emitted as a result of energy changes of electrons.*

Therapeutically, gamma sources are used more than any other form of radioactive emission. Examples include radium (although this has tended to be replaced by others), cobalt and caesium.

Gamma rays are a form of electromagnetic radiation of very short wavelength – they are often shorter than typical X-rays. They can be represented as $^0_0\gamma$, where no change in either atomic mass A or atomic number Z occurs, which in fact indicates the loss of energy that almost invariably follows the emission of another particle or particles. This may be shown thus:

$$^A_Z \longrightarrow X + {}^0_0\gamma \quad \text{where } {}^A_Z x \text{ is an atom in an unstable state.}$$

As indicated above, no change of atomic mass A or atomic number Z has occurred.

X-rays

These are sometimes called Roentgen rays and are produced for medical applications by machines. As mentioned above, they are a form of electromagnetic radiation having the same nature as gamma rays, but produced differently. The essential step in the production of X-rays is the heating of a filament to produce electrons, which are then accelerated to bombard a metal target to produce the X-rays. (Refer to Figs. 12.17 and 14.2.)

The voltages used to accelerate the electrons in X-ray machines may be in the range 20 000 to 200 000 volts, but are about 80 000 (80 kV) for a typical diagnostic machine.

The voltage used determines the minimum wavelength of the X-rays produced, and the wavelength in turn will determine the penetrating power of the radiation. Long wavelengths may be absorbed almost entirely by the skin, whereas some short wavelengths will penetrate very deeply – some so deeply that they pass right through the body.

This variable penetration leads to diagnostic use, since the emerging rays are used to affect a photographic film which, when developed, will show shadow-type picture of bones etc.

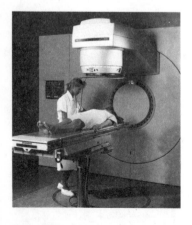

Figure 14.2. A linear accelerator. (Courtesy of Medical Applications P/L)

Others

Two other forms of radioactive decay (positron emission and electron capture) exist, but these need not concern us here.

Comparison of α, β, and γ decay

Figure 14.3 illustrates the effect that an electrostatically charged plate exerts on each of these types of decay.

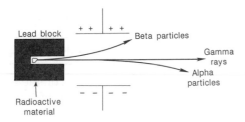

Figure 14.3. The three common types of nuclear radiation, from a mixture of different radioactive materials. (From Nave & Nave: *Physics for the Health Sciences*, 3rd Ed. Philadelphia. W.B. Saunders. 1985.)

The alpha particles, being positively charged, are deflected towards the negatively charged plate. The beta particles, being negatively charged, are deflected towards the positively charged plate and the gamma rays, being electromagnetic radiation and carrying *no* charge, are not deflected.

These and other properties are summarised in Table 14.1.

Formation of New Nuclei

So far we have spoken essentially of natural decay of nuclei. It is now possible to form new nuclei by the means discussed below and these new nuclei may then undergo decay. This is sometimes called *artificial radioactivity*.

The formation of new nuclei is usually effected by means of bombardment by other particles. The particles used may be:

1. *Neutrons*

$$^{27}_{13}\text{Al} + ^{1}_{0}\text{n} \longrightarrow ^{28}_{13}\text{Al}$$

This isotope is radioactive and thus decays:

$$^{28}_{13}\text{Al} \longrightarrow ^{28}_{14}\text{Si} + ^{0}_{-1}\text{e} \qquad \text{(i.e. it is a } \beta\text{-emitter)}$$

Other examples are:

$$^{238}_{92}\text{U} + ^{1}_{0}\text{n} \longrightarrow ^{239}_{92}\text{U} \longrightarrow ^{239}_{93}\text{Np} + ^{1}_{-0}\text{e}$$

$$^{239}_{93}\text{Np} \longrightarrow ^{239}_{94}\text{Pu} + ^{0}_{-1}\text{e}$$

and

$$^{239}_{94}\text{Pu} + 2^1_0\text{n} \longrightarrow {}^{241}_{94}\text{Pu} \longrightarrow {}^{241}_{95}\text{Am} + {}^{0}_{+1}\text{e}$$

2. *Other nuclei*
(For example, helium nuclei, i.e. alpha particles).

$$^{239}_{94}\text{Pu} + {}^4_2\text{He} \longrightarrow {}^{242}_{96}\text{Cm} + {}^1_0\text{n}$$

$$^{242}_{96}\text{Cm} + {}^4_2\text{He} \longrightarrow {}^{245}_{98}\text{Cf} + {}^1_0\text{n}$$

What has all this to do with the student nurse? The answer is that the isotopes used in various medical applications are prepared in this way. One of the essential functions of the Australian Nuclear Science and Technology Organisation reactor at Lucas Heights, for example, is to prepare the isotope $^{60}_{27}\text{Co}$, commonly known as cobalt-60, which is used for the treatment of cancer. This is achieved by the nuclear reactions between a neutron and $^{59}_{27}\text{Co}$.

$$^{59}_{27}\text{Co} + {}^1_0\text{n} \longrightarrow {}^{60}_{27}\text{Co}$$

More will be said of this isotope shortly.

RADIOACTIVITY AND PEOPLE

Radiation and Matter

When alpha and beta particles and gamma rays collide with matter:

1. They lose energy to the matter, which is converted to heat, which is given off to the surroundings (it is this heat that is thought to cause rock to melt in the earth's interior).
2. They may also lose energy as light. One instrument used to detect radioactivity, called a **scintillation counter,** takes advantage of this effect.
3. Ionisation can occur, as indicated in Table 14.1. This involves the removal of electron(s) from an atom or molecule to form an ion (which is positively charged). Ionisation results from collisions by particulate radiation or from the energy supplied by wave radiation.

The **Geiger-Müller counter** makes use of this principle. It detects the presence of radiation and measures contamination levels by identifying the number of interactions occurring in a specific time or volume.

The ability of these three types of radiation to ionise matter is of particular relevance to our present studies. It is this capacity that gives rise to the harmful effects of radiation on the human body, by ionising (and eventually destroying) the organic molecules that make up the cells of the body. However, we are able to take advantage of the capacity of this radiation to destroy cells of the body in therapies that destroy abnormal cells.

The beneficial or harmful effects of radiation on people result not only from ionisation but also from the 'freed' electrons (beta particles, or those produced by radiation), which may interact with ions or molecules present in the body, creating changes in these. The energy sometimes available from gamma radiation may also cause electrons to be removed from atoms. These electrons may transfer energy as they proceed, so that even more electrons are knocked off other atoms. These effects can wreak havoc in living tissue as molecules and compounds are changed, causing possible alterations in structures, genetic material and functioning of cells. Furthermore, the numerous changes that can occur are completely unpredictable in the uncontrolled situation.

Particles such as alpha particles, which are larger and more highly charged, will be involved in more interactions in a given volume compared to the very much smaller, more penetrating radiation of beta rays, for example. The latter will be involved in fewer interactions in a given volume but the damage will be spread throughout a larger volume because they travel further. This effect is accentuated by the fact that this kind of radiation possesses much higher energy. Such considerations are most important in selecting the correct form of radiation to treat a particular region, whether it be a cancerous tumour of the lung or a skin cancer on the face.

Factors Affecting the Extent of Radiation Damage

The extent of the damage caused to the human body depends upon five factors:

1. The amount of radiation absorbed by the body
This is commonly expressed in **grays** (the former unit being the **rad,** where 1 gray, or Gy = 100 rads), defined thus:

A **gray** is equivalent to the absorption of one joule of energy for each kilogram of body tissue.

The effects of exposure of the body to a single dose of radiation are given in Table 14.2.

However, *small* doses of this ionising radiation, to which the body is exposed many times, can be very serious. Many people who worked on radioactivity research and such developed cancer, sometimes as long as 40 years after the initial exposure to radiation. Marie Curie and her daughter both died of leukaemia

TABLE 14.2   Effect of exposure to a single dose of radiation

Dose (sieverts*)	Probable effect
0 to 0.25	No observable effect
0.25 to 0.50	Small decrease in white blood cell count
0.50 to 1	Lesions, marked decrease in white blood cells
1 to 2	Nausea, vomiting, loss of hair
2 to 5	Haemorrhaging, ulcers, possible death
5 +	Fatal

*sievert = gray × RBE (relative biological effectiveness of a particular type of radiation)

as a result of exposure to this radiation. Similarly the incidence of leukaemia among survivors of the nuclear bombing of Hiroshima and Nagasaki was found to be very high.

Note the terminology used here. These weapons were originally called 'atom bombs' and people spoke of 'splitting the atom'. However, it could be said that an atom is split every time an ion is formed! Thus the preferred terminology is 'nuclear' weapons or bombs, 'nuclear' reactions, etc., because all these reactions (unlike normal chemical reactions) involve the *nucleus* of the atom concerned.

2. The type of radiation
Alpha rays are stopped by the skin, beta rays penetrate about one centimetre, but gamma rays penetrate in the same way as X-rays.

The total biological effect is expressed as **dose equivalent** (in sieverts), calculated by multiplying the dose by a 'quality factor' for the type of radiation involved:

$$\begin{array}{ccc} \text{dose equivalent} = & \text{dose} & \times \text{quality factor} \\ \text{(sievert)} & \text{(gray)} & \text{(RBE)} \end{array}$$

(RBE is the relative biological effectiveness of a particular type of radiation).

where the quality factor = 1 for γ and β radiation and X-rays and the quality factor = 15 for α radiation and high-energy neutrons.

3. The chemical nature of the radiation
The chemical nature of the isotope involved (and thus the chemical properties of the element involved) is of particular importance. As a contrast, let us consider krypton-85 and strontium-90.

Krypton-85 is produced during nuclear reactions and is released into the atmosphere during the reprocessing of nuclear fuels. However, krypton is a very unreactive and chemically inert element. Once in the atmosphere, it affects the skin and lungs, but, being chemically unreactive, it does not pass to other parts of the body nor does it accumulate in the body.

On the other hand, although strontium-90 is also formed in nuclear reactions, it 'follows' calcium, i.e. because strontium is chemically very similar to calcium, it tends to go where calcium goes. Thus strontium-90 tends to enter bones, where it accumulates and where its radiation can cause bone cancer and leukaemia.

The other common example of this accumulation is iodine-131 which, like other iodine isotopes, enters the thyroid gland.

4. Oxygen concentration

It has been found that large concentrations of oxygen at the time of irradiation will increase the amount of damage occurring. This is an important consideration in radiotherapy, since tumour cells, for example, that have been well oxygenated are easier to treat, but cells that are low in oxygen are less susceptible to destruction. In addition, tumour cells usually have a higher level of metabolic activity than surrounding cells and thus require larger quantities of oxygen. As a consequence, tumour cells will take up more oxygen, which aids in their irradiation. In such radiation treatments, it is important to be careful to destroy the more highly oxygenated tumour cells and to leave normal cells that are lower in oxygen alive to form possible centres of regrowth.

5. Radiosensitivity

Some tissues and organs in the body may react differently to radiation – some may be more susceptible than others.

Cells with high sensitivity to radiation include self-renewing systems such as the glands of the intestine, which divide rapidly and regularly, and non-specialised cells in the ovaries, testes, bone marrow, lymph, etc.

Cells with medium sensitivity include cells that individually have long lives and need a stimulus to undergo cell division, e.g. those of the liver, kidney, mature bones, etc.

Cells with low sensitivity include fixed postmitotic cells that have lost all or most of the ability to divide and are highly specialised. These are the most resistant to radiation, such as those of the brain, muscle and spinal cord.

Most of the tissues and cells of the body can be fitted somewhere between these levels.

Effects of Radiation

On the cell

The production of ions can lead to chemical reactions which will be unpredictable: for example, irradiation of water can produce H^+ and OH^-; some ions are powerful oxidising or reducing agents that cause further chemical interactions; some ions will interact with each other, with oxygen, with organic molecules, etc. Cell poisons or abnormal products may be produced as a result of these chemical reactions.

Effects of these reactions and abnormal products may include:

1. Alteration of organic compounds leading to changes in their structure and thus in the behaviour of cells, e.g. DNA and RNA may be altered to create immediate effects or effects that don't occur until the cell undergoes division – effects that may not be evident for years.

2. Cells may be sterilised by early 'aging', in which case the cell never attempts to undergo division.

3. Outright death of the cell may occur or eventual death as a result of the changes described.

Genetic effects

Genetic alterations can also result from radiation. By causing changes in the chromosomes of plants and animals, mutations can be produced, and this effect is considered to occur in human beings. Children of radiographers, for example, show an increased frequency of congenital defects, as do children of survivors of Hiroshima and Nagasaki. This effect can occur even at very low levels of exposure in some circumstances. There appears to be no absolutely safe maximum dose or threshold below which these effects will not occur.

The effects of radiation on the reproductive system are of concern to female nurses because so many of them are of child-bearing age.

The genetic alterations involved are gene mutations (changes) and chromosome aberrations (breakages, abnormal interchanges between chromosomes, etc.). Direct evidence of genetic effects in humans is rather limited.

The doses required to produce permanent sterility are relatively high. In men, the most radiosensitive cells in the reproductive system are the unspecialised germ cells and the spermatozoa (sperm) in the seminiferous tubules that are not fully mature. Mature sperm cells are relatively resistant to radiation. Since a man produces sperm over a large span of his life, it means that if all the immature sperm present are destroyed at some specific time, he may produce more later. This assumes that active sperm-producing cells (spermatogonia) still exist. In women, the problem is rather different, since they have all their unspecialised germ cells, oocytes (primitive ova or eggs), early in life, and these cannot be replaced if they are lost. It follows that radiation can cause permanent reduction in reproductive potential. Data on human ovaries suggests that a single whole body dose of three sieverts will lead to permanent sterility.

The radiation damage to a fetus depends upon the stage of pregnancy at the time and the size of the dose. (Relative proportions of radiosensitive cells vary during pregnancy. They are very high in the embryo and decrease with specialisation Also once some structures are fully formed, they are more resistant.)

It is considered wise not to assign pregnant nurses to patients with radiation sources on or in the body.

Radiation sickness

This is a general reaction that may occur during a course of radiation treatment, but it is not as common or severe as it used to be. Improved radiation techniques, new types of equipment (using megavoltages) and better patient care have contributed to this reduction. The reaction of an individual to radiotherapy will vary with his or her own susceptibility, the dose used, the locality being radiated and exposure times. The patient may exhibit fatigue, weakness, nausea, vomiting, headaches and diarrhoea, with other problems developing later on.

In general, the first organ system to manifest radiation effects is the haemopoietic system (blood cell system), which has highly radiosensitive cells. Bone marrow depression may occur, resulting in insufficient blood cell production, which is a very serious toxic effect. The next system to be affected is the gastrointestinal system, which also has some highly sensitive cells, with other organ systems following.

The reaction is usually relatively mild because the situation is controlled, whereas more serious radiation sickness may occur as a result of accidents or such things as nuclear weapons, where exposure is uncontrolled. The effects in these situations may range from mild to extremely severe (known as acute radiation syndrome) through to death. Since it is not likely that the nurse will have any contact with the more severe exposure, we will not discuss it here but suggest that the interested reader refer to specialised texts that deal with extensive effects and their causes.

Skin reaction

This warrants a separate mention since most radiation in therapy and in accidents passes through or to the skin surface. In fact, this was a very limiting factor before the use of megavoltage, which produces maximum dosage below the skin surface. However, the skin reaction is still important, in terms of sensitivity of the individual patient's tissues and the effects observed and felt by the patient. The characteristic effect is **erythema** – 'redness', occurring after a varied interval of time (weeks, months or years, depending on the situation); its severity, depending on dose, controlled or accidental, time of exposure, etc.

The reactions are not very strong or common with the better radiation techniques and associated patient care. Other responses of the skin following damage to the most actively growing basal cells may or may not include loss of hair, some residual pigmentation, itching, temporary dry peeling, the more severe (but less likely these days) blistering and scaling, and the very rare necrosis of tissue (death of tissue). The loss of hair is not always permanent, but depends on the severity of the reaction and damage.

It is of great importance for the nurse to realise that all forms of irritation – mechanical, thermal or chemical – must be avoided at the sites of therapy, since they will increase the severity of reactions, in the same way as sunburn would be affected. Some of the things to be avoided include hot-water bottles or heating pads, razors, most talcum powders, zinc oxide adhesive, certain creams, lotions or ointments (any of which contain heavy metals that can give rise to secondary radiation), and tight clothing. The treatment area is generally marked on the skin by the therapist and is not usually washed, since washing involves towelling and soaps, which irritate. Note that the therapy marks must not be removed since they are the therapist's guide to the area.

Remember that avoidance of such irritants must also involve the patient whenever possible. The nurse should explain the situation to the patient so that he or she understands what is being done (or not being done) and why. This allows the patient to assume a degree of responsibility for his/her care, and this will not only help to make the treatment effective but may contribute to the patient's well-being.

Some of the effects of radiation are less common or highly specific to the irradiated site, such as cataracts in the eye.

Exposure of Human Beings to Radiation

We have already seen the effects of exposure to a single dose of radiation (Table 14.2). We will now look at some typical radiation exposures in the United States (Table 14.3). This data is used here because it is readily available and because it includes the effects of nuclear power plants, which do not exist in Australia.

Some comments about this data are appropriate:

1. It may be seen that of the total ionising radiation received by a person in the US in each year, two-thirds comes from natural sources, but varies from place to place. Cosmic radiation, for example, is much more intense at high elevations because

TABLE 14.3 Typical radiation exposures in the United States

Sources	Millisievert per year
Natural	
A. External to the body	
1. From cosmic radiation	0.50
2. From the earth	0.47
3. From building materials	0.03
B. Inside the body	
1. Inhalation of air	0.05
2. In human tissues (mostly $^{40}_{19}K$)	0.21
Total from natural sources	1.26
Man-made	
A. Medical procedures	
1. Diagnostic X-rays	0.50
2. Radiotherapy X-rays, radioisotopes	0.10
3. Internal diagnosis, therapy	0.01
B. Nuclear power industry	0.002
C. Luminous watch dials, TV tubes, industrial wastes	0.02
D. Radioactive fallout	0.04
Total from man-made sources	0.67
Total from natural and man-made sources	1.93

(From Masterton: *Chemical Principles.* 5th Ed. Philadelphia. Saunders College Publishing. 1981.)

much of the screening effect of the atmosphere is diminished. In Denver, Colorado, for example, the level of exposure to cosmic radiation is twice the national average.

2. X-rays account for the largest exposure to man-made sources of ionising radiation. A single dental X-ray is equivalent to 200 microsieverts and a chest X-ray is 500–2000 microsieverts. These figures can increase if the X-ray is not taken properly whether through the inexperience of the operator or a faulty machine.

X-ray machines (fluoroscopes) used to be provided in shoe shops so that people could check on the fitting of new shoes. This practice ceased when the danger was appreciated and, similarly, excessive clinical use of X-rays as a diagnostic tool is to be avoided.

3. The exposure of people to radioactive fall-out amounted to about 300 microsieverts (in the year prior to the nuclear test ban treaty in 1963). Much of the present radiation from this source comes from the testing activities of countries such as France and China which have continued the testing of nuclear weapons in the atmosphere.

4. Overall, exposure to radiation from nuclear power plants is very low – about two microsieverts/year, but is higher near a plant. However, it has been calculated that a person sitting on the fence of a nuclear power plant for a year would receive only 50 microsieverts of radiation and that a person standing at the gate of the Three Mile Island plant for the first two weeks after the

March 1979 accident would receive about 800 microsieverts – less than the radiation from a single chest X-ray. However, the effects of the Chernobyl accident are much more extensive.

The above remarks are not meant to imply that the authors support nuclear power plants – it is not our function here to comment on such issues. We simply wish to make comparisons and emphasise the importance of being informed and the need to treat all isotopes and X-rays with the utmost respect.

5. In the case of an area contaminated by fallout, the fallout over dams would mean that people who drink water, whether as water or in tea or coffee, will be ingesting radioactive material. Similarly, people who drink milk from cows which have grazed on contaminated pasture can ingest iodine- 131 in the milk. This effect has already been observed.

6. Biological concentration is also important. In each step in a food chain, concentration of radioactive isotopes can occur. Thus if cows eat grass with a very low concentration of strontium-90, the concentration increases as the cow eats and processes a lot of grass and the strontium-90 is increased even further in milk. People who then drink such milk will ingest strontium-90 and can increase the concentration again through accumulation if they continue to ingest it.

Half-life

Radioactive material (whether naturally or artificially radio-active) decays in a logarithmic fashion, as shown in Fig. 14.4.

What is meant here is that the mass of the isotope decays most rapidly at the beginning of its life. This means that to attempt to define the total life of an isotope is rather pointless. For this reason, the half-life is used.

The half-life(t) (of any mass of radioactive material is the time required for half of the mass of material to decay. This is illustrated in Fig. 14.4. The isotope used ($^{15}_{8}O$) has a half-life of two minutes. Thus, if we start with 20 milligrams of material:

At the beginning we have 20 mg
After 2.0 minutes (one half-life) we have 10 mg
After 4.0 minutes (two half-lives) we have 5 mg
After 6.0 minutes (three half-lives) we have 2.5 mg
After 8.0 minutes (four half-lives) we have 1.25 mg and so forth.

The reader will observe that in the first two minutes, ten milligrams of material decayed. However, in the last two minutes listed (i.e. from six to eight minutes) only 1.25 milligrams

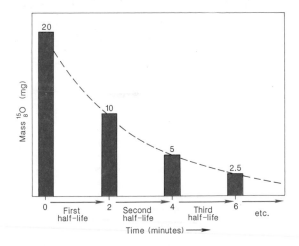

Figure 14.4. Decay of 20 mg of $^{15}_{8}O$. For each half-life, the quantity is reduced by one-half. (From Brescia, *Chemistry: A Modern Introduction*. 2nd Ed. Philadelphia. W.B. Saunders. 1978.)

decayed. Thus *the rate of decay is constant in relation to the mass present, but the actual mass that decays decreases.*

Half-lives range from millionths of a second to billions of years:

Half-life

(a) $^{214}_{84}Po \longrightarrow {}^{210}_{82}Pb + {}^{4}_{2}He$ 1.64×10^{-4} sec

(b) $^{238}_{92}U \longrightarrow {}^{234}_{90}Th + {}^{4}_{2}He$ 4.51×10^{9} years

Table 14.4 lists the half-lives of some common radioactive isotopes.

Note: The term 'biological half-life' is also used in this context. The biological half-life is defined as the time taken for half the radioactivity to disappear from the body, on a purely chemical and biological basis. Both the physical and biological half-life affect any internal isotope, so that treatment and diagnosis is often arranged in terms of the 'effective' half-life, a combination of these two half-lives. The effective half-life is particularly important in choosing radioisotopes that will be injected or ingested directly into the body and that will either remain in the body for a prolonged period, or must be eliminated by the body through various processes. The faster the level of radioactivity of the particular isotope is reduced and the sooner a stage is reached at which the level presents absolutely no risk or danger to the patient's cells or to the people treating or caring for the patient, the more useful the isotope. That is, providing there is sufficient time for the objective(s) of diagnosis or treatment to be completed.

TABLE 14.4. Radioisotopes commonly used in diagnosis and therapy

Isotope	Application	Half-life
^{182}Ta (tantalum)	Low dose rate treatment	115 days
^{192}Ir (iridium)	Low dose rate treatment	74 days
^{137}Cs (caesium)	Low dose rate treatment	30 days
^{60}Co (cobalt)	Low dose rate treatment	5.26 years
^{203}Hg (mercury)	Brain scans	47 days
^{197}Hg	Brain and kidney scans	65 hours
^{99}Tc (technetium)	Brain, lung, kidney, bone, liver and thyroid scans and cardiovascular blood pool	6.0 hours
^{113}Ir	Brain, lung, liver scans and cardiovascular blood pool	1.73 hours
^{131}I (iodine)	Cisternography, lung, thyroid, liver and kidney scans, cardiovascular blood pool	8.06 days
^{133}Xe (xenon)	Lung scans	5.27 days
^{125}I	Thyroid scans	60 days
^{123}I	Thyroid scans	13 hours
^{198}Au (gold)	Liver scans	2.70 days
^{75}Se (selenium)	Pancreas scan	120 days
^{85}Sr (strontium)	Bone scan	65 days
^{87}Sr	Bone scan	2.8 hours
^{18}F (fluorine)	Bone scan	110 mins.

Note: The half-lives quoted are those for the particular isotope listed and used for these purposes in each case.

CLINICAL USES OF RADIOISOTOPES

Radiation has a number of specific roles in medicine:

1. It can be used as a diagnostic aid – as a radiotracer to locate growths, etc.

2. It can be utilised therapeutically to destroy tumour growths.

3. It can be used as a palliative measure – to relieve pain for periods of time in advanced cancer, e.g. metastatic cancer of the breast to the bone (the site of the cancer is the breast but it has affected the bone nearby).

4. It is also employed in medical research.

Radioisotopes in Diagnosis and Research

These have been found to be most useful in a wide range of applications as a diagnostic tool in medicine, to study the functions of specific organs and to measure such quantities as blood volume, circulation rate, red blood cell turnover, cardiac output, lung blood flow, hormone concentrations, and to locate tumours and lesions within the brain, kidneys, liver, lungs, bone, pericardium, etc.

Some of the advantages of radioisotopes include:

1. They can be tagged to (attached to or combined with) specific units, e.g. red blood cells, compounds such as serum proteins, enzymes, hormones, etc. Substances labelled with a radioisotope, such as radioiodine (^{131}I)-labelled human serum albumin, or sodium chromate ^{51}Cr-labelled blood cells, behave physiologically like their unlabelled counterparts. This means their behaviour, role and concentrations in the body will be unaffected by the radiotracer and thus can be studied, measured or followed by scanning techniques or detectors.

2. Some radioisotopes are chemically similar to specific body substances, for example, sodium and iodine. They can be utilised to fill the same roles, and thus the substance or its behaviour can be more easily tested or studied.

3. Some radioisotopes will seek certain areas of the body, and this facilitates studies of those areas. For instance, with strontium-85, active bone formation can be identified as can osteomyelitis (bone infection) and neoplasms.

4. They can be given orally or by injection and only minute doses (e.g. one nanogram, equalling 10^{-9} of a gram) are required, so that the body is exposed to a minimum level of radiation and cell damage should not occur. It also follows that the risk to the staff caring for the patient is minimised. Those isotopes with very short half-lives are to be preferred in such applications.

Note: It would be easy to say here that no risk exists to the patient or the caring personnel, but in the interests of scientific accuracy this would be incorrect in the strictest sense, since *some* risk almost invariably exists, no matter how slight that risk might be. However, the risk with diagnostic isotopes has been reduced to such an extent that, providing all instructions are followed, no real danger should exist.

5. Extremely small amounts of radioactivity can be detected accurately by detectors and cameras or scanners. The most popular detector of radioisotopes is the scintillation counter or scanner.

As an example, iodine-131 has been used as a check on thyroid activity. If a solution of sodium iodide containing a small quantity of iodine-131 is drunk by the patient, the iodine (with the iodine-131 tracer) goes to the only part of the body that utilises iodine – the thyroid gland. The ability of the thyroid to assimilate the iodine can be determined by placing a Geiger counter close to the thyroid gland in the lower neck, to measure the quantity of radiation being emitted.

A 'normal' thyroid gland will absorb about 12 per cent of the available iodine in the space of a few hours.

In this type of procedure, the concentration of iodine-131 used is very low, so that the patient is not subjected to harmful levels of radioactivity.

6. Some radioisotopes can be utilised to test for the functioning of glands through blood tests. No radioisotope is given to the patient. Instead it is added to a serum or blood sample that has been taken from the patient. One thyroid test uses the radioisotope (triiodothyronine) T_3 in this way to test for thyroid function.

Criteria for choosing a suitable radioisotope include:

- Its ability to emit beta (can be detected in excreta) or low-level gamma radiation (easily detected outside the body).
- The minimal dose required for detection.
- The shortness of its half-life.
- The ease with which it is eliminated from the body and time required for elimination.

Radioimmunoassays (RIA)

This technique involves radiotracers and is very highly sensitive to minute amounts of hormones, drugs and many other substances.

As an example, these methods can be used to provide an early indication of pregnancy or to detect substances that indicate a particular disease is in evidence, in the early stages of that disease. A small sample of blood, urine, or tissue, etc., is used for the assay.

Positron emission tomography (PET)

This interesting recent advance in nuclear medicine represents a combination of conventional radioisotope tracer scans with the mapping capabilities of X-rays, MRI and ultrasonic techniques. Its greatest application so far has been in brain metabolism studies, where this technique has been able to differentiate between the brain activity involved in talking as distinct from listening to music. It offers great potential in brain activity research. Other applications include studies of various types of cancer, including improving the effectiveness of treatments; management in epilepsy, Alzheimers disease and other dementias; clinical evaluation of movement disorders; detection of coronary artery disease and other cardiac applications, to name but a few.

Precautions

Since the quantities used in diagnosis or study of a patient are so minute, they do not usually represent a significant exposure hazard in ordinary nursing care. The care of the patient may not alter greatly, despite the presence of the isotope. The precautions necessary will depend on the test, the dose, how the body handles the isotope (i.e. where it goes, how widely distributed it is within the body, whether it is excreted and how, etc.), and, of course, the particular isotope being used.

All that may be required is the careful handling and disposal of some of the patient's body fluids or wastes, such as blood, urine, vomit, sweat and faeces. For example, iodine-131 circulates in the blood and is excreted in the urine. Therefore, these fluids should be handled carefully and, in the case of urine, for example, collected and disposed of according to the institution's procedures and policies.

RADIATION THERAPY

The main aim of the use of radiation in therapy is to destroy malignant tumours or cells while leaving surrounding tissues relatively unharmed. The concept of treatment is based on tumour cells being more sensitive to radiation (since these cells are usually dividing more rapidly than others, they are generalised in function and often immature) and slower to recover than healthy cells after damage. This provides the obvious advantage of destroying or damaging more abnormal cells than normal cells. If treatment is also based on an intermittent programme with a short rest period between sessions, damaged normal cells are more likely to recover than any damaged abnormal ones.

Radiation treatment may be utilised alone or in combination with other forms of treatment such as drugs or surgery. Its overall objective may be active (to destroy all abnormal cells) or palliative (to relieve discomfort, or to prolong life in a terminal situation).

The most successful treatments occur on tumours that are located in areas where fairly large doses can be given, e.g. those on the skin or mucous membranes, or body cavity areas with access to the outside of the body. Treatment of tumours deep within the body (such as the pancreas) are the least successful since account must be taken of the large volume of normal tissue that would be affected as the rays pass through it.

External Applications of Radiation

These involve the use of either X-ray machines (linear accelerators) or radioisotopic sources.

X-ray therapy
This can be used for the treatment of skin cancer or deep-seated cancers.

Radioisotopes
These are used in:

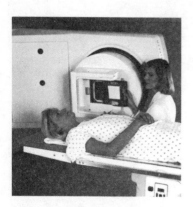

Figure 14.5. The type of machine used for cobalt radiation therapy. (Courtesy of Medical Applications P/L.)

1. **Teletherapy** (distance therapy) in the form of 'bombs': for example, high intensity sources of cobalt-60 or sometimes caesium-137 (only the gamma radiation is used). The source is enclosed in a protective housing or casing called a 'bomb' (e.g. a cobalt bomb').

The patient is set at a fixed distance from the source, which may be stable or may rotate around the patient to reach all areas of growth and distribute the radiation entry evenly (Fig. 14.5).

This technique is used to irradiate and destroy deep cancers in the body as it causes less destruction to overlying skin. Examples in which this treatment is suitable are in tumours of the brain, oesophagus and the lungs.

Another advantage of this treatment is that it causes less radiation sickness than X-rays.

Note: The patient is not radioactive since the source of radiation is outside and separate from the body. The patient is transferred to the radiotherapy department for the treatment and then returns to the ward or goes home, leaving the source behind. Therefore no special precautions regarding the radioisotopes themselves will be necessary in the ward or home areas.

2. **External moulds** containing radioisotopes, e.g. cobalt-60 and radioactive strontium (which is particularly valuable in treating carcinomas of the lips, ears, scalp, mouth, etc.) are applied to the skin surface. Protective moulds may sometimes be bent to fit certain positions or shapes in relation to the tumour. It should be remembered that the isotope itself is not in direct contact with the skin, so that when the encasing container is removed from the area, no radioactive material is left behind.

In this case the patient has the radiation source actually on his body and thus specific and more extensive precautions must be taken (discussed in general later in this chapter).

Internal Applications of Radiation

These involve the implantation of selected radioisotopes into the body. They may be implanted directly into the tumour, into the region adjacent to the tumour or into the circulation. This means the patient actually has the source of radiation (i.e. the radioisotope) within his or her body until it is removed or until it is no longer sufficiently radioactive. As before, it requires very important precautions to be taken by the nurse and others in contact with the patient until the source is removed or until no really hazardous radiation is emitted (see under 'safety', below).

The three major types of internal therapy are:

1. Intracavity therapy

This involves placement of the radioactive isotope into a cavity of the body to irradiate adjacent or nearby carcinomas, in the bladder, uterus, maxillary sinus, etc. In this case the isotope is usually encapsulated by some material which is used to contain it and may be used to regulate the types of radiation that will be utilised, i.e. particles or rays.

These implants may be permanent or temporary. Examples of temporary, removable implants include radium-226, cobalt-60, iridium-192 and tantalum-182; and examples of permanent implants include gold-198, radon-222 and iridium-192. Temporary implants usually have long half-lives and will still be radioactive on removal, for example – radium-226 has a half-life of approximately 1600 years. Permanent implants have short half-lives: that of radon-222 is about 3.85 days.

The devices used for encapsulation are varied in shape and size but include capsules, plastic tubes, beads and even balloons (Fig. 14.6), which are placed into position with the aid of instruments (speculum, cystoscope, needle-colloidal gold-198 into thorax, etc.), but usually without surgery. It is interesting to note that when a balloon is used, generally in treating the bladder, it is filled with a liquid form of radioisotope after placement.

This intracavity technique is found to be particularly successful in cancer of the uterus and bladder. However, it can cause some irritation to immediately adjacent tissues and, for example, excess mucous production can occur.

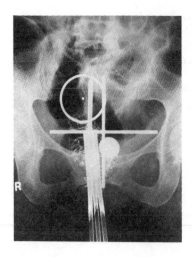

Figure 14.6. A radiograph demonstrating radium sources. The circle and the cross are markers to assist the radiographer. The three channels at the bottom of the photograph are used for the introduction of the sources. (From Mackay, et al. *Illustrated Textbook of Gynaecology* (Fig. 35.38). Sydney. W.B. Saunders. 1991.)

2. Interstitial therapy

In this case the radioisotopes can be surgically implanted directly into the malignant tumour tissue or region for example, a gland – and are commonly contained in needles, beads, seeds, ribbons or catheters. Depending on the position of the tumour, its size, shape and type and also on such factors as the desired level of dose, an appropriate isotope and container will be selected. For example, cobalt-60 encased in gold or silver needles can be used to treat cancer of the cervix.

Irradiation may also be accomplished without the use of containers. The radioisotope, which is made up into a solution, can be injected directly into the tumour and adjacent tissues. For example, colloidal gold-198 solution is very suitable for this type of treatment. It can also be injected into the pleural cavity, where it will precipitate on to the surfaces for irradiation. Also, a radioisotope in solution may be taken orally by the patient – usually in situations where the isotope, such as radioactive iodine, is specific to the tissues requiring treatment, such as the thyroid gland.

Examples of the isotopes commonly used in interstitial therapy are cobalt-60, iodine-125, tantalum-182, caesium-137, gold-198 and iridium-192.

3. Systemic therapy

This involves the use of radioisotopes, which are administered intravenously to treat certain disorders such as myelogenous (bone marrow) leukaemia, in which case sodium phosphate (phosphorus-32) is utilised.

It is important to be aware that the body's pattern of distribution, metabolism and excretion of unsealed isotopes (i.e. not in containers) varies. Some isotopes are excreted in urine, others in faeces; some are excreted rapidly, some slowly; and others are metabolised rapidly by organs, such as the liver and spleen. It thus follows that considerable variation exists in the time that hazardous radiation is present in the patient's body, and the particular body fluids or wastes that are contaminated. It should be remembered that the half-life will also affect the length of time that radiation will present a problem.

Safety

There are three cardinal factors controlling radiation exposure — time, distance and shielding.

1. Time

The fundamental and obvious consideration here is that the less time spent in the radiation field the better, since the exposure is then smaller. In nursing care, careful planning will be required to ensure the maximum number of patient needs are met in the time exposure permitted. It will be easier to keep track of and maximise time if all equipment and supplies are prepared and obtained before nursing care is commenced. Organisation of staff will be needed to ensure rotation of nurses' duties in the care of a patient receiving internal therapy or in operating rooms where implants are being done.

2. Distance

Once again it is obvious that the greater the distance between the nurse and the source, the smaller will be the exposure to radiation. This is governed by an inverse square law, with which some readers may be familiar. This relationship tells us that *the intensity of radiation received from a source decreases as the square of the distance* (See Fig. 14.7).

If the intensity of radiation received one metre from the

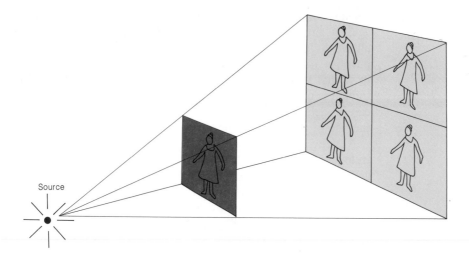

source is R units, then:

- The intensity of the radiation received two metres from the source will be $R/2^2 = R/4$.
- The intensity of the radiation received three metres from the source will be $R/3^2 = R/9$.
- The intensity of the radiation received four metres from the source will be $R/4^2 = R/16$, and so on.

In general, then, we see that the level of radiation decreases very rapidly as distance increases.

It should also be remembered that the type of radiation (i.e. using alpha, beta or gamma rays) will affect the implications associated with distance.

The implications of this for the nurse include planning the patient's care ahead of time, so that the care requiring direct patient contact or closeness to the patient is carried out first with a gradual movement away from the patient as soon as possible. At all times it should be remembered that the greater the distance the nurse can maintain from the patient in carrying out any particular task, the better. Visitors may need instruction as to where they can sit or stand and for how long. Placement of the patient in the ward will also be affected. However, with thought and planning the patient can still have human contact, even if only from the doorway.

3. Shielding

Reduction in radiation exposure can be achieved by the interposition of a radiation-reducing material between the source and the person involved. One of the most commonly used materials is lead, and this material is usually required for gamma emitters,

Figure 14.7. Inverse square law. If the distance is doubled, the intensity of radiation is now $1/2 = 1/4$. Similarly if the distance is tripled, the intensity of radiation is now $1/3 = 1/9$.

because of its high density and consequently its effectiveness against gamma radiation. It should be emphasised again that although lead is one of the best materials available for the purpose, it will only *reduce* the gamma radiation passing through it, so that adequate protection can be obtained only if a sufficient thickness of lead is used. The effectiveness of the shielding used can be determined satisfactorily for any given radiation only by the use of appropriate monitoring instruments.

Lucite and aluminium can be used with beta emitters. Indeed, lead should *NOT* be used against beta emitters because gamma radiation may be produced.

A number of misconceptions exist regarding the use of certain shields, particularly lead aprons. Many people believe that the lead apron will give them complete protection against isotopic sources, but this is not the case. The lead apron is intended for use in diagnostic radiology and is effective against these lower energies. It is questionably effective against the therapeutic isotope iodine-125 but is virtually transparent to higher gamma energies. The sense of false security that such devices can tend to confer could lead to more time being spent near radioactive sources than is absolutely necessary. One should always check with the officer in charge of radiation safety regarding shielding.

In operating rooms where implants are being done, devices such as lead barriers of various shapes and sizes are being used, together with forceps with extra long handles, etc.

Lead boxes are available for the collection of sources that have been removed from patients or for transporting sources to operating rooms.

General Policies and Methods which Minimise Radiation Risks

1. Institutions that have radiotherapy units usually employ a radiation safety officer, and have specific policies, guidelines and procedures related to the use, handling, storage and disposal of radioactive materials and for coping with accidents, radiation disasters in the community, etc., all of which must meet stringent government requirements.

2. The nurse should make sure that he or she fully understands the treatment and nursing care situation and fully plans the patient care before proceeding to the patient. A knowledge of the acute emotional and psychological effects on the patient of his or her disease and treatment is of the utmost importance in the care of these patients.

3. All spills or leaks of radioactive material and loss of sealed sources are notifiable, so that the nurse always needs to

know how or where to contact the radiation safety officer or authority.

4. Remember that **unsealed** sources of radioactivity in the body provide **two** hazards:

• Emissions from the patient's body; and
• contamination of one or all body fluids and products, such as urine, vomit, sweat, drainage and faeces. In turn these may contaminate clothes, bed-linen or surfaces such as floors.

These must all be handled gently to prevent inhalation and disposed of according to the prescribed requirements of the institution, in conjunction with any requirements for collecting specimens. Usually contaminated clothes, linens, materials used to wipe up spills, etc., are collected in designated bags and will be removed by radiation staff to be disposed of or kept until no longer contaminated.

5. **Under no circumstances must radioactive sources ever be touched with bare hands.** This includes those in sealed containers, since a leakage could occur, so that:

• Appropriate gloves *must* be used, usually lead lined in the case of strong sources such as those in sealed containers. In the case of diagnostic doses, spills of body excreta may require only rubber or plastic gloves.
• The use of elongated forceps keeps sources at a greater distance.

6. Film badges provide a useful check on the exposure to which *you* have been subjected and it is in your interests always to wear them when required to do so and to co-operate with the authorities in this means of monitoring exposure.

7. A patient using an external or internal radioactive source may require isolation.

8. Always clearly indicate the type of source being used at any time, by using signs and/or labels. Clear instructions help to spread communication and prevents both contamination and misunderstandings.

9. Always give clear instructions to patients and visitors.

10. Ensure that full training is given to both direct staff (nurses, etc.) and to indirect staff (floor sweepers, meal attendants, etc.).

11. All staff must pay particular attention to personal hygiene.

12. Always keep containers readily available or in the ward for sealed sources which are removed or lost from the body.

13. Regularly check therapy sites to ensure that implants are in place.

14. Patients who are being discharged with sources still in place must be given detailed and explicit instructions.

Finally, the use of radioactivity has proved to be an indispensible diagnostic and therapeutic tool. The nurse who seeks to understand all that has been written above will be more effective to patients, colleagues and associates, and the general public.

REVIEW

1. Answer the questions posed in the introduction to this chapter.
2. If you were drawing up a nursing plan for a woman who has a radium implant in the uterus, what precautions and care specifically related to this treatment would you include and why?
3. Consider a patient who has received a diagnostic dose of a radioisotope. What information would be needed to enable you to care effectively for this patient?
4. Imagine that another patient who is to receive cobalt therapy comes to you to seek information and reassurance. What would you say?
5. Outline the changes that occur during:
    (a)   alpha decay;
    (b)   beta decay; and
    (c)   gamma decay.
    How is gamma radiation used in therapeutic applications?
6. What are the effects of ionising radiation on human tissue?
7. List the factors that affect the susceptibility of tissue to radiation.
8. Why is the half-life of a radioactive isotope an important factor when considering the use of radiation in diagnosis and treatment?
9. What are some of the clinical uses of radioisotopes?
10. If radioactive isotopes are capable of causing damage or even death to human beings, what factors enable these substances to be used to treat tumours?

15

Environmental and occupational health

OBJECTIVES

After studying this chapter students should be able to:

1. List the main components of atmospheric pollution and describe the effects of each on the human body.
2. Describe the formation of temperature inversions and discuss the hazards associated with these.
3. List some of the diseases caused by water pollution and comment briefly on each.
4. Distinguish between ionising and non-ionising radiation and the effects of each on people.
5. List and briefly describe some of the factors that affect the toxicity of poisons.
6. List some of the chemical elements that are harmful to humans and describe their effects.
7. Detail the toxic effects of various pesticides and herbicides on people and outline the special problems associated with their use.
8. Describe some of the effects of such substances as asbestos and food additives on the body.

INTRODUCTION

When problems, potential or otherwise, related to the health and welfare of a community are reported, they are of concern to the nurse for three reasons.

Firstly, since the nurse is a member of a community, anything that affects the health of that community as a whole, or subgroups of it, may affect the health of the nurse.

Secondly, the nurse is actively involved in the promotion and care of the health of the community and its members by virtue of his or her chosen profession.

Thirdly, we are all aware, or should be aware, of the very large number of contacts among the peoples of the world in this day and age. Whether these contacts are available through cycles in nature such as the water cycle, through ease of transport and movement, through personal contact or through the exchange of goods on the world market, it follows that what happens in one locality in the world no longer occurs in isolation, but can have very extensive effects. The spread of various infectious diseases such as tuberculosis and smallpox in the past is a good example. Today we find things such as insecticides showing up in the diet of people who have never used them or sometimes never even heard of them, such as the Eskimos or other isolated groups.

This chapter seeks to discuss some of the health hazards of modern living that are perhaps less obvious. We are becoming aware of some of these, since we hear and see comments and discussions in the media about pollution levels in the atmosphere, water pollutants, insecticides and other toxic substances, and occupational hazards such as asbestos and silica.

This is such a broad area that we can but alert the practising nurse to some of the problems, the potential dangers of some substances, of noise, etc., without even touching upon factors such as stress (in the sense in which the term is commonly used). One of the problems in discussing such topics is to decide at what point some of these factors become problems. Let us look at some examples.

Firstly, let us consider noise. At what level does noise become a problem? To many of the readers of this book, the sounds emanating from an amplified rock group may be quite acceptable (mentally, perhaps, rather than physiologically!), but to others these sounds may constitute noise or, at least, a volume level that is not acceptable.

Audiologists and related professions have consistently expressed concern at the permanent hearing damage that may be caused as a result of high volume levels. This seems to be particularly unfortunate when it is the hearing of young people that is under discussion.

(While on this subject, it is perhaps also appropriate to mention that the ultra violet lights used in some discos give off UV radiation of dangerous wavelengths – dangerous in the sense that it can burn out the retinas of the eyes.)

Secondly, at what point does the level of intake of artificial colourings and flavourings become serious in young children (if current suggestions about these subjects are correct)? When the children become so hyperactive that they have to be taken to a general practitioner or a paediatrician? And how is hyperactivity determined? And for which children, since some seem to be more disposed to hyperactivity than others? When should the community nurse advise a mother to decrease her child's intake of cordials, ice-blocks, etc.?

Thirdly, problems arising from smog and other air pollutants have already been referred to in earlier chapters. Even while this book was being writtien, one high school had to advise students who were asthmatic not to take part in a fund-raising run. The students who did run were advised to cease running if they felt distressed in any way, because of the high pollution levels on that day.

Thus we are discussing problems that are both real and controversial, in that it is debatable as to whether some of these things do, in fact, constitute hazards and, if so, when?

Within this text we have not assumed the responsibility of discussing all aspects of the following topics, but we feel that we should introduce the reader to a few health hazards in the hope that it will encourage the reader to delve more deeply into these areas. We would recommend that this be followed up by further reading of reliable media reports, of specialised texts and of journal articles. It should also be mentioned that some of the information in this chapter may be less relevant to the trainee nurse than to the practising occupational health nurse or the community nurse.

The following is an outline of some of these health hazards under purely arbitrary headings, since many are interrelated. All of these factors influence human beings in one way or another, whether directly or indirectly, through biological cycles or food chains.

ATMOSPHERIC POLLUTION

We have previously discussed the composition of 'pure' air and turn now to discuss the real air of so many industrialised cities of the world – air that is much less than clean (Fig. 15.1).

It is appropriate at this stage to define what we mean by the term 'pollutant'. A **pollutant** is any substance that contaminates the environment to such an extent that it adversely affects *people or* things that they value. We will essentially be concerned with the direct effect of pollutants upon people.

A number of substances contribute to what we refer to as smog. These include:

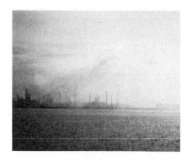

Figure 15.1. Air pollution. (Courtesy of NSW State Pollution Control Commission.)

1. Carbon monoxide (CO), hydrocarbons and nitrogen oxides produced by motor vehicles.

2. Particulate matter and sulfur oxides produced by industry and power plants, and the burning of fossil fuels such as coal.

3. Fluorides.

4. Carbon dioxide (CO_2), water (H_2O) and nitrogen (N_2), none of which are of concern in relation to the health of people at the moment.

Let us now look at each of these more closely.

Carbon Monoxide

This gas is produced by the incomplete combustion of carbon and its compounds. It competes with oxygen to combine with the haeme group of the haemoglobin molecule to form **carboxyhaemoglobin**. Furthermore, it is able to combine with the haeme group more strongly than oxygen (more than 200 times as much) and thus *reduces the oxygen-carrying capacity of the blood.*

Levels of carboxyhaemoglobin above five per cent of total haemoglobin are likely to cause headache, drowsiness, fatigue (which can lead to syncope, i.e. fainting), coma, respiratory failure and, of course, death (at concentrations of about 50 per cent). The actual blood concentration of carbon monoxide gas necessary to reach lethal levels is less than 0.1 per cent.

It is considered that levels of carboxyhaemoglobin as low as 1 per cent can cause distress, and it is noteworthy that the effects of carbon monoxide are exacerbated by exercise. Smokers are considered to have carboxyhaemoglobin levels as high as 6 per cent. It has been suggested that this may have a strong link with heart disease, as well as brain disease and degeneration, since the brain and the heart are the two organs in the body most requiring oxygen.

Hydrocarbons

Petrol consists of a mixture of hydrocarbons (compounds of hydrogen and carbon) having formulas which include C_4H_{10} through to $C_{14}H_{30}$. Some of these compounds are not burned fully in car engines and thus emerge unchanged from the exhaust. Other hydrocarbons are released into the atmosphere by refineries as part of the processing of crude petroleum.

These account for only about 15 per cent of the annual release of hydrocarbons into the atmosphere, the remainder (essentially methane, CH_4) being released by marshes, swamps, etc. However, the concentration is very high in urban areas, so that cities in particular suffer from the effects of hydrocarbon release.

The main offending pollutants resulting from and associated with hydrocarbon activity are produced by photochemical oxidation, that is by an increase in the oxygen content of some substances by the action of light (hence the term 'photochemical smog'). This produces **ozone**, which is irritating and toxic to the pulmonary system, and a substance called **peroxyacyl nitrate** (abbreviated, to PAN), which has been linked with chronic respiratory disorders. Apart from the damage that these cause to plants, which in the Los Angeles district of the USA has been extensive, their toxic nature has been established to the satisfaction of many scientists.

Oxides of Nitrogen

The first of these is **nitrous oxide** (N_2O), which is not man-made, is inert and not harmful. It is also known as laughing gas and is used as an anaesthetic.

The second is **nitric oxide** (NO) and is rather toxic. The main problem with this gas is that it reacts with oxygen in the atmosphere to produce nitrogen dioxide (NO_2).

The third of these is **nitrogen dioxide**, which is highly toxic and contributes directly and indirectly to photochemical smog. Some readers will recall nitrogen dioxide as the brown gas produced when nitric acid reacts with some metals and other substances. It is also involved in the reaction that produces PAN.

Many nitrogen oxides are produced by natural means and by the burning of fossil fuels. These compounds react with water to produce acids such as nitric acid, which are not pleasant in their effect on human tissue. Most of the effects seem to be observed in the respiratory tract (although eye and nasal irritation is also suffered). Respiratory distress is usually followed (in very severe cases) by pulmonary oedema and death, several hours after exposure.

The effects of current atmospheric levels of nitrogen oxides are unknown, but it seems reasonable to conclude that our health is not improved by them!

Oxides of Sulfur

Most of the **sulfur dioxide** (SO_2) and **sulfur trioxide** (SO_3), released directly into the atmosphere is generated by man. However, a large proportion also enters the atmosphere by oxidation of naturally produced hydrogen sulfide (H_2S, commonly known as rotten-egg gas).

Atmospheric sulfur dioxide is rapidly converted to sulfur trioxide, which dissolves in water to form **sulfuric acid**. The effects of this gas are thus very similar to that described for nitrogen oxide.

Gases such as nitrogen dioxide and sulfur trioxide contribute to the formation of 'acid rain', which has severely polluted some rivers of countries like Sweden to such an extent that fish can no longer live in them. The effects of oxides of sulfur can be observed in the areas around Mt Lyell, near Queenstown, Tasmania. Here all the vegetation has been stripped from the countryside by these pollutants to produce a 'moonscape'.

Concentrations as low as 1.6 ppm (parts per million) of sulfur dioxide will cause bronchiolar constriction (which is reversible). Above this level, observable respiratory distress occurs.

As well as the production of sulfuric acid, chemical reaction produces sulfates, which are severe irritants. Concentrations of sulfates as low as 0.002 ppm (that is, atmospheric concentration levels) are known to cause problems for some people, particularly asthmatics.

The combined effects of bronchiolar constriction and irritation are more likely to cause problems, and more rapidly, in those people who are either susceptible to, or are suffering from, lung disorders such as asthma, bronchitis, emphysema, etc.

Fluorides

These are released into the atmosphere by industry (e.g. by brick factories, aluminium smelters) and have been shown to have harmful effects on plants and on the grazing animals that consume these plants. Dairy cattle are thought to be particularly at risk. The symptoms are bone malformations, lameness and loss of teeth.

The effects upon the human body are not known at this stage.

Particulates

Particulates in the atmosphere are solid (smoke, grit, ash and dust) and liquid (droplets or aerosols). These sometimes include living materials such as viruses, bacteria, moulds and the spores of these, which will be treated separately.

If these particles are small enough to pass through the respiratory tract to the alveoli of the lungs, they can cause bronchitis and similar illnesses by interfering with the ciliary 'beat' (a mechanism by which millions of tiny hairs [or **cilia**] move backwards and forwards to remove unwanted matter), and thus obstruct the removal of harmful materials in the bronchioles. The possibility of a synergistic effect (i.e. when two factors taken together cause a much greater effect than would have been expected) also exists, with all the carcinogenic implications of this.

In conclusion, the combined effects of these pollutants have the potential to increase the incidence of not only lung disorders, but other problems as well. These include neurological changes such as learning and behaviour problems, which have been reported in children whose schools are beside major roads. The extremely high levels of gases from car exhausts (together with the effects of lead additives) have been suggested as the possible offenders.

Temperature Inversion: The Mass Killer

Normally, the temperature in the lower atmosphere (say up to 8–15 km) falls as the altitude increases, which means that the warmer air closest to the surface of the earth rises, because it is less dense (remember the discussion of convection in Chapter 2). This means that pollutants are often carried to higher altitudes and are therefore dispersed more readily from the earth's surface.

On occasions, however, a different situation can occur. The air closest to the ground becomes cooler than the air above it, usually because heat is lost by conduction and radiation to the cooler ground surface underneath. The creation of this cooler layer of air close to the ground, with a warmer layer above it, is called a temperature inversion. The inversion may be a few tens of metres deep or it may be several thousand metres deep. It is dependent upon still air so that no exchange of cool air (which, because of its high density, stays closest to the ground) and warm air takes place. The pollutants that are present are then trapped with the cool air in a layer immediately above the earth's surface.

A number of catastrophes resulting from a combination of air pollution and temperature inversion have been documented and include:

- The Meuse Valley, Belgium (1930) – 60 people died.
- Donora, Pennsylvania, USA (1948) – 20 people died and 6000 became ill.
- Poza Rica, Mexico (1940) – 22 people died and 320 were hospitalised.
- London (1952) – approximately 4 000 people died (in excess of the deaths normally expected for the five days involved).

Obviously, pollution is now a very sensitive issue and authorities are rather reluctant to talk about recent cases of sickness and death resulting from it. However, there would appear to be little doubt that people are still dying from these factors, although it is sometimes difficult to establish a direct link between such factors and deaths and illness at the time. Some of those people most likely to be affected may already be suffering from emphysema, for example, and this may be given as the official cause of death.

RADIATION

Radiation from the sun is essential to our existence. Without it we would all instantly freeze to death. The radiation we receive is infra-red radiation. Together with the infra-red we also receive ultra-violet radiation, which causes sunburn (whether clouds are present or not!) and **actinic keratoses**. These are horny growths that are caused by excessive exposure to the sun and may become malignant.

Ionising Radiation

As we have already seen, this term is used for radiation that removes electrons from atoms to form ions. Proteins, enzymes, hormones or genes may be changed, causing illness or death, depending on the extent of the exposure and the intensity of the radiation.

The effects can be:

- carcinogenic – cancer causing;
- mutagenic – causing a permanent transmissible change in genetic material;
- teratogenic – causing deformity of an embryo.

Nuclear weapons produce ionising radiation. Isotopes have been previously discussed; radioactive ones such as iodine-131 (taken in by cows after nuclear fallout and passed on in milk) accumulate in the thyroid gland and damage surrounding tissue. Strontium-90 'follows' calcium (i.e. 'whither thou goest I will go') and thus accumulates in bone tissue and may cause leukaemia.

X-rays also produce ionising radiation. It is claimed that radiographers have an average lifespan five years less than the general average for the rest of the population. The restriction on the use of x-rays for pregnant women and in the genital region generally is most welcome.

Non-Ionising Radiation

One obvious example is microwaves. Many a busy person would be lost without a microwave oven. Australian standards are stringent in the amount of permissible leakage of microwave radiation from these, but periodic testing is essential. Microwaves are being used increasingly in industry for drying.

Some Russian research leads to the claim that exposure to microwaves results in disturbances of the circulatory, nervous and respiratory systems, with behavioural alterations being quite common. More research is needed to determine the validity or otherwise of such claims but these devices must be treated with the greatest respect.

One cannot be too careful, particularly those people of child-bearing age, because the type of damage that may be caused may not be observed for many years and, for some, this may be too late.

WATER POLLUTION

Pollution of water supplies is thought to be responsible for more human illness than any other environmental influence (Fig. 15.2).

Hazards in water supplies that affect humans can arise from direct contamination or poisoning.

Direct Contamination

Direct contamination by bacteria, etc., causes diseases such as:

1. Cholera
This disease is caused by ingestion of a bacterium (*Vibrio cholerae*) commonly found in contaminated water supplies as a result of contact with human and/or animal excreta. Victims suffer from extreme diarrhoea, resulting in rapid fluid depletion and death for the vast majority of untreated patients. The bacteria are passed with the stools and must be ingested for the disease to be transmitted. The disease is now generally restricted to Asia, particularly India.

2. Schistosomiasis
This is caused by **Schistosomes**, which are blood-flukes, and is second only to malaria among serious tropical diseases. The larvae of schistosomes (called **cercaria**) enter human bodies through the skin when people swim, work or are otherwise immersed in contaminated water. The larvae enter the blood-stream and affect tissues such as the liver, lungs and kidneys. The

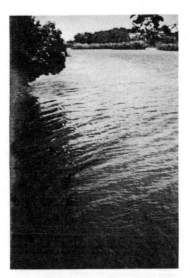

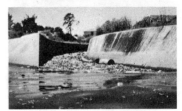

Figure 15.2 (a and b). Water pollution. (Courtesy of NSW State Pollution Control Commission.)

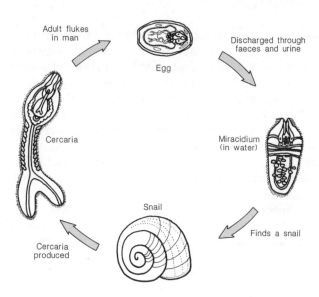

Figure 15.3. Life cycle of the schistosome. (From Cree & Webb: *Biology Outlines.* Sydney. Pergamon Press. 1984.)

eggs of the schistosome leave the affected human bodies through faeces and urine and go through other stages (Fig. 15.3).

It is estimated that over 100 million people throughout the world are afflicted with schistosomiasis – in Africa, Asia and parts of Latin America.

Once again, water supplies are involved.

3. Typhoid

This disease is transmitted by the ingestion of contaminated food or water. Bacteria are passed from a carrier in faeces and urine. Thus, contamination of water supplies normally occurs when sewage and sanitation systems are poor. Food contamination usually arises as a result of poor hygiene which, if it occurs in combination with an asymptomatic carrier in the food industry, can have devastating results.

Other diseases are transmitted in this way. These include viral diseases such as poliomyelitis and hepatitis.

The purity of a water supply is usually given as a coliform count (*Escherichia coli*, or *E. coli*, is used as an indicator organism for faecal contamination), but no assessment of viral content is indicated, nor are some treatment plants effective in destroying viruses.

From the above discussions, the importance of water supplies with satisfactory treatment plants becomes apparent. Furthermore, the contamination of these supplies can occur so easily if proper facilities to remove sewage from homes do not exist or are inadequate, and if satisfactory pollution control plants are not available to treat sewage prior to its disposal.

In some areas, situations exist in which other types of sewage disposal methods (such as soak-away or pump-out septic systems or deep pits) are located too close to a water supply. When this is coupled with septic systems that are functioning inefficiently, so that inadequately treated effluent is being discharged, contamination often follows. The contamination may occur during times of heavy rainfall when the ground is waterlogged and effluent can seep to the surface and form part of the runoff, with contamination of soil occurring along the way.

This is all not in the realm of idle speculation, or something which only happens elsewhere – ground contamination has been reported in areas of Sydney only 12 km from the General Post Office. Furthermore, in one such area (in which one of the authors lives), the *E. coli* counts reportedly could not be measured on some occasions because the counts were so high. This can present a danger to children especially, since they often love to play with soil and mud.

The disposal of sewage from large cities is an increasingly difficult problem. It was welcome news that the main Sydney sewer outlets are to be extended out to sea on the continental shelf. This followed public outcry that some of the finest beaches in the world were contaminated by sewage effluent whenever an onshore wind was blowing, with consequent fear of infections.

The other means of contamination which is worthy of mention is that resulting from poisons (which we will discuss in more detail later in this chapter), such as pesticides and herbicides, metals, etc. Such contamination can arise from direct spraying and leaching of soils, and some mining methods that involve the use of cyanides. Once again, the runoff from such areas tends to find its way into rivers which then become contaminated. A body of water in one of our capital cities became contaminated with cyanide in this way, resulting in a major fish kill.

Contamination can also occur by waste disposal from boats and ships, oil spillages from ships, wrecked ships (particularly those with hazardous cargoes, such as nuclear waste), and waste disposal from industry, particularly the chemical industry.

NOISE

This can be defined as *unwanted sound or sound levels*. However, such a definition is, of necessity, subjective – it depends on who doesn't want the sound.

Noise can damage hearing, cause other adverse effects on general health and behaviour, and interfere with our ability to communicate with each other. Have you ever tried to conduct a telephone conversation near a busy road, near someone who is using a motor mower, or a jackhammer or other machinery? Or

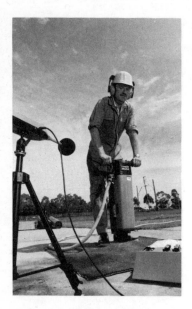

Figure 15.4. The use of acoustical ear muffs assists the operator by reducing noise and protecting hearing. (Courtesy of NSW State Pollution Control Commission.)

perhaps you have simply tried to talk to someone under such circumstances. Some of these points have already been referred to in Chapter 12.

General city noise may be sufficient to damage hearing permanently, if exposure is continuous. Advancing age is often blamed but is not necessarily the main reason for reduced hearing. Hearing loss is often the result of accumulated exposure to noise.

A substantial number of researchers in this area believe that other effects resulting from exposure to noise are more serious than impaired hearing. These include anxiety and stress, the latter being manifested by increased heart rate, blood vessel constriction, digestive problems, etc. The emotional effects on people are not measured easily, but it is clear that work efficiency is decreased.

Furthermore, it would seem that these effects (and others, such as an increase in irritability) may also affect ability to cope with daily living experiences. It should also be pointed out that the noise does not have to be loud to give rise to anxiety and stress – it can be something that is intermittent but perhaps relatively constant, such as a crying baby, a dripping tap or even the buzzing of a blowfly.

Quieter machinery is certainly one effective way of reducing noise. Acoustic materials will help to absorb noise, but if these measures are not available, sound reduction becomes a matter for the individual. The use of earplugs or earmuffs (or even better, a combination of these) will reduce noise substantially and protect one's hearing (Fig. 15.4). Removing the source of the noise, or oneself from the source, is the most effective way to reduce noise, but it is not always possible. Therefore, reducing the level of the noise with various devices and/or increasing the ability to cope with the noise may be the only alternatives.

Table 15.1 shows the effects of different types of noise. A combination of earplugs and earmuffs can reduce noise by 40 to 50 decibels. Thus the noise from a jet flying overhead can be reduced to the noise of an air-conditioning unit.

The reader is reminded that the decibel scale is a logarithmic one. Thus a reading of 20dB does not represent a sound twice as loud as one which gives a reading of 10 dB, but ten times as loud, and 30 dB is 100 times as loud.

POISONS AND TOXINS

In this section we are going to have only a brief look at this subject. The reader who seeks detailed information should consult authoritative literature on the subject.

The definitions of these terms tend to vary somewhat but, in general usage, the term **poison** refers to a substance that brings about death or ill-health *rapidly* (but the situation is then confused further by the term 'slow poison'). **Toxins**, on the other hand, are often seen as *slow-acting*, sometimes because of the incubation period of the bacteria involved. The adjective 'toxic' is used more widely, however. For our purposes and for the sake of simplicity, we will define the terms poison and toxin as referring to *any substance which, either directly or indirectly, is detrimental to one's health* (Fig. 15.5).

In discussing these, we will be mentioning a number of poisons some of which are quite exotic, but it should be remembered that many ordinary household substances are poisonous and have an unenviable record in the deaths and distress they have caused. These include:

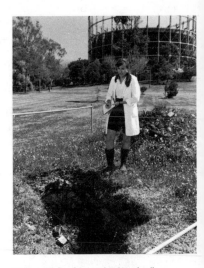

Figure 15.5. An examination of soil pollution. (Courtesy of NSW State Pollution Control Commission.)

- Drain 'unblockers' and oven cleaners.
- Cleansers of almost all types, detergents and disinfectants.
- Turpentine, kerosene, petrol and lighter fluid.
- Paints.
- Such diverse things as insect repellants, iron tablets, medicinal drugs, shampoos, mothballs and perfume.

Toxicity

Another difficulty to which we have already referred is that of *degree*. The boundary between 'toxic' and 'non-toxic' substances is not clear. For example, is cigarette smoke toxic? Toxicity also tends to depend upon such factors as the following:

1. How much of the substance is taken in.
In some cases, a substance may be harmless, perhaps even beneficial, in small doses, but be toxic in large doses. One example is the fluoride compound which is added to water supplies to help prevent dental decay. The same compound is used in toothpaste and in dental treatments in very small quantities to achieve the same effect. Similarly, alcohol is present in cough mixtures and is safe in very small doses, but is toxic in large doses.

It must be remembered that a *threshold level* exists for most substances – there is a level of intake below which no detrimental effects to one's health occur, as illustrated by the two examples above. In some cases in fact, a small quantity of a substance is essential to life, but a large amount is toxic, for example, vitamins A and D. The latter should never be given freely or without proper medical supervision.

However, it is not known whether even a minute trace of

TABLE 15.1 Sound levels and human responses

Sound intensity factor	Sound level, dB	Sound sources	Effects — Perceived loudness	Effects — Damage to hearing	Effects — Community reaction to outdoor noise
1 000 000 000 000 000 000	180–	• Rocket engine	↑	↑	
100 000 000 000 000 000	170–				
10 000 000 000 000 000	160–			Traumatic injury	
1 000 000 000 000 000	150–	• Jet plane at takeoff	Painful		
100 000 000 000 000	140–		Injurious	Injurious range: irreversible damage	
10 000 000 000 000	130–	• Maximum recorded rock music	↓ ↑		
1 000 000 000 000	120–	• Thunderclap / • Textile loom / • Auto horn, 1 metre away			
100 000 000 000	110–	• Riveter / • Jet flying-over at 300 metres	Uncomfortably loud		
10 000 000 000	100–	• Newspaper press	↑ ↓	Danger zone; progressive loss of hearing	
1 000 000 000	90–	• Motorcycle, 8 metres away / • Food blender / • Diesel truck, 80 km/h, 15 m away	Very loud		Vigorous action
100 000 000	80–	• Garbage disposal	↓ ↑	Damage begins after long exposure	
10 000 000	70–	• Vacuum cleaner			Threats
1 000 000	60–	• Ordinary conversation / • Air conditioning unit, 6 metres away	Moderately loud		Widespread complaints
100 000	50–	• Light traffic noise, 30 mctres away	↑ ↓		Occasional complaints
10 000	40–	• Average living room / • Bedroom / • Library	Quiet		No action
1 000	30–	• Soft whisper	↓ ↑		
100	20–	• Broadcasting studio	Very quiet ↓		
10	10–	• Rustling leaf	↑ Barely audible		
1	0–	• Threshold of hearing			

(From Turk & Turk: *Environmental Science.* 3rd Ed. Philadelphia. Saunders College Publishing. 1984.)

some substances may convert a normal cell into a cancer cell and start a chain reaction, which may then be fatal.

The *rate at which substances enter the body* can also be important. In the case of lead poisoning, for example, a relatively large single dose may be tolerated without serious or fatal result, but a much smaller dose repeated over a period of months accumulates and can cause serious or fatal intoxication.

2. The means of entry into the body

A toxic substance is able to enter the body in four different ways:

1. By ingestion into the gastrointestinal tract.
2. By inhalation into the lungs.
3. By absorption through the skin.
4. By direct entry into the bloodstream, i.e. by a puncture wound such as a snake or spider bite, or via an injury that allows the entry of toxins, or toxin-producing organisms such as *Clostridium tetani*, which causes tetanus.

As an example, mercury (as the *element*) is regarded as not being particularly toxic if swallowed, but is highly toxic if the vapour is inhaled or if mercury salts are ingested.

Safety Note: While current medical opinion does support the view that mercury is not particularly toxic if swallowed, it is the strong belief of the authors that the metal should be treated at all times as being dangerous if it is swallowed, since the vapour of mercury metal crosses cell membranes easily and could thus travel quite happily from the gastrointestinal tract to the lungs. As vapour it may then be passed to the brain and cause both neurological and psychiatric effects such as tremors, emotional instability, excessive sweating, depression and irritability.

Other substances, such as benzene, are toxic whether drunk, inhaled or absorbed through the skin.

3. The individual

Individuals exhibit considerable variation in their susceptibility to toxic substances. An amount that is fatal to one person may have much less effect on another. These differences may arise from such factors as the level of physical activity of the individual, the different rates of metabolism between one individual and another and the quantity of adipose tissue present in the individual's body, since this may act as a store or reservoir for some poisons (e.g. DDT).

4. Other factors

Some substances that are toxic have a much greater effect in the presence of other substances. The toxicity of carbon tetrachloride is a case in point. This substance was used for many years as a dry-cleaning agent, for removing grease in garages and on stove-hoods, for cleaning carpets and as a spotting agent for stains. The people using this substance inhaled the vapour, unaware of the hazards involved. It was found that the toxicity of this substance is increased in any individual who has been drinking alcohol, and is often fatal in such cases. It is a very nasty substance, which is best completely avoided as it attacks both the liver and the kidneys. Today, many newer compounds are available for the same purposes.

It has also been found that the risk of lung cancer as a consequence of exposure to asbestos is greatly increased for a smoker compared to a non-smoker. According to a report of the National Health and Medical Research Council (*NHMRC Report on the Health Hazards of Asbestos*, 1981), the risk for a smoker may be as much as 100 times greater.

One other factor worthy of mention is the rate at which the body *eliminates* or disposes of a substance. If a substance accumulates as a result of slow elimination of that substance by the body (or, indeed, failure to eliminate it at all), the effects on the body are likely to be much more significant (e.g. strontium-90, arsenic).

Toxic Elements – Non-Metals

Arsenic
This element has been known both as a therapeutic agent and as a poison for some 2400 years. The discovery of penicillin brought about the end of arsenic compounds for treatment purposes other than for some tropical diseases.

Arsenic is found in the atmosphere, in soil and in water, and is a by-product of the smelting of some ores such as those of lead, zinc and copper. In the process, it can be released into the environment. Some of its compounds are used as pesticides and herbicides, and others are used as food additives for poultry and other livestock. The average daily human intake is about 900 µg.

This element is a cumulative poison, causing vomiting and abdominal pains before the onset of death. It may cause bronchitis and dermatitis, and it is thought to be carcinogenic to some tissues (e.g. parts of the gastrointestinal tract and the bladder, but particularly the skin, often as a result of handling weed killers and such).

It may also affect the circulation, the kidneys, the central nervous system, the blood, the liver and general metabolism. Metal workers exposed to arsenic show an increased incidence of lung cancer closely correlated with exposure time – the longer the time of exposure, the greater the incidence of lung cancer amongst these workers.

Arsenic tends to accumulate in some food chains (e.g. fish and shellfish), although human poisoning does not appear to have occurred as a result of this – as yet.

Selenium

This element occurs in some metallic ores and is used in the manufacture of metal alloys and in the rubber industry. It is also used in the treatment of some skin disorders such as dandruff. Some of its compounds are very highly toxic, that is, they can be toxic at quite low concentrations. It has also recently been established that a very small quantity of selenium is necessary for adequate nutrition. The element itself, when existing as part of protein molecules and thus available to biological systems, is an anti-oxidant, is essential to some enzymes and is known to stabilise membranes. In drinking-water the maximum permissible level appears to be about 0.01 ppm.

Selenium irritates the eyes and upper respiratory tract. It is also thought to cause gastrointestinal, liver and kidney problems; pneumonia; and cancer of the liver. However, some selenium compounds are now considered to be *anti-cancer agents*.

For example, one compound of selenium containing sodium and oxygen (in particular concentrations) has been found to reduce the incidence of skin and liver tumours when fed to rats that have been exposed to carcinogenic agents.

It should be noted at this stage that the effects of some elements tend to depend on:

1. The *concentration* of the substance involved.
2. The *form* in which the element is involved – as the element itself or as the compound – and if the latter, which compound.

Toxic Elements – Metals

As a matter of convenience, the metals are given in alphabetical order rather than in the order of their relative toxicity.

Barium

This metal and its compounds are used in many industrial applications, such as the purification and manufacture of alloys. Some of these compounds when ingested are highly toxic, causing vomiting and diarrhoea, which may be associated with various types of internal bleeding. They may also affect the central nervous system leading to convulsions, etc.

It should be noted that it is the barium ion (Ba^{2+}) which is the culprit in such cases. Thus it is the highly *insoluble* barium sulfate which is administered as a 'barium meal' to enhance contrast in X-ray work in the gastrointestinal tract. This compound is comparatively harmless, since very little of it dissolves.

Beryllium

This metal is used in the aircraft industry and for making special alloys (e.g. for computer components and car brake-drums). Exposure to fumes or finely divided dust of beryllium salts causes **berylliosis**, otherwise known as beryllium disease. It usually involves the lungs and sometimes the skin, subcutaneous tissues, lymph nodes, liver and other organs.

It has been found that beryllium has caused cancer in animals, but the position with humans is not yet clear.

Cadmium

Cadmium is a metal that 'follows' zinc, i.e. it tends to be found associated with zinc ores, of which the most common is zinc sulfide. It is also found associated with lead and is almost as bad as lead and mercury in terms of its toxicity. It has many industrial applications, such as cadmium plating and in the manufacture of nickel-cadmium batteries. The combustion of coal and other fossil fuels releases cadmium into the environment.

Cadmium *accumulates* in the body, particularly in the liver and kidneys. Symptoms of mild exposure are vomiting, diarrhoea, nausea and colitis (inflammation of the colon). More severe exposure may lead to hypertension, heart malfunction, emphysema and death, usually due to massive pulmonary oedema. Carcinogenic properties have been suggested, and while the evidence with animals is convincing, the position with humans is not clear.

The tendency of cadmium to accumulate makes it a particularly dangerous element.

Chromium

This element is an essential micronutrient and is used extensively in industry, for plating metals and as an additive in steel manufacture, to harden the steel or to make stainless steel.

Chromium forms a number of different ions, both directly from the element and in combination with oxygen. The latter ions (chromates and dichromates) cause irritation of the eyes and upper respiratory tract, and the ions of the metal have been known to cause lung cancer. Chromium (with a valency of six), in particular, has been associated with cancer in both humans and animals. It has also been found to cause dermatitis.

Copper

Copper is used extensively in domestic applications (copper water pipes, hot-water tanks and electric cable) and many industrial ones, and is necessary for bone, blood, blood vessel and nerve tissue formation because of its occurrence in several enzymes. One of these assists the formation of haemoglobin from iron. It is thus an essential **micronutrient**.

Toxic effects tend to be associated with direct exposure to salts of the element, e.g. ingestion of copper sulfate. It is the Cu^{2+} ion which is the culprit in this case. While small quantities tend to cause vomiting, thus relieving the problem, larger quantities can be fatal. Fumes of the metal can also have temporary effects on metal workers engaged in welding, smelting and galvanising. Some people are more susceptible to the effects of copper for genetic reasons, because of an affliction called **Wilson's disease.** Some of the characteristic effects of this complaint are brain, liver and eye damage.

Mention has been made of the fact that copper pipes are used to carry drinking-water. As a result of this, the copper concentration in the water does rise slightly, but this is not normally a problem. It does become a problem where water is drawn only infrequently from taps connected to copper water services. However, we do need a certain amount of copper to survive, as it is a component of some enzymes.

Iron

This element requires no introduction to the reader. It is essential to the body in the manufacture of haemoglobin, cytochrome and many enzyme systems. Excessive intake, however, may interfere with enzyme activity. Fatalities are rare in adults (other than in suicide cases), but can occur in children, particularly in one- to two-year olds. As little as one or two grams of iron may cause death, but more commonly two to ten grams are ingested in fatal cases. The problem of accidental poisoning in children usually arises from careless storage of iron tablets. The underlying cause is a lack of knowledge and respect for iron as a drug with a toxic level. This applies equally to attitudes towards the use of other elements such as zinc, and vitamins A and D. Because they are sold without prescription and, especially, since the increase in interest in health and health foods, minerals and vitamins are too frequently seen as being without danger. Therefore, tablets are commonly left within reach of children. In addition, adults are not always familiar with dosage restrictions for children.

Lead

Lead is used extensively in domestic and industrial applications. Fumes of lead compounds arise from a number of different sources, including lead 'anti-knock' compounds in petrol, such as tetra-ethyl lead. This has unfortunate consequences in cities and large towns.

The use of lead in white paint has now largely ceased, since babies chewing paint from cots and from other sources used to be poisoned by the lead compounds in the paint. However, exposure can still occur where old cots or houses are, or have been, renovated. If the original paint contained lead, new paint used over it may chip off; or lead paint flakes made available during removal may be ingested. Particles may be inhaled during the sanding of lead paint surfaces. Degeneration of the central nervous system is one of the significant consequences of lead poisoning, together with effects on the blood and the digestive system.

Symptoms include loss of weight, anaemia, stomach cramp ('lead colic'), constipation and mental depression. In children, irritability and convulsions may be observed.

Choice Magazine (Journal of the Australian Consumers Association) September 1983, p. 17, makes a number of significant points regarding lead poisoning:

- Vegetables grown in the inner-city area of London may contain so much lead that they are unsafe for children and pregnant women. Up to one-third contain more than the British government's recommended maximum safety level.
- Not much difference exists between root and leaf vegetables, whether washed or unwashed.
- This last point is significant in that many people believe that washing vegetables and fruit will remove all poisons from them.
- It is believed that motor vehicle exhausts contribute most of this lead.

(As an aside, it is believed by some that the fall of the Roman empire was caused by lead – well partly, anyhow! The theory is that the Romans' drinking vessels and water pipes contained a high proportion of lead. This caused lead poisoning, which affected the mental faculties of the ancient Romans. Perhaps Nero became unstable through no fault of his own!)

It should also be mentioned that some countries are not fussy about the lead content of the solder used in food cans, and this constitutes a definite health hazard.

Manganese

This element is used in some industries, e.g. the steel industry. Compounds of this element occur in very small amounts in body tissue. Manganese poisoning can result from the absorption of dust of manganese and its salts. Symptoms include inflammation of the respiratory system and mental disorders.

Mercury

Reference has already been made to this element and the varying levels of toxicity resulting from different means of its introduction to the body (i.e. it is not as harmful if swallowed but lethal if inhaled, damage to the central nervous system being one of the effects).

Many of the compounds of mercury are highly toxic (the effects of the hatters of yesteryear have already been mentioned). One of the main sources of danger with mercury arises from its misuse in school science laboratories and other laboratories where spills occur. Mercury is very volatile, i.e. it changes into a vapour very easily, so that mercury spills result in a high mercury vapour concentration, which can lead to mercury poisoning.

The symptoms of mercury poisoning include:

1. In the *acute* form, arising from ingestion of compounds of mercury (i.e. releasing mercury ions): vomiting, bloody diarrhoea and damage to the whole gastrointestinal tract. Emphysema and haemorrhage often follow. High mercury concentrations have been found in fish in many parts of the world, which has led to the banning of fishing in some areas at various times. This occurred in Japan in the 1950s, when 121 people were poisoned and 46 died. Bread made from flour that had been treated with a mercury fungicide caused the deaths of some 500 people and the hospitalisation of more than 6500 others in Iraq in 1971.

2. In the *chronic* form, due to inhalation of mercury vapour, absorption through the skin and ingestion of some mercury salts: discoloured and sore gums which bleed easily, loose teeth, tremors and lack of coordination.

Mercury is used in dental fillings (amalgams, which are alloys of mercury and are apparently safe), in thermometers and sphygmomanometers, in wallpaper glue, as a fungicide, and in agriculture.

Nickel

This element is also used for the plating of steel and in alloy manufacture (e.g. for coins), as well as other extensive applications.

It is a micronutrient, being an essential constituent of some enzymes, but is toxic in large quantities. Respiratory disorders, dermatitis and lung cancer have been associated with poisoning by this element. One of the main culprits as far as cancer is concerned is nickel (with a valency of two), apparently mainly in association with nickel refining.

Tin
This metal is also used extensively in various applications, an obvious one being tinplate.

It too is an essential micronutrient, but some of the organic compounds formed from tin are toxic, the degree of toxicity being variable. The central nevous system is affected by these compounds.

Vanadium
This metal is not well known but has a number of industrial applications, such as the production of steel alloys designed to withstand high temperatures.

Poisoning by compounds of this metal usually occurs via the lungs. Symptoms include respiratory tract irritation, inflammation of the lungs, conjunctivitis and anaemia.

Zinc
Zinc is widely used for many applications. Zinc-plated (galvanised) steel is used in the manufacture of tanks to store drinking water. It is an essential micronutrient, since it is a constituent of many enzymes. One such enzyme is carbonic anhydrase, which is important in the removal of carbon dioxide from the body.

Zinc also plays an important role in protein synthesis and in cell division. Zinc salts are often poisonous when absorbed by the human body, resulting in a chronic poisoning similar to that caused by lead.

Pesticides and Herbicides

Pesticides are chemical substances utilised to control organisms that may affect the health of people – either directly or indirectly. The organisms involved are insects, vermin (rats, mice, etc.), roundworms and fungi.

Herbicides are chemical substances used to remove weeds and other unwanted plants in agriculture and horticulture.

It is not our function in this text to debate the wisdom or otherwise of the use of these chemicals, but we wish to point out some of the hazards associated with their use. The controversy over the long-term effects of such chemicals as agent orange may not be fully settled for some years, but it highlights some of the potential dangers involved. However, because of the lack of long-term evidence, the question of genetic mutations will not be discussed.

A large variety of these chemicals is used today and includes the following groups of compounds:

Rat poisons

These include anticoagulants, which cause death by internal bleeding, and more toxic substances such as strychnine derivatives and cyanides. Most are lethal to human beings.

Chlorinated hydrocarbons (organochlorines)

These include such compounds as DDT (**D**ichloro**d**iphenyl**t**richlorethane) and other similar compounds referred to as DDE and DDD. Some of these compounds have a long residual life and are relatively non-biodegradable and so remain in the environment for decades. Even some of the more modern insecticides such as dieldrin have not completely disappeared after two and a half years. These compounds are used for borer and white ant control and as insecticides.

While these substances are toxic, many eventually break down into compounds that are even more toxic, such as polychlorinated biphenyls (PCBs). They are all hazardous if swallowed, absorbed through the skin or inhaled as vapours or spray mists. For this reason they should never be sprayed inside houses or on walls.

Recent studies in the USA have shown that some of these compounds can migrate. Pesticides used for termite control under concrete slabs have permeated into dwelling spaces, and eggs from free-range hens were found to be contaminated with heptachlor, which had been used to treat the poultry owner's house for termites, 18 months before.

Once again, *Choice Magazine* makes a number of points ('Pest Control Companies', September 1983, p. 28, and 'De-Bugging the Family Pet', November 1983, p. 10):

- The Western Australian press has reported people suffering symptoms of organochlorine poisoning from heptachlor being sprayed inside wall cavities, on outside walls and under floors.
- Symptoms include a disfiguring skin rash, liver damage, sensitivity to light, headaches, nausea, vomiting, and nose and throat irritation. Breast milk of nursing mothers can also be contaminated.

Note: The residual action of organochlorines in undisturbed soil lasts lor at least 25 years.

- Japanese researchers have found chlordane in two seals

caught in Antartic waters in 1983. One of these also had DDT
and PCB in its body.

• It should be pointed out here that the spraying of houses
  inhabited by children and pets can be highly dangerous, since
  they are unaware of the danger and are less careful.

Unfortunately, indiscriminate overuse of some of these
compounds has led to contamination of rivers and lakes.

PCBs were responsible for farm animal feed contamination
in the state of Michigan, USA, and many people may have
suffered some degree of poisoning through eating contaminated
meat, eggs and milk.

Finally, there has been a worldwide spread of these compounds. As an example of this, DDT has been found in breast
milk and in the tissues of Eskimos.

It must not be inferred from this that the authors necessarily
condemn all use of these compounds – we wish only to alert
readers to some of the hazards associated with their use.

Organophosphates

These include common garden sprays such as malathion and
some insecticides. These are rapidly degraded in the environment, but are similar to nerve gases and can thus be lethal to
human beings. The need for protective clothing and goggles and
even a respirator is essential – the alternative may be too morbid
to contemplate.

The effect of these gases is to interfere with the action of
acetylcholinesterase, causing massive release of acetylcholine at
synapses. This, in turn, leads to convulsions, tremors in involuntary muscles and death. These organophosphates are generally
more toxic than organochlorines, and while they do not accumulate in the body they can have a cumulative effect on acetylcholinesterase (also known as cholinesterase). In general, where
recovery from organophosphate poisoning occurs, it tends to be
quicker than is the case with organochlorine poisoning.
Organophosphates are easily absorbed through the skin, and are
toxic if inhaled, absorbed or swallowed.

These compounds are widely used on fruit and vegetables.
Limits of these pesticide residues in fruit and vegetables are set
by the National Health and Medical Research Council
(NHMRC). However, numerous problems exist with monitoring
these limits, and with the lack of standardisation in testing for
residues and conflicting advice given to consumers.

For example, the Australian Consumers' Association (in
1983) found the levels of the organophosphate fenamiphos in
some celery from a supermarket to be double the NHMRC limit.
Furthermore, results published by the NHMRC for 1980 samples showed organophosphate levels to be high in a number of

foods, such as onions, beans and strawberries. Remember the cumulative effects are of particular concern in this case.

These compounds are also used in pets' flea collars, washes and medallions.

Their potential dangers to children and pets should be considered, particularly in the washes which are supposed to dry on the animal's coat.

Carbamates

These include compounds such as baygon. These are less harmful to people and less persistent in the environment, but must be used with care. They are also anti-cholinesterase compounds and are used in flea collars and medallions.

Pyrethroids

These include the pyrethrins commonly used in household insect sprays. They are rapidly broken down after application and have a low toxicity to human beings. However, they can cause allergic reactions and dermatitis.

Large concentrations can cause vomiting, nausea, headaches and other problems associated with the central nervous system.

Drugs used to treat roundworms

Various types of chemicals are used for this purpose. It appears that they may not be harmful to human beings, but this should not be assumed.

Fungicides

These are also variable in nature and thus may be harmful. Some are similar in their effects on humans to chlorinated hydrocarbons and are best treated with considerable respect.

Herbicides

Some are low in toxicity, but others such as **paraquat** are known to have caused several deaths. One, 2,4,5-T, apart from other effects, is known sometimes to contain an impurity (dioxin) which is teratogenic, i.e. it causes physical defects in developing embryos, and also causes a skin disease called chloracne. The infamous substance known as agent orange was used in the Vietnam war to destroy vegetation and expose the hiding places of the Viet Cong. It is a mixture of 2,4,5-T and 2,4-D, and contains dioxin.

Pesticides and herbicides which are not compounds of carbon

These include compounds of elements such as mercury, arsenic and copper, together with compounds such as sodium chlorate. These are generally highly toxic to a large number of organisms, including humans. Their use is best avoided if possible.

Some final comments

1. Research to date has been insufficient to be too definite on levels, cumulative effects, thresholds, doses, migration effects and long-term genetic effects.

2. Unfortunately, there is a lack of standardisation of testing programmes and surveys, methods of handling and the registration of pesticides and herbicides; and a lack of consistency in the information released to the public. As recently as 1983 one state still issued a pamphlet that listed DDT, for example, as having low toxicity!

3. The general public still seems to harbour the idea that if a small quantity performs a given function satisfactorily, then a large quantity must be even better. There is an obvious need to keep the public better informed.

4. In Australia, we still do not take carcinogenic potential into proper account (particularly in comparison with the USA, where if a compound is suspected of being carcinogenic its use is banned). The onus here still seems to be on the consumer to prove ill-effects, rather than on the manufacturer to demonstrate that the compound in question is safe beyond doubt. In some cases, it appears that companies may have withheld information on these effects from the public. Unfortunately, it is often not until many workers have suffered adverse effects from such chemicals that any action is taken.

Perhaps we should once again ask the question: is it better to be cautious (overcautious?) and refuse to allow the use of any product where any doubt exists as to its effect on humans (and animals in some cases), or should it be used until its direct effect on humans is known? People usually do not want to be guinea pigs, but once a product is on the shelves it is harder to get it withdrawn.

5. It has been shown that some pests have become more resistant to the effects of pesticides. This tends to exacerbate the problem.

6. It seems that the whole community must take responsibility for the use of these products. Fruit and vegetable growers tend to use pesticides in response to our wish to eat fruit and vegetables unblemished by spots, even though the flavour and quality may not be impaired by spots. The price is high – the extensive use of pesticides – and the blame must be shared.

Asbestos

Asbestos is a family of complex silicates of calcium, magnesium and other metals, and is fibrous in nature. Various types of asbestos give rise to different types and degrees of problems.

It is used in building materials ('fibro'), in the manufacture of automotive parts (gaskets and brake-linings), in the manufacture of heat and fire-resistant materials, vinyl asbestos flooring materials, rubber, plastics, adhesives and cements, paints, sealants, and gaskets and filters used in the production of beverages.

The inhalation of these fibres (and the possibility exists that a *very small* number of these fibres can be harmful) leads to lung scarring or **asbestosis**, which is associated with various types of cancer of the lung, particularly **mesothelioma** – a malignant tumour found in tissue linings. The first documented case of asbestos-related mesothelioma outside South Africa (where extensive mining of blue asbestos has occurred) was reported in 1962 in an ex-miner from Western Australia.

The risk also involves workers' families, since the dust can be carried into the home. People who have spent some time in asbestos workers' homes, or even in the neighbourhood of asbestos mines and plants, may ingest asbestos fibres from the air in these localities.

Asbestos was used in some schools in New South Wales in ceilings for assembly halls and classrooms until quite recently. This has posed problems: workers refuse to remove them because of the risk to themselves; the government is concerned about cost; parents are concerned about their children and threaten to remove them from schools until something is done, and so forth. At the time of writing. the saga continues.

A National Health and Medical Research Council (NHMRC) report entitled *Report on the Health Hazards of Asbestos*, published in June 1981, yields the following points:

1. The International Agency for Research on Cancer (IARC), in a 1977 monograph concluded: 'It is not possible to assess whether there is a level of exposure in humans below which an increased risk of cancer would not occur'. The agency considered both the results of experiments with animals and epidemiological evidence (studies that may provide links between exposure to asbestos and the incidence of cancer).

2. Both the number of fibres in a specific volume of air and the length of exposure are important, together with other factors such as smoking, which greatly exacerbates the problem.

3. The main asbestos-related diseases have a delay or lag period, which may be 20 years or more, depending on the exposure. After this time, symptoms may appear and even progress, although exposure may have ceased.

4. The inability of researchers to identify a threshold does not mean that one does not exist – some people in urban areas

have been found with asbestos fibres in their lungs but no sign of asbestos-related disease. Also, asbestosis (fibrosis of the lung) has occurred without cancer, and mesothelioma without a history of exposure to asbestos, or indeed without the presence of asbestos fibres in the tissue around it.

Food Additives

BHT and BHA

The effects of these chemicals in foods is important. They are **anti-oxidants**, i.e. they are added to foods containing fats and oils to prevent these from oxidising and becoming rancid. Examples of these foods are fried foods such as doughnuts, potato chips, hamburgers, fried chicken (note that fast food outlets are involved) and salad dressings. Some people suffer from strong allergic reactions to these chemicals.

Nitrates and nitrites

These are added to meats in quite large amounts to retain colour, and in smaller amounts to preserve them.

Some infants suffer from a disease (methaemoglobinaemia) that limits the oxygen-carrying capacity of the blood, if food containing these additives is consumed. Hence baby foods do not contain nitrates and nitrites, which means that babies may suffer from this affliction only by eating adult food containing these compounds.

These additives are able to form compounds called **nitrosamines** in the oesophagus and stomach, by reaction with compounds called secondary amines found in cereals, tea, beer, wine and other foods. Some nitrosamines are known carcinogens. These were banned in Norway in 1973.

Unfortunately, the evidence of long-term effects of these and many others of the thousands of food additives used today is inadequate, and 'experts' differ in their opinions regarding these additives.

Artificial colourings, flavourings and preservatives

At the beginning of this chapter, reference was made to cordials, which contain artificial colourings and flavourings as well as preservatives These have been associated very strongly with hyperactivity in children, to such an extent that a marked decrease in hyperactivity is observed in many children when these drinks are removed from their diets. Others would argue that hyperactivity is a 'parent phenomenon' and has nothing to do with flavourings. Some allergies have also been associated with artificial colourings and flavourings.

There are so many different food colourings, flavourings and preservatives on the market that space in this text precludes a discussion of them all. It will be sufficient to observe that examination of the shelves of any food shop will reveal an abundance and wide range of foods containing these substances. The effects, especially long-term, cumulative or synergistic, are relatively unknown.

General conclusion

Many of the points we have raised in this chapter are of special concern to the occupational nurse, but the community nurse may also be involved. Furthermore, as responsible citizens with direct concern for, and interest in, the general health of the community, it should indeed be of concern to all. We cannot escape our important responsibilities to our children, and their children after them.

Some of the concluding points in the pesticide and herbicide section regarding potential long-term and cumulative effects have a general application in a wide variety of situations. Unfortunately, groups with vested interests so often manage to gag informed debate and prevent action being taken.

However, the nurse can, and indeed must, play a part by being vigilant on such matters, particularly where babies and young children are concerned.

REVIEW

1. List the main ingredients of atmospheric pollution and their effects on people.
2. What is a temperature inversion and in what way does it constitute a hazard?
3. Distinguish between ionising and non-ionising radiation and their effects on people.
4. List some of the diseases caused by water pollution and comment briefly on each.
5. Briefly outline some of the hazards associated with noise.
6. What are some of the factors affecting the toxicity of poisons?
7. List some of the chemical elements that are toxic to humans.
8. Comment on the effects on the human body of some pesticides and herbicides.
9. What are some of the particular problems associated with asbestos and the human body?
10. Describe the effects of some food additives on people.
11. Identify ways in which a nurse and the nursing profession can be active in the promotion of health care in the community with regard to potential environmental hazards.

16

Genetics and heredity: the blueprint of life

OBJECTIVES

After studying this chapter students should be able to:

1. Describe mitosis and meiosis and distinguish between them.
2. Discuss the two main factors influencing the development, growth and maturity of an individual.
3. Define terms such as dominant, recessive, homozygous, heterozygous and incomplete dominance, and apply an understanding of these to genetic problems and situations.
4. State Mendel's laws.
5. Define sex-linkage and apply an understanding of this to the genetic transmissions of afflictions such as haemophilia and colour blindness.
6. Define mutations and describe the types of mutations that can occur.
7. Discuss genetic engineering and eugenics.
8. Describe amniocentesis and its use.
9. Discuss the benefits of skilled genetic counselling.

INTRODUCTION

It is said that the best laid plans of mice and men often go astray. This is equally true of the propagation of human beings. Why do things sometimes go haywire? How are some diseases genetically transmitted? What has happened to the genetic plan for growth when a child is born without fingers or without an arm? What problems may arise as a result of a mother having Rh-negative blood?

These are the kinds of questions we seek to answer in this chapter. Our task is to help provide the basis of knowledge that the nurse will need in order to understand the implications of genetics. She will then be able to direct inquirers to seek specialised counselling and to understand the advantages of investigative techniques. Techniques such as amniocentesis can provide some information regarding abnormalities in the growing fetus. The community nurse, for example, is often the first 'port of call' for some people and it is important that he/she be able to give correct advice and know where to send people for further help.

To provide the background knowledge and understanding necessary to achieve these aims, we need to look at the animal cell, cell division, genes, chromosomes and inheritance patterns.

ANIMAL CELLS

Most living cells are about the same size and are microscopic. Thus, unicellular animals are themselves microscopic, but larger animals simply have more microscopic cells. All animals begin life from one or two cells. A unicellular animal does not grow by division, but a multicellular animal grows by constant division of its cells until the required size is reached. The size of the animal and the number of cells will be genetically determined.

An animal cell of average size, such as a red blood cell, is about 8 µm (i.e. eight millionths of a metre) in diameter. It may be argued that cells could grow larger than they do before they divide. In the case of the red blood cell, it would have considerable difficulty in negotiating some of the very fine capillaries through which it must pass in the course of its day's work. However, there is an even more compelling reason why *all* cells are restricted in size:

If a cell were to become too big, its surface area would be too small compared to its large volume. The surface area of the cell membrane would be too small to allow enough food and oxygen to enter the cell and to allow for the passage of the larger quantity of waste products out of the cell.

A typical animal cell is shown in Fig. 16.1. We, as human beings, are made up of such cells, although it must be remembered that as highly sophisticated animals – at least in terms of structure – we have many cells in our bodies that are highly specialised to perform particular tasks; for example, blood cells, nerve cells, brain cells and muscle cells.

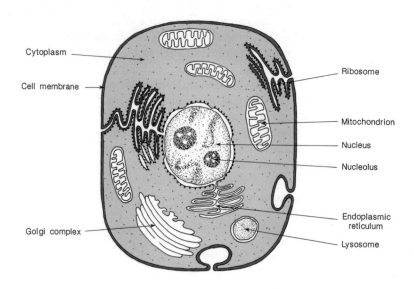

Cytoplasm

Cell membrane

Ribosome

Mitochondrion

Nucleus

Nucleolus

Golgi complex

Endoplasmic reticulum

Lysosome

Figure 16.1. A diagram of an animal cell when viewed under an electron microscope. (From Cree & Webb: *Biology Outlines* Sydney. Pergamon Press. 1984.)

We will now review those aspects of cell physiology that are particularly relevant to the understanding of genetics and inheritance.

Cell Division

Cell division is not only the means by which an animal grows, it is also the means by which it can eventually pass on its genetic material. This material contains the information necessary for the growth and development of a new individual and thus the preservation of a species.

The division of a cell involves that cell splitting into two parts in a process called **binary fission.** The original cell is often called the *parent* cell and the two new cells the *daughter* cells. (We are unaware of the existence of any non-sexist terms to replace this!) Prior to this division, short, thick strands called **chromosomes** become visible in the nucleus.

Chromosomes contain the genetic information that is passed from one generation to the next, and in this type of cell division, called **mitosis,** the number of chromosomes in the daughter cells is identical to that in the parent cells. This means that the parent and daughter cells have identical **genotypes** or genetic constitution – identical numbers of chromosomes and identical information carried on those chromosomes. This information is considered to be carried by a compound called DNA (deoxyribonucleic acid).

Note that mitosis occurs in all body cells except those giving rise to **gametes** (the cells involved in sexual reproduction – sperm and ova).

When we speak of genetic constitution or genetic code, we are referring to the presence of **genes,** which are the units of heredity (simply, the transmission of genetic information to offspring). A gene may then be defined simply as a unit of *inherited material*. Genetic information determines so many parts of our make-up, from the colour of our eyes and hair to the way we walk. As mentioned above, this genetic information is carried in molecules of DNA and, as a result, some authors now define genes in terms of molecules of DNA, rather than as units of inheritance. For the sake of simplicity, we have retained the latter definition.

Mitosis

During this type of cell division, the nucleus of the parent divides into two identical nuclei, after which the cytoplasm of the cell divides. Mitosis is a continuous process, but for convenience is described as having seven phases, as shown in Fig. 16.2.

1. **Interphase:** This is the resting stage of the cell between cell divisions and constitutes much of the cell's life. Note that no chromosomes are visible at this stage, but the genetic material exists as a structure called the **chromatin network,** a network of fine threads spread throughout the nucleus.

Just prior to mitosis commencing:

- Each chromosome is duplicated.
- Each chromosome is connected to its replicate or identical duplicate at one point called the **centromere.**
- Each of these sister or identical chromosomes is known as a **chromatid.**

2. **Early prophase:** In the early part of the prophase stage, long, threadlike, duplicated chromosomes appear. These duplicated or doubled chromosomes (twice the usual number of chromosomes) contain two identical complete sets of genes.

3. **Late prophase:** In the later part of the prophase stage, the chromosomes shorten and become thicker, thus becoming visible as chromosomes. As we have pointed out already, the two strands of a chromosome are called chromatids *and* are held together at a common point called the centromere. Furthermore, the nuclear membrane (the membrane around the nucleus itself) breaks down and disappears into the cytoplasm.

4. **Metaphase:** During metaphase, the chromosomes line up on the equator of the cell (i.e. in the central part of the cell) on

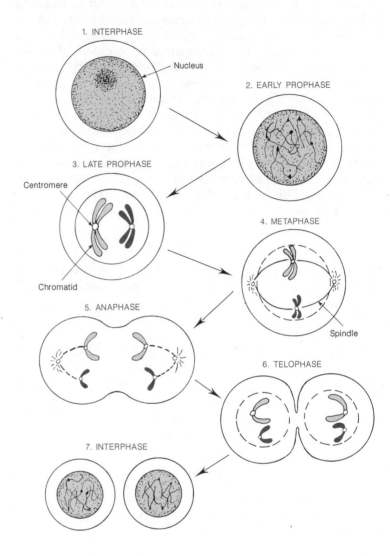

Figure 16.2. Stages of mitosis. (From Cree & Webb: *Biology Outlines.* Sydney. Pergamon Press. 1984.)

a fibrous protein structure which has formed at this stage, called the **spindle**.

5. **Anaphase:** At this stage the chromatids separate from each other, perhaps because of a shortening of the protein fibre attached to the centromeres. The separation of the chromatids, with one of each pair moving to each side of the centre, creates a situation where each half of the cell now has the original number of chromosomes. The stage is now set for the final act of this drama, the separation of the two halves of this cell.

6. **Telophase:** This is the last stage of mitosis, during which

the cell membrane pinches inward, forming a groove around the equator, new nuclear membranes begin to form, chromosomes and spindle fibres disappear, the chromatin network reappears and the cells complete the final separation.

7. **Interphase:** The new daughter cells, with the same number of chromosomes as the parent, now enter the resting stage described above for the parent cell, and mitosis is complete.

Cell differentiation and specialisation
The process of mitosis enables an organism to grow by cell multiplication. As well as growth, a developing fetus, for example, undergoes cell specialisation, in a process called differentiation. Although each cell has received an identical genetic code, each cell will use only that part of the genetic information that it requires to perform its specialised task. Thus we have cells in the pancreas that produce a hormone, insulin, while nerve cells conduct electrical impulses.

Sexual Reproduction

Some cells differentiate to form special sex cells called **gametes**. The female gamete is the ovum (plural ova), which is formed in the ovary. The male gamete is the sperm, which is formed in the testis (plural testes). When an ovum is fertilised by a sperm, a **zygote** is formed, which can develop into a complete and mature human being. The cell division that forms gametes is called meiosis, which is discussed below and is different from mitosis.

Chromosome number
We have already seen that, in mitosis, each new cell has the *same* number of chromosomes as that of the parent cell.

Chromosomes in all parts of the body exist in pairs, with the two chromosomes lying very close to each other. These pairs of chromosomes should be clearly distinguished in the student's mind from the two strands of one chromosome that are called **chromatids** and are formed only during cell division.

The two chromosomes of a pair are *identical* (or almost identical) in form and in the basic genetic information they carry. These chromosomes are described as being *homologous* chromosomes (homo means 'the same').

The 46 chromosomes normally carried in each cell of a human being are thus arranged as 23 pairs. The word 'normally' is included because, as we shall soon see, things sometimes go wrong. A cell with a complete set of homologous chromosomes is said to have the diploid number, i.e. $2 \times 23 = 46$ (since di- means two).

In the type of cell division that we are going to look at now, meiosis, each of the four gametes produced by the parent cell will have *half* the number of chromosomes or the *haploid* number – 23 (as illustrated in Fig. 16.3).

Figure 16.3 A comparison of mitosis and meiosis.

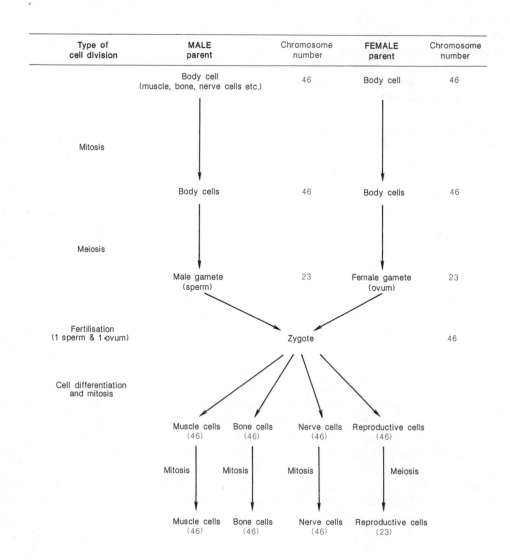

Type of cell division	MALE parent	Chromosome number	FEMALE parent	Chromosome number
	Body cell (muscle, bone, nerve cells etc.)	46	Body cell	46
Mitosis				
	Body cells	46	Body cells	46
Meiosis				
	Male gamete (sperm)	23	Female gamete (ovum)	23
Fertilisation (1 sperm & 1 ovum)			Zygote	46
Cell differentiation and mitosis				
	Muscle cells (46)　Bone cells (46)	Nerve cells (46)	Reproductive cells (46)	
	Mitosis　Mitosis	Mitosis	Meiosis	
	Muscle cells (46)　Bone cells (46)	Nerve cells (46)	Reproductive cells (23)	

Meiosis

It has been stated that the diploid number in human beings is 46 (horses have 66 and cats 38, by way of comparison), but for convenience (in Fig. 16.4) we are going to consider cells with a diploid number of chromosomes of four. Let us now look at the stages of meiosis. Stages 1 to 6 show the first division, to produce *two* cells; and stages 7 to 9 the second division, to produce *four* cells.

Stage 1: This is a resting stage (or interphase) between cell divisions. No chromosomes are visible. Near the end of this stage, duplication of chromosomes occurs and each chromosome

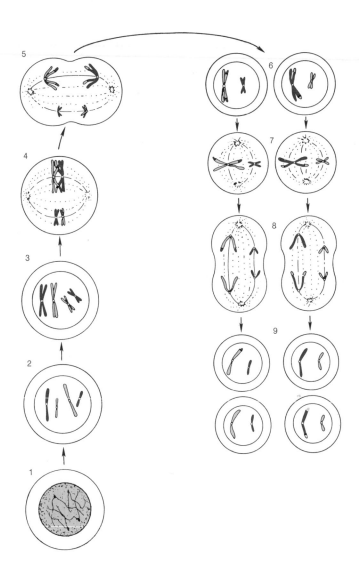

Figure 16.4. Meiosis for a cell in which the diploid number is 4. One set of chromosomes is shaded (female derived) and the other is not (male derived). The inner circle represents the nuclear membrane. The small white circle in the middle of the chromosome is the centromere. The dotted lines represent the spindle. On the right, (9) shows the four cells derived by meiosis from the parent cell in (1). This parent cell would be in the ovary or testis. (From Cree & Webb: *Biology Outlines*. Sydney. Pergamon Press. 1984.)

now consists of two joined identical strands, once again called chromatids.

Stage 2: Chromosomes are now visible and have become short, thick and coiled.

Stage 3: In this stage, the duplicated chromosomes may be seen to be arranged in their homologous pairs. That is, (unlike mitosis at a similar stage) the members of each pair of chromosomes come together and lie next to each other in an intimate association, often intertwining. This process of pairing is known as **synapsis**.

Stage 4: Crossing-over may now occur. The closeness or intimacy of the intertwined association of the coiled chromatids leads to some entanglement. As a result, breakage may occur, particularly as the independent chromosomes segregate, causing some pull on the entangled chromatids. Furthermore, at various places along the chromatids, as they lie side by side, cross-union may occur with the non-sister homologous chromatid (i.e. a chromatid derived from a male and a chromatid derived from a female on a chromosome pair). As a result some chromatids lose part of their original material and gain a piece from a non-sister chromatid. This type of exchange process contributes to genetic variability in a species and, more specifically, to variability in offspring from the same parents.

Crossing-over may occur at several points along the chromatids, depending on their length and other factors. In human egg cells for example, two or three points at which crossing-over has occurred are usually observed on each pair of homologous chromosomes (Fig. 16.5).

Also, during this stage the nuclear membrane disappears, spindles are formed (as in mitosis) and chromosome pairs line up on the equator of the spindle at random. As an example, both 'white' chromosomes may line up on one side and both 'black' chromosomes on the other, or they may not. Thus it is a completely random arrangement.

Stage 5: The chromosomes are now completely segregated.

Stage 6: The first division is now complete and the nuclei reform, two daughter cells having been formed.

Figure 16.5. Double crossover. Two chromatids in the tetrad cross over twice, exchanging segments between the A and C loci. (From Arms & Camp: *Biology.* 2nd Ed. New York. Saunders College Publishing. 1982.)

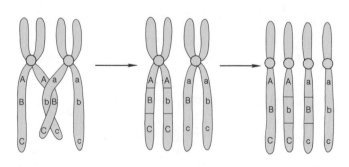

A comparison between mitosis and meiosis is useful at this stage:

- Mitosis would now be finished. The chromatids would have separated, one going to each of the daughter nuclei, so that each daughter nucleus would have two pairs or four homologous chromosomes.
- In meiosis, however, we have reached the stage where we have two daughter cells each containing unseparated chromatids, since only the homologous pairs have separated; each cell has four chromosomes or two pairs of chromatids.

Stage 7: In each of the two new cells the second division commences, with the disappearance of the nuclear membrane, spindle formation, lining up, etc., as before.

Stage 8: The chromatids now separate, in preparation for the final division in which the new cells will have *two* chromosomes only (the haploid number), compared to the *four* chromosomes (the diploid number) of the parent.

Stage 9: The second division is complete and we now have four cells, each with the haploid number of chromosomes – two.

It is important to note that the genetic composition of each of the four cells is different (which we have endeavoured to show graphically in Fig. 16.4). In the human case, the four cells would each contain the haploid number of chromosomes (23), with a very large number of variations in the genetic information transmitted in each case.

Thus, the result of fertilisation of human cells (in the mother, for example) by cells from the other parent (the father, whose cells have been formed by the same process) will have some characteristics that are similar and others that are different. The offspring may all look similar, but will still be different. This is not surprising, since there are eight million ways in which the 23 chromosomes of a mother and the 23 chromosomes of a father can combine!

When any daughter cell that has been formed by meiosis is fertilised by a sperm cell, the resulting cell or zygote will contain 46 chromosomes – 23 from the mother and 23 from the father. Therefore, every homologous pair of chromosomes in a cell will have one chromosome from the mother and one from the father. This will result in genetic variations (in addition to those caused by crossing-over) occurring in the gametes from which the new offspring are formed. As was explained in stage 4, the homologous pair of chromosomes separate at random between nuclei, giving rise to this variation. The four daughter cells formed in meiosis may thus have some chromosomes from the original mother and some from the original father, or all from one or the other.

We now have a general picture of how the basic physiological process of inheritance works. However, this has told us only how the genetic material moves from one generation to the next, but nothing of how it is expressed in the individual or the individual's offspring, or of gene activity as such.

GENETICS, INHERITANCE AND VARIATION

In the development, growth and maturity of an individual, two factors are particularly important.

The first is **heredity**, which simply consists of those traits passed on to offspring by parents, as has already been pointed out. The messengers or factors that carry this information are genes, which, in turn, are carried by chromosomes and passed on in every cell division, whether mitosis or metosis.

The other factor is **environment**. This consists of all the external factors in one's life such as home, food, education, relationships, etc.

Therefore the mature individual has been (and still is) influenced by all the environmental factors around him or her and these, together with genetic factors, account for all the traits of an individual.

Sometimes both genetic and environmental factors can be involved in the determination of one particular trait. As an example, our height is determined both by genetic factors and environmental factors, such as the food we eat.

The influence of the environment on the individual is a whole field of study in itself, so that only brief mention of this has been made here as the other contributing factor in determining the characteristics of any individual. The sum of all the characteristics making up any individual is called the phenotype. This includes size, shape, colour, body temperature, cellular respiration, diet type, weight, etc.

Patterns of Inheritance

An Austrian teaching monk named Gregor Mendel carried out some breeding experiments with pea plants, from which he derived some basic principles of inheritance. These were published in 1866.

Mendel laid the foundations for the study and development of genetics and inheritance.

There has been considerable alteration to, and development of, his original laws, mainly because human beings are much more complex individuals than Mendel's peas! Furthermore, new methods of study and technological development have led to greater penetration into this field of study. However, to understand and appreciate something of the complexity of the human being, it is easier if one first examines the simpler situations from which the laws were developed.

Mendel studied different traits in plants, such as height, colour, texture of seeds and so forth. Initially, he crossed plants that differed by only one characteristic. Furthermore, he used only those plants which he knew to be 'pure'. Pure plants were those he had bred for many generations to ensure that the trait he wanted to study was faithfully reproduced from one generation to the next. Thus tall plants would keep on reproducing tall plants over many generations.

The principle of dominance

As a result of Mendel's experiments, it has been found that:

1. Each trait is controlled or determined by at least one pair of genes (one gene on each chromosome of a homologous pair) at identical locations.

2. Most traits in human beings are controlled by several pairs of genes on the same homologous pair or on different pairs.

3. Alternative or contrasting forms of the same trait are **alleles** of one another. As an example, height in plants is controlled by the genes for tall plants and the genes for short plants, and these are alleles of one another (Fig. 16.6).

4. Two or more alleles for a given trait can exist in the same cell. If the pairs of genes are identical, they are known as **homozygous** genes for that trait. If not they are known as **heterozygous** genes.

5. When two members of any given pair of hereditary units are different (i.e. a chromosome pair contains dissimilar genes or alleles at a specific location), competition exists for expression in the individual. The result is that one gene may mask or conceal the other one to produce a particular trait. The one that is shown or manifested is described as being **dominant** and the hidden one as **recessive**.

6. The dominant one is always expressed in the phenotype, while both will be present in the **genotype** (which shows the genes actually present – see below).

These principles may be illustrated by looking at the result of crossing a pure tall pea plant with a pure short pea plant. P_1 represents the pure parents, F_1 the first generation and F_2 the second generation.

Mendel explained this in the following manner.

If we represent the dominant pair of genes for tallness by TT, and we represent the recessive pair of genes for tallness by tt, we are then crossing TT (pure tall) with tt (pure short):

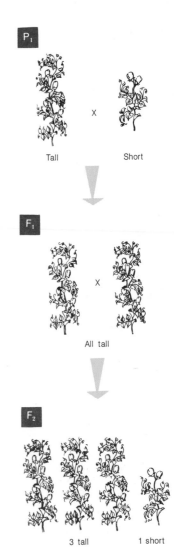

Figure 16.6. A cross between a tall pea plant and short pea plant results in tall offspring. The short trait shows up in the next generation. (From Otto et al. Modern Biology. First Canadian edition. Toronto. Holt, Rinehart & Winston of Canada. 1982.)

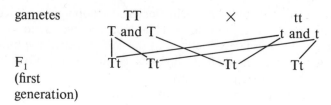

gametes   TT   ×   tt

F_1
(first
generation)

Since T is dominant and t is recessive, the plants will all be tall.

(*Note:* Offspring resulting from a cross between parents that are genetically different are called *hybrids.*)

If two F_1 individuals are then crossed,

Tt   ×   Tt

gametes   T and t   T and t

We obtain the four possible offspring in the second (F_2) generation from the four possible combinations of these gametes, as shown in Table 16.1.

Note that Table 16.1 shows the use of a **Punnett square,** in which the gametes for one parent are shown horizontally and the gamets for the other parent are shown vertically on the side. It is then possible to work out all possible random combinations of gametes, particularly where multiple traits are being studied, as we shall soon see. The traits of the resultant offspring can then be determined.

The result of this cross is three tall plants and one short.

TT, Tt and tt are called **genotypes,** because they show which genes are present.

TT and Tt genotypes will both yield tall plants, since T is dominant and t recessive. Because of this, they are described as having the same phenotype or appearance – tall.

A different phenotype is produced by tt, and the plants which have this genotype will be short.

The genotype ratio, TT : Tt : tt, is thus 1 : 2 : 1. Since TT and Tt both produce the same phenotype (tall), however, the phenotype ratio is 3 : 1. That is:

TT, Tt, and Tt all give rise to tall plants – a total of 3,

and tt gives rise to short plants – a total of 1,

so that the ratio of tall : short = 3 : 1.

This (3 : 1) is called a **Mendelian ratio** and is still important in simple situations today. If we have a sufficient number of progeny, for any particular trait that is completely dominant, there will be three chances out of four that the dominant trait will show up in the offspring. The idea of complete and incomplete dominance will be discussed shortly.

It should be noted that these ratios are approximate, but

TABLE 16.1

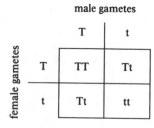

	male gametes	
	T	t
T	TT	Tt
t	Tt	tt

female gametes

become more accurate when the sample size is increased. This accounts for the odd results sometimes observed in small samples. As an example, two brown-eyed parents may have three blue-eyed children, despite the fact that brown eyes, B, is dominant over blue eyes, b.

Since each child is blue-eyed and blue eye colour is recessive, the genes for eye colour must be bb, with one b coming from each parent. However, since the parents are brown-eyed, their genes for eye colour must be Bb in each case. It is thus more likely that the children will be brown-eyed (either BB or Bb), but may be blue-eyed (bb). The ratios measured over a large population of such crosses would give a brown to blue ratio of three to one, but this may not show up in a small group such as a single family.

Some other monohybrid crosses

Hybrid crosses are those between parents whose genetic make-up is different. Monohybrid crosses are those between parents whose genetic make-up differs with respect to the one characteristic under consideration.

The first example concerns the presence of horns in cattle. In cattle, the polled (hornless) condition is due to a dominant gene, while the recessive gene causes horns to appear. The reason why two polled cattle have a calf that develops horns can be seen in Table 16.2. Note that P represents the dominant gene for polled cattle and p represents the recessive gene (which may give rise to horns).

Since the calf is horned, it must carry the genotype pp, i.e. homozygous horned. The only way in which the calf can have this genotype is by obtaining one p from *each* parent. Thus each parent must have one p present in its genotype. However, each can have only one p since they are polled, and the only way in which they can be polled is by having the dominant gene P present. Thus the genotype of each parent must be Pp.

The second example concerns the white belt produced around the body of pigs by a dominant gene B, while the recessive gene b gives rise to a body in which the white belt is not present. What would be the expected result of a cross between a plain coloured boar with a homozygous white-belted sow?

The boar would have to have a genotype of bb, since the white belt caused by the dominant B gene is absent. Thus the boar is homozygous plain coloured – bb.

The sow is stated to be homozygous and white-belted. Thus the two genes have to be identical and have to be the dominant gene for white-belted pigs, B. Thus the genotype of the sow is BB.

The result of this cross (see Table 16.3) is that all the offspring are white-belted, since they all have the dominant gene B present in their genotypes.

TABLE 16.2

		sperm (male)	
		P	p
eggs (female)	P	PP	Pp
	p	Pp	pp

TABLE 16.3

		sperm (male)	
		b	b
eggs (female)	B	Bb	Bb
	B	Bb	Bb

That is, the pigs are all heterozygous white-belted.

Incomplete dominance

Relatively few genes in complex organisms display a pure dominant-recessive relationship to their alleles. The commonest situation is one in which the dominance of one gene over another is incomplete. In other words, the trait is dominated by both alleles. The following example illustrates this concept.

red flowers RR × white flowers rr
F_1 first generation : all pink Rr
F_2 generation

TABLE 16.4

male gametes

	R	r
R	RR	Rr
r	Rr	rr

female gametes

pink Rr	×	pink Rr
RR Rr		Rr rr
red pink		pink white

i.e. red : pink : white $= 1 : 2 : 1$.

This is illustrated in Table 16.4.

Note: 1. Genes remain unchanged during meiosis. They do not blend in any way but remain segregated as discrete units; only their effects can result in a blending or mixture of offspring.

Each gene segregates in a pure form unaffected by association with its contrasting allele. Chance alone determines which chromosome (with the genes it carries) will travel to which gamete, and which gamete of one parent will combine with which gamete of the other parent.

In other words, since homologous paired chromosomes separate randomly during meiosis, and the chromatids are eventually distributed randomly among the gametes, chance determines whether any one gamete has obtained a chromosome from the mother or the father. The same then applies to the gene on that chromosome and thus chance equally determines which allele for any given trait a particular gamete receives.

2. Another exception to the dominant-recessive relationship arises when *only one* gene for a particular trait is present. That allele is then the only one which will be expressed in the phenotype, regardless of whether it is dominant or recessive. Examples will be discussed later, in sex-linked genes.

Multiple gene inheritance

When Mendel investigated the inheritance of two or more traits simultaneously, such as seed colour and shape, he found that the situation was much more complicated. The number of possible combinations of gametes could increase to produce greater variations in offspring, particularly in genotype.

The number of variations that can occur in the inheritance of more than one trait is dependent upon the genetic relationship between the characteristics. For example, if the pairs of genes for two particular traits are found on different chromosome pairs, they will be inherited independently of each other, as we have already seen. We have also seen that they will be inherited randomly because of the pattern of distribution of chromosomes in meiosis. Therefore great potential for various combinations exists. However, if one member of each pair is linked (i.e. found on the same chromosome) they will be inherited or distributed among the gametes together, or as a single entity. The same reasoning will then follow for the other two members of the pairs found on the matching homologous chromosome.

This will lead to less variation, the overall pattern then observed being the same as for single traits.

Below is an example of multiple trait inheritance, in which seed colour and shape (whether or not it is wrinkled) is considered. These characteristics are independently assorted, or non-linked, which means that the two characteristics act completely independently of each other. Thus:

seed colour alleles: yellow	— dominant	— Y
green	— recessive	— Y
shape alleles: round	— dominant	— R
wrinkled	— recessive	— r

Thus the possible genotypes, in homozygous parents, of these independent traits are:

round yellow	RRYY
wrinkled yellow	rrYY
round green	RRyy
wrinkled green	rryy

Mendel found that when he crossed homozygous round yellow (RRYY) peas with homozygous wrinkled green (rryy) peas, the first (F_1) generation were all round yellow. That is:

parents	round yellow	$\times$	wrinkled green
	(RRYY)		(rryy)
gametes	Ry and Ry		ry and ry
	RrYy	RrYy RrYy	RrYy

(F_1) first generation : all round yellow (RrYy)

If these self-pollinate (i.e. are crossed with each other):

round yellow $\times$ round yellow

(F_2) round : wrinkled : round : wrinkled
      yellow   yellow   green   green

Mendel's results

315 : 101 : 108 : 32

i.e. (approx)

9 : 3 : 3 : 1

These results of Mendel's work may be derived from a consideration of Table 16.5.

Table 16.5 The F$_2$ from a cross of two F$_1$ individuals in a dihybrid cross.

		Male gametes			
		RY	Ry	rY	ry
Female gametes	RY	RRYY round yellow	RRYy round yellow	RrYY round yellow	RrYy round yellow
	Ry	RRYy round yellow	RRyy round green	RrYy round yellow	Rryy round green
	rY	RrYY round yellow	RrYy round yellow	rrYY wrinkled yellow	rrYy wrinkled yellow
	ry	RrYy round yellow	Rryy round yellow	rrYy wrinkled yellow	rryy wrinkled green

(From Cree & Webb: *Biology Outlines*. Sydney. Pergamon Press. 1984.)

Multiple gene inheritance is a term that is also used to describe the situation where one characteristic is determined by several pairs of independent genes, but where these pairs may or may not be on the same homologous chromosome pair. Each set of genes makes a contribution to the expression of a particular characteristic independently of the other set(s). Each set of genes would produce only a small effect if taken separately from the others but produces a large effect when taken with the others.

Skin colour is a good example, as this type of control provides for many degrees of variation in the phenotype, and the results are readily observable in human skin colouring. Usually, no pair is completely dominant. In the skin colour example, at least two pairs of genes are known to be involved, two of these genes being responsible for production of quantities of pigmentation and their alleles causing no pigmentation whatsoever. This then gives rise to a wide variety of degrees of pigmentation because of the additive effects of the two genes and their alleles.

Other known examples of multiple gene inheritance are height, weight and intelligence.

An example of particular relevance to nursing is that of the **Rh factor** in the blood. One of the unfortunate consequences of problems with the Rh factor is haemolytic disease of the newborn (HDN), otherwise known as *erythroblastosis fetalis*. We will now take a brief look at the origins of HDN.

In one survey in New York, it was found that 85 per cent of the population was Rh+. This means that this 85 per cent have an antigen on the erythrocytes (red blood cells) of their blood called the **Rhesus factor** or Rhesus antigen (named after the Rhesus monkey on which many early experiments were carried out). This antigen reacts with particular antibodies, which are formed in the blood if the blood is injected with the blood of the Rhesus monkey or with most human blood.

For the reader who is not familiar with this terminology, antibodies are proteins that are formed by the body when certain substances foreign to the body gain access. This mechanism provides the body with natural protection against invaders (antigens), such as bacteria and viruses. The antibodies that are formed attack these antigens and seek to destroy them. Furthermore, antibodies tend to remain in the bloodstream and confer immunity against further attack. This is the principle of inoculation, whereby the body builds up its concentration of antibodies to the particular antigen following an injection of that antigen. These antibodies will then provide immunity against that particular antigen in future exposures. This idea will be explained in greater detail below in the discussion of the Rh factor.

It has been found that the genetic basis for inheritance of the Rh antigen is one of the two most complex in the human body. For our purposes, we will characterise the system by simply assuming the existence of two alleles, R and r, R being the dominant allele. It then follows that:

1. an Rh-positive (Rh+) individual possesses the Rh antigen and is thus either homozygous RR or heterozygous Rr; and

2. an Rh-negative (Rh−) individual lacks the Rh antigen and is thus homozygous for the recessive allele r, i.e. is rr.

The inheritance of Rh factor then follows the basic rules for simple recessive characteristics.

Now let us consider an Rh − woman having children (Fig. 16.7).

1. In her first pregnancy, she may supply an r allele and her partner an R allele, so that the genotype of the fetus will be Rr and the phenotype Rh+. Note that if her partner is also Rh−, no problem will occur.

2. During the birth process, some Rh+ red blood cells from the fetus become mixed with the Rh− cells of the mother. It should be borne in mind that one drop of Rh+ blood is all that is necessary for antibody formation.

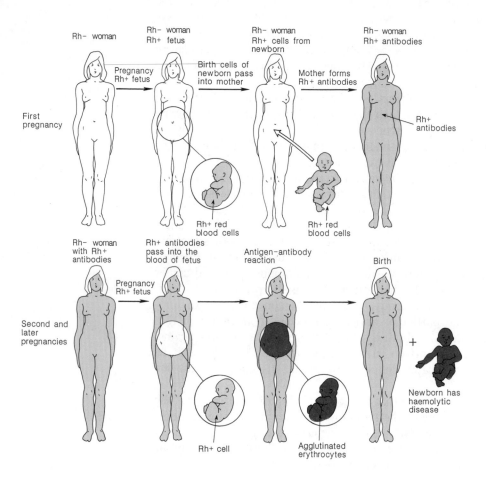

Rh– woman

Rh– woman
Rh+ fetus

Rh– woman
Rh+ cells from
newborn

Rh– woman
Rh+ antibodies

First
pregnancy

Pregnancy
Rh+ fetus

Birth cells of
newborn pass
into mother

Mother forms
Rh+ antibodies

Rh+
antibodies

Rh+ red
blood cells

Rh+ red
blood cells

Rh– woman
with Rh+
antibodies

Rh+ antibodies
pass into the
blood of fetus

Antigen–antibody
reaction

Birth

Second and
later
pregnancies

Pregnancy
Rh+ fetus

Newborn has
haemolytic
disease

Rh+ cell

Agglutinated
erythrocytes

Figure 16.7. The steps leading to HDN. An Rh – woman is exposed to the Rh + antigen on conception. If she then develops Rh + antibodies and produces an Rh + fetus, in a subsequent pregnancy the antibodies may be carried in her circulation through to the new fetus, destroying red blood cells in the fetal circulation and causing the premature death of the fetus or the birth of a child with HDN.

3. As a result of this, the mother forms anti-Rh antibodies (antibodies that attack Rh+ blood), and these are maintained in the bloodstream.

4. For all subsequent pregnancies, any fetus that has Rh+ blood will have its blood attacked by the anti-Rh antibodies in the mother's bloodstream, causing agglutination (sticking together) of the red blood cells of the fetus. The child then suffers from HDN. Many infant deaths still occur from this disease, despite the fact that it can normally be prevented by means of an injection that inhibits antibody formation in the mother. This is an area in which the nurse in the community can actively promote health care. The recommendation that prospective parents or women of child-bearing age should know their blood types and seek some form of pre-natal care is of benefit not only to the parents but also to their children.

Mendel's Laws

From the results of his experiments, Mendel proposed two postulates which are now known as Mendel's laws.

Mendel's first law: The law of segregation

This states that when gametes are formed, pairs of factors (or genes) segregate (or separate), because the chromosomes on which they exist separate, in such a way that each gamete receives only one gene from each pair of genes.

Mendel's second law: The law of independent assortment

This law states that the segregation of each pair of genes is completely independent of the separation of other pairs of genes on other homologous chromosomes. This means that the genes for skin colour may separate quite independently of the separation of the genes responsible for, say, eye colour, hair colour, shape of the foot or disposition to baldness.

However, some characteristics are linked by virtue of being on the same chromosome, e.g. colour blindess and haemophilia (bleeder's disease). In this case, the genes for colour blindness and those for haemophilia do *not* separate independently of each other, if both are present.

Summary of Simple Inheritance Patterns

1. If the parents are both homozygous for a given trait, whether dominant or recessive, that trait will appear in the offspring and be passed on.

2. If the parents are each homozygous for dissimilar traits, the phenotype of the offspring resembles the dominant parent but the genotype, which will be heterozygous, has genes for both traits from the parents.

3. If the *parents are heterozygous for a given trait*, the offspring will display the characteristic given by:

- phenotype – dominant : recessive = 3 : 1
- genotype – 1 homozygous dominant
  – 2 heterozygous
  – 1 homozygous recessive

(Disorders due to recessive genes are usually transmitted in this way.)

4. If one parent is heterozygous (the phenotype will show the dominant trait), and one parent is homozygous for a recessive trait, the offspring will have:

- phenotype – dominant and recessive genes in a 1 : 1 ratio
- genotypes – those that display the dominant trait have a heterozygous genotype.
    – those that display the recessive trait have a homozygous genotype.

5. Some characteristics are determined by more than one gene.

Sex-Linkage

In humans, the female has 44 ordinary chromosomes and two *similar* sex chromosomes (XX) – one X from the mother and one X from the father. The male also has 44 ordinary chromosomes but has two *dissimilar* sex chromosomes, X and Y – the X from the mother and the Y from the father. If genes are carried on the female (*X*) chromosome and have no corresponding gene on the male sex chromosome, (*Y*), then these genes are *said to be sex-linked*. Some 30 traits are known to be sex-linked. However, these are all X-linked (linked to the X chromosome), with one exception. The only known Y-linked gene in humans produces the H–Y antigen, a protein which is found on male cells only and is associated with the production of male characteristics. The Y chromosome acts rather like a dominant gene to produce maleness when it is present. When it is not present, a female develops.

One example is colour vision, which is controlled by a gene on the X chromosome. Sometimes, this gene does not impart colour vision to a new individual satisfactorily. This is because of a mutation (we will discuss these in the next section). The gene is normally dominant, but is recessive in the mutant or abnormal form.

If we then represent the normal chromosome by X and the chromosome that carries the mutant gene for colour vision by Ⓧ, we then have (with respect to colour-blindness):

XX – normal female.
XⓍ – a female who has normal vision but is carrying an abnormal recessive mutant gene as well as the normal dominant gene.
XY – a normal male.
ⓍY – a colour-blind male (some 8 per cent of Australian males are colour-blind).
ⓍⓍ – a colour-blind female. This is rare.

It can be seen that whenever the male receives an X chromosome with a gene for a trait that is not carried on the Y chromosome, it will always be expressed in the phenotype. This was pointed out earlier in exceptions to the dominant-recessive relationship. Furthermore, since the male never receives his X chromosome from his father, any abnormalities that the father carries in his X genes will not pass to the son but will go to any daughters.

In a similar way, let us now consider haemophilia. This affliction also occurs as a result of a gene carried on an X chromosome, and normally affects males only. (Remember that the affected form is recessive.)

Now since a male transmits an X chromosome to each of his daughters and a Y chromosome to each of his sons, all the daughters of a haemophiliac male will be carriers (while not being affected themselves), and the sons will not be affected. The reason that sons of haemophiliacs are never affected is that an X-linked trait is never transmitted from father to son, the son receiving his X chromosome from his mother.

If a carrier female marries a normal (with respect to haemophilia) male, we see that half of the sons, on average, will be affected and half of the daughters will become carriers like the mother (Table 16.6).

Note that it is extremely unusual to find a female who is a haemophiliac, because her father would need to be a haemophiliac and her mother would need to be a carrier. Statistically, this is not very likely.

It is interesting to note also that Queen Victoria was a haemophilia carrier and her healthy carrier daughters introduced this affliction genetically into the Russian and Spanish royal families. Queen Victoria's son Edward II was lucky and did not inherit the gene for haemophilia and thus it was not transmitted down to his descendants, including the present British royal family.

Another example of sex-linked disorders of the same type of pattern is Duchenne's muscular dystrophy.

TABLE 16.6

(carrier female X $\widehat{X}$ gametes)

	X	$\widehat{X}$
X	XX	X$\widehat{X}$
Y	XY	$\widehat{X}$Y

normal male gametes

Mutations

These are permanent changes in the hereditary material of cells. They may arise from:

1. Changes in particular genes.
2. Changes in the structure of a chromosome.
3. Changes in the number of chromosomes in a cell.

Some changes occur in body cells (or *somatic* cells) but these disappear with the death of the individual. Changes that occur in gametes, however, may be passed on from generation to generation.

Causes of mutations

These may be classified under two main headings:

1. Natural or spontaneous causes. The example of Queen Victoria and her introduction of the haemophilia gene into other royal families falls under this heading, since this great queen underwent *spontaneous mutation*. This is evident from the fact that her parents, Edward, Duke of Kent, was a normal male (with respect to haemophilia) and Victoria, Princess of Saxe-Coburg, was a non-carrier female.

2. Agents that create a change – agents known as **mutagens** or mutagenic agents. These agents increase the frequency of occurrence and/or the rate of increase of mutations in genetic materials. The mutagens may be genetic, physical or chemical.

The reasons why mutations occur or suddenly seem to appear is not well understood. Some of the consequences of these factors are such things as cleft palate, webbed fingers, missing limbs, etc.

Genetic factors: These are sometimes called mutator genes, which increase mutation rates, in one locality or several.

Physical factors: These include some of the types of radiation we have already discussed (gamma rays, X-rays and ultra-violet rays), high temperature and possibly sound.

Three important mutagenic sources form what is described as 'background radiation'. These are:

- Cosmic rays (radiation from outer space consisting largely of charged particles).
- Radioactive elements in the crust of the earth.
- Radioactive elements ingested as food.

Experimentation with bacteria, mice, *Drosophila melanogaster* (fruit-fly) and other organisms has given us a great deal of information to confirm that radiation causes mutations in these species. The evidence in the case of humans is not as clear, but is surely sufficient to make us very careful, particularly younger people of child-bearing age.

Chemical factors: Some reference has already been made to the possible mutagenic effects of substances such as tar, smoke, smog, some food additives (such as sodium nitrate and sodium cyclamate), mustard gas, formalin, carbolic acid, caffeine, pesticides and some solvents. The evidence that mustard gas is a powerful mutagen is compelling, but the evidence is much less so for substances such as caffeine. However, the possibility does exist and it would seem that care in the use of such substances is indicated. Some chemicals may be particularly dangerous because of synergistic effects.

Of even greater significance in today's society is the effect of drugs. Without even discussing the possible genetic effects of hard drugs, so many disasters have occurred with prescribed drugs that the patient who is wary of taking any drugs at all is entitled to our sympathy and respect. One outstanding example is thalidomide, which led to horrific deformities after it was prescribed for pregnant women.

Types of mutations

1. **Point mutations or gene mutations:** These are by far the most common type of mutation and occur when a DNA molecule is changed in some way, in a single gene.

Point mutations may:

(a) Affect the production of one amino acid in a protein, by leaving it out of the protein, or by including the wrong amino acid. Examples of the latter include sickle-cell anaemia and albinism. In the case of albinism the enzyme (protein) involved in the pigment melanin is affected and the individual then lacks melanin in the skin, eyes and hair.

(b) Affect the production of a whole protein as in haemophilia (normal blood coagulation requires the presence of a particular protein known as antihaemophiliac globulin).

This type of mutation is commonly spontaneous and often reversible – the mutation might be such as to revert back to the original form at some time.

Other examples of point mutations include:

- Mutations caused by *dominant* genes:
    achondroplasia (a type of dwarfism), gout
    Huntington's chorea (degeneration of nerve tissue)
- Mutations caused by *recessive* genes:
    cystic fibrosis,
    alkaptonuria
    phenylketonuria

2. **Chromosome structure:** This type of mutation arises by virtue of the loss of pieces of chromosomes or whole chromosomes, or the transfer of a piece of chromosome to another chromosome, perhaps with an odd type of recombination. Note that if this occurs during mitosis, gross deformity or death may result, but this is *not* normally passed on to other generations.

Deletion is the loss of part of a chromosome and is normally fatal in the homozygous state.

Duplication of parts of chromosomes may occur.

Inversions change the sequence or order of genes on a chromosome, which affects its ability to pair with its unchanged partner during meiosis.

Translocations are exchanges involving two or more chromosomes, as discussed under 'crossing-over'. This is one important cause of Down syndrome (or trisomy 21). The latter term has come into use because chromosome 21 is involved. In this case an exchange of chromosome segments occurs between chromosomes 21 and 15. A small piece of 15 is transferred, but a major portion of 21 is transferred to produce a very long 15. The result is a gamete with one smaller 21 chromosome and a 15 with a very long piece of 21. This means that two abnormal 21 chromosomes exist (together with an unaltered 21 – making effectively three 21s all told), within an overall framework of 46 chromosomes. This contrasts with another type of Down syndrome in which the individual has 47 chromosomes (instead of the usual 46) three of which are 21s.

3. **Chromosome number** (a) One of the two chromosomes in a set is lost. If this is an X chromosome, for example, the individual is left with only one X chromosome, called XO. This is one type of an affliction known as *Turner's syndrome* and affected females have impaired intelligence (with respect to some particular skills, such as space-form perception and mathematics), are short in stature and usually sterile.

(b) One or more chromosomes are added to the usual 46. Examples include:

- *Klinefelter's syndrome*, in which afflicted males have XXY, XXYY or XXXY, instead of XY. Their limbs are longer than normal and their testes do not develop – they are thus sterile. They look outwardly male, but commonly exhibit some female characteristics, such as highly developed breasts.
- *Down syndrome* (formerly known as mongolism) in which children have an extra chromosome – 47 instead of 46 – because they have three chromosomes instead of the normal two in the 21 position, as previously discussed. Such children suffer from moderate to severe mental retardation, physical retardation and other characteristic facial features.

Effects of mutations

1. The vast majority of mutations have either damaging or neutral effects. Most point mutations are damaging. Mutations may produce phenotypes which are incompatible with the environment, and these do not survive unless outside intervention is able to sustain or prolong life. Examples are haemophilia and diabetes mellitus.

However, mutations are also responsible for the great genetic variability which can be of advantage to the survival of a species.

This is more easily observable in plants, but mutations occur in human beings which contribute to such observations as race formation.

2. The majority of new mutations in diploids are recessive, with less than one per cent being completely dominant.

3. In natural populations, such as humans, many different forms of the same chromosomes exist because of the presence of different alleles. These are described as *polymorphisms*. This means that several distinct forms exist within one species. One example is human blood groups, which are separate and distinct within the one species.

4. One form of polymorphism is called *balanced* polymorphism. This is a mechanism by which variations arise because the heterozygote condition (where the paired genes for a specific trait are not identical) is favoured. Examples include eye colour and sickle-cell anaemia. Sickle-cell anaemia occurs in up to 4 per cent of the population in parts of Africa, with about 30 per cent of the population being carriers. However, it seems that people with this condition are more resistant to infection by a particularly virulent form of malaria (falciparum malaria). It appears that people with sickle-cell anaemia are more able to remove the parasite from the blood by phagocytosis than is the unaffected population.

5. The *multiple-factor* or *multifactorial theory* puts forward the idea that a given trait may be affected by many genes, with or without the effects of the environment. Mutations may also require the alteration of more than one pair of genes. Abnormal traits which may be inherited in this way include spina bifida, some common forms of congenital heart disease, cleft lip and cleft palate, congenital club foot, congenital dislocation of the hip, some psychiatric disorders (such as schizophrenia and manic-depressive psychosis), hypertension, diabetes mellitus, rheumatoid arthritis and peptic ulcers.

FUTURE DIRECTIONS IN GENETICS

Genetic Engineering

Human beings have been practising selective breeding for as long as they have been using dogs, horses and plants. For example, they have bred horses like the Clydesdales to do heavy work, and race horses for speed.

The term 'genetic engineering' appears to have arisen, with all its ethical implications, when scientists foresaw the possibility of determining sex before conception by selecting the appropriate sperm. The whole idea of artificial insemination ('test-tube babies') may be an example of genetic engineering to some extent.

More strictly speaking, this term is used to refer to another technique (introduced in 1974) in which the genes of micro-organisms are manipulated by deliberate recombination of DNA.

This technique has come to be known as recombinant DNA research and has been defined by the British Health and Safety Regulations (1978) as:

'The formation of new kinds of heritable material by the insertion of nucleic acid molecules produced by whatever means outside the cell, into any virus, bacterial plasmid, or other vector system so as to allow their incorporation into a host organism in which they do not naturally occur, but in which they are capable of continued propogation.'

The following are a few comments that have been made by professionals about recombinant DNA research:

- has made contributions in basic genetic research;
- has been used in such practical applications as the commercial production of insulin;
- has been subject to careful controls by the scientific community, because of its concern in such matters;
- has *not*, to date, attempted to interfere with the genetic makeup of human beings;
- should not, present any threat to the community and the human beings within it.

Eugenics

This is the study and control of procreation as a means of improving hereditary characteristics of future generations, and is of two types.

1. Positive eugenics: This is concerned with optimal reproduction of people having 'desirable' or 'superior' traits.
2. Negative eugenics. This involves prevention of reproduction by people having 'undesirable' or 'inferior' traits.

In the earlier part of this century, laws were passed in several countries in Europe and many of the states of the USA permitting the sterilisation of 'defective' persons. These laws were later repealed because of doubts regarding the relative contribution of genetics and the environment.

One may also well ask:

Which *are* 'desirable' and 'undesirable' traits?

Who determines the desirability of various traits?

What of the rights of an individual human being? Shouldn't these be protected?

Thus, the ethical issues surrounding such techniques and studies are as important as they are complex.

Genetic Counselling

This rather new area was handled until recently by medical practitioners who may not have been expert geneticists, or academic geneticists who may not have had training in counselling techniques.

When people are faced with problems that may be genetic, or partly genetic, in origin, they deserve to be given accurate information and skilled counselling in order to make the best decision in a difficult situation. They may also require informed advice so that they may be fully aware of the means by which future problems may be avoided, or handled in the light of their own religious, ethical, philosophical and moral constraints.

While it is not the function of, say, a community nurse to attempt to offer genetic advice or counselling, he/she may be the first person who is approached on such matters. In most cases, referral to the appropriate clinics in that particular state may be the best course of action. In New South Wales for example, genetic counselling clinics exist at the Prince of Wales Hospital and the Royal Alexandra Hospital for Children. Furthermore, most obstetricians would be able to provide a referral to a genetic counsellor.

Amniocentesis

This technique involves the removal of fluid from the amniotic cavity surrounding a developing fetus. It is then possible to examine fetal cells to determine the sex of the fetus and chromosomal abnormalities that it may possess. It is also possible to determine some 30 genetic disorders biochemically.

Thus, if any problems exist, the parents have the opportunity of making a decision regarding the pregnancy or the future offspring, and thus can be better prepared for future action.

REVIEW

1. Mr Smith has had a lawsuit brought against him by his girlfriend. He has denied paternity of her daughter and refused to pay support. He charges that Ms Jones' daughter's real father is a Mr Brown.
   Knowing the following data, would you say that Mr Smith has a good chance of winning this case? Blood group O is recessive to groups A and B.

	Blood Group
Mr Smith	AB
Ms Jones	O
Child in question	O
Mr Brown	A

2. A man, who has no history of haemophilia in his family, seeks your advice. He is married to a woman whose brother and maternal uncle both have haemophilia. He wants to know if there is any need to be concerned about any children he might have. Should he seek professional aid before starting a family?

   From the information given, construct a chart showing the inheritance pattern which exists in this family. What information have you obtained regarding the genetic inheritance possibilities of his children? What advice would you give?

3. A man has just been told he has Huntington's chorea. His wife has no family history of the disorder nor does she show any symptoms. They have four young children.

   He is told that Huntington's chorea is a genetic disorder in which symptoms do not usually arise until middle age. Unfortunately it is an autosomal dominant disease.

   With the aid of punnet squares discuss the various possibilities of the children's genetic inheritance patterns for Huntington's chorea.

4. Phenylketonuria is a genetic disease in which a liver enzyme, phenylalanine hydroxylase, is not synthesized. As a result mental retardation occurs due to CNS damage. A test can be done on babies to detect this abnormality which allows early treatment to begin.

   Following is a pedigree of a family, some of whom have phenylketonuria. What pattern of inheritance is depicted by this chart?

   Why might there be a higher incidence of genetic problems in this family group?

Square = male, unaffected
Circle = female, unaffected
Circle or square with dot = carrier
Dark blue circle or square = affected person
Double lines (═══) indicate a consanguineous (blood) relationship or kinship

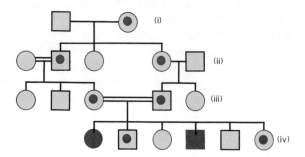

Units of measurement

Much of the day-to-day activity of the nurse is taken up with measurement of one kind or another — temperature, blood pressure, urine output, fluid intake and weight and height measurements, to name but a few. The importance of accurate measurement and recording of information cannot be over-stressed and will be frequently mentioned.

Measurements will essentially be of two main types:

1. *Quantitative* measurements, into which category all of the above quantities would fall. The determination of those is essentially *objective*, in that the quantities involved are measured using instruments and do not normally depend on any judgment on the part of the observer.

2. *Qualitative* measurements, which are probably not measurements in the sense in which we normally use the word, are descriptive. These are *subjective* in that they tend to depend very much on an observer's judgment, for example the colour of a patient's skin, whether a patient 'looks better' or 'seems to be better or worse', or a description of a patient's state of shock as absent, mild, moderate or severe.

Quantitative Measurements

Measurements have no meaning simply as numbers. Even the statement that a patient's temperature is 38.4° implies the unit 'degrees Celsius'.

Thus, *any quantitative measurement has to have a unit*. This is a quantity adopted as a standard of measurement. The *standard* of any unit is the means by which the unit is standardised so that it will be consistent wherever it is used.

The standard kilogram is given by the mass of a particular platinum-iridium cylinder which is kept in Paris and against which each country's standard is periodically checked.

The standard metre is now defined as the distance which light travels in $1 \div 299\ 792\ 458$ seconds. Another way of saying this is that 299 792 458 metres is the distance travelled by light in one second.

The standard second is given by the time which a caesium atom takes to undergo 9 192 631 770 vibrations.

These are examples of the standards used for three of the fundamental or *base units* in the international system (Système International or SI), which is now used in Australia. In this system very large numbers, such as the two above, do not have divisions indicated with a comma, but with a space. The base units are the *fundamental* or *foundation units* of the system and all other units in the system should be derived from them for continuity. While names may change with the language used, the symbols have been internationally agreed upon by all participating countries.

The seven SI base units are listed in Table A.I.1.

TABLE A.I.1 SI fundamental or base units

Quantity	Unit	Symbol
length	metre	m
mass	kilogram	kg
time	second	s
electric current	ampere	A
temperature	kelvin	K
luminous intensity	candela	cd
amount of a substance	mole	mol

A number of other units, called *derived* units, are also of interest to nurses. These units are derived from the base units and represent a combination of two or more of the base units. These units broaden the field of measurement and are listed in Table A.I.2.

TABLE A.I.2 SI derived units

Quantity	Unit	Symbol
area	square metre	m^2
volume	cubic metre	m^3
density	kilogram per cubic metre	kg/m^3
force	newton	N
pressure	pascal	Pa
energy	joule	J
potential difference	volt	V
resistance (electrical)	ohm	Ω
frequency	hertz	Hz

Some countries have retained some of their older units for everyday use, often because the SI unit is not seen as appropriate for some purposes. For example, the second is often impractical as a unit because it is too short; the cubic metre is a very large unit, appropriate for building sand but not for units of blood or urine output; and the Celsius temperature is more convenient than the kelvin temperature. The non-SI units of interest to nurses are listed in Table A.I.3.

TABLE A.I.3. Non-SI units

Quantity	Unit	Symbol
mass	gram	g
capacity	litre	L
time	minute	min
time	hour	h
temperature	degree Celsius	°C

Some of the units are too big or too small for particular applications. This led to the development of an agreed system of multiples and sub-multiples, based on powers of ten and designated by standard prefixes. The important ones used in nursing are indicated with an asterisk (*), but the full list is given for the sake of completeness in Table A.I.4.

TABLE A.I.4. Prefixes and their values

Prefix	Symbol	Meaning	Value Factor
exa	E	one million teras	10^{18}
peta	P	one thousand teras	10^{15}
tera	T	one million million	10^{12}
giga	G	one thousand million	10^{9}
mega*	M	one million	10^{6}
kilo*	k	one thousand	10^{3}
hecto	h	one hundred	10^{2}
deca	da	ten	10
deci*	d	one tenth	10^{-1}
centi*	c	one hundredth	10^{-2}
milli*	m	one thousandth	10^{-3}
micro*	µ	one millionth	10^{-6}
nano*	n	one thousandth of a millionth	10^{-9}
pico*	p	one millionth of a millionth	10^{-12}
femto*	f	one thousandth of a pico	10^{-15}
atto	a	one millionth of a pico	10^{-18}

Scientific Notation

In Table A.I.4, we have used scientific notation in the Value Factor column, once again for convenience. One of the numbers we have used (p. 136) is called Avogadro's number and has the value:

602.2 × 1 000 000 000 000 000 000 000
or
6.022 × 100 000 000 000 000 000 000 000

Since this is clumsy, we use the more convenient scientific notation for this number, 6.022×10^{23}. It is conventional to have just one integer in front of the decimal point, as shown.

If the number is, say 0.004276, we express it as 4.276×10^{-3}.

Some Important Units

International Unit
This is defined as the amount that produces a specified biological effect and is internationally accepted as a measure of the activity of the substance, e.g. vitamins.

Metre
The metre is used to measure distance, length, width, etc. Since this is a rather large unit in which to measure wound or dressing sizes, the centimetre (cm) is often used in nursing as well as in everyday life. Note that 1 metre = 100 cm.

Kilogram and Gram
These are units of mass — the amount of matter contained in a body. This is not quite the same as weight, which is actually a force – the force of attraction between the body and the earth. When people speak of weighing 67 kg, they are really speaking of a force and should refer to 67 kg force. However, for all practical purposes, we know what they mean!
Note that 1 kg = 1000 g, and 1 g = 1000 mg.

Kelvin and Degrees Celsius
While it is true that the unit of temperature on the SI scale is the Kelvin, people have been measuring temperatures on the Celsius scale for a long time now and change will no doubt be slow in coming. The size of the units involved would be rather awkward in recording human temperatures and would certainly leave greater room for error.
Two simple rules show the connection between these units:

- To convert a kelvin temperature to Celsius temperature, *subtract* 273.
- To convert a Celsius temperature to a kelvin temperature, *add* 273.

American books still often use the old Fahrenheit scale. To convert such temperatures it is probably easiest to use a conversion scale such as that in the inside cover of Solomon and Davis' physiology text (see biliography). However, for those who want to use conversion formulae, the following are applicable:

$$C = 5/9 \{F - 32\}$$
$$F = 9/5C + 32$$

where C is the Celsius temperature and F is the Fahrenheit temperature.

The Mole
This concept is discussed in some detail in Chapter 6, where its application is considered. *The mole is equal to the formula mass (or molecular mass of a substance expressed in grams).* For an explanation of the term 'formula mass', see p. 137.
It is most important for the nurse to become familiar with the mole, the millimole and so forth, because the concentration of various solutions with which the nurse frequently works are expressed in millimoles per litre. These include drug solutions, blood, urine and many of the body's other fluids.

Litre
This unit is still used in lieu of the cubic metre, a large and cumbersome unit which is not suitable for most nursing and many everyday applications. The millilitre (mL) is used very frequently when speaking of liquid drug dosages, small quantities of fluids such as urine, etc. Note that 1 litre = 1000 mL.

Pascal

For similar reasons the pascal (Pa) and the kilopascal (kPa) are slow to gain acceptance. Part of the reason for this is that instruments for measuring blood pressure (sphygmomanometers), still tend to be graduated in the old units, which are mm of mercury (Hg). Similarly, medical people still tend to speak of the pressure of cerebrospinal fluid in terms of centimetres of water.

To change a reading of pressure in millimetres of mercury to kilopascals, multiply by 0.133.

Joule

This is an example of a newer unit which is gaining acceptance and is gradually replacing the old unit of energy which was the calorie.

$$1 \text{ calorie} = 4.184 \text{ joules.}$$

The old dietary calorie is, in fact, a kilocalorie.

Thus one dietary calorie = 1000 calories = 4.184×1000 joules = 4.184 kilojoules (kJ).

Others

Many other units, such as the decibel, the rad, a half-life, etc., have been used in this text and are defined when they are first used. Any reader wishing to look up any such units is referred to the index at the back of the book.

Significant Figures

While it is probably inappropriate to enter into a detailed discussion of this matter here, one point should be made: *When any calculation is performed involving two or more numbers, the answer can be no more accurate than the accuracy of those numbers.*

When we divide 10 mL by 7.0, our calculator might come up with 1.4285714 mL. The answer quoted is rather meaningless in terms of accuracy, since both of the numbers with which we started had two significant figures only. Thus the answer we should give is one with only two significant figures also, that is 1.4 mL. It may be convenient at times to stretch this to 1.42 mL, but any further digits are absolutely meaningless.

Rules to Follow

1. In the SI system commas are not used to space digits in numbers; spaces are used, together with a decimal point if necessary.
• If five or more digits are used in any number on either side of the decimal, groups of three digits are to be used.

e.g.

$$23\ 847\ 981\ 264$$
$$63\ 651\ 904$$
$$17\ 072$$
$$28.803\ 937$$
$$7\ 902.492\ 638$$

Note that a comma may be used instead of the decimal point and that the decimal point may be on the line or at mid-letter height. For example:

$$27.50 = 27,50 = 27\cdot50$$

Note also that the only variation to the spacing rule above occurs when sums of money are involved, e.g. $10250.75

- In four-digit numbers, the space may be omitted: thus 1234 or 1 234 are both acceptable.

   2. The singular form of unit symbols is always used, e.g. 27 km, not 27 kms.

   3. Full stops are not used at the end of abbreviations, so that 317 g is correct, but 317 g. is not.

   4. A space is always left between the number itself and the symbol for the unit. Thus 317 g is correct, but 317g is not.

   5. A zero is always used before the decimal for any numbers less than one, i.e. 0.50 mL is correct, but .50 mL is not. This is most important for drug dosages, as errors can result from lack of clarity about the decimal point.

   6. In all verbal communications, the term 'zero' is used, not 'nought'.

Finally, these units are part of the nurse's 'tools of trade'. The nurse's attention to detail in listing quantities correctly, with a proper regard for the units involved is *critical* to is avoid unnecessary errors which, in some cases, could be hazardous to life.

The microscope

Microscopes have many uses and are invaluable tools in medical practice. This is a brief introduction to these instruments.

The Compound Light Microscope

These instruments have one or several **objective lenses**, near to the specimen or object being viewed. If several objectives are present they usually have different magnifying powers and are contained in a rotary head. These lenses form a magnified image of the specimen.

Further magnification of the specimen occurs by means of an **eyepiece** or **ocular lens** (which may also be interchangeable). through which the operator views the specimen.

The magnification factor of the microscope can then be determined by multiplying the power of the ocular lens by the power of the objective lens.

The resolving power of a microscope, on the other hand, is the ability of the lens system to show fine detail. This is measured in terms of the ability of the lens system to resolve or separate fine lines or dots. While we do not need to concern ourselves with mathematical expressions of resolving power, we do need to understand the concept.

One way of achieving this is to visualise a car approaching on a straight country road, at night. When the car is close, we can clearly see both headlights, but when the car is a great distance away, the two headlights fuse into one, and we 'see' only one light. This is because our eyes are not capable of resolving or separating the two lights, until the car is closer. Just as our eyes are limited in their capacity to resolve the images of the headlights, so lens systems of microscopes are limited in their capacity to separate or resolve dots or lines.

Other parts of a microscope of significance are:

1. *A light source.* On earlier models, this often consisted of a mirror which reflected and concentrated light on to the axis of the lens system. On most modern microscopes the light source is built in to the base of the instrument.

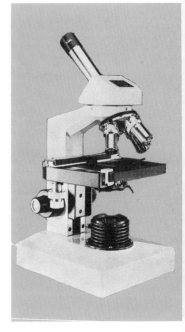

Photograph A II.1 The compound light microscope. (From Villee, et al. *Biology*, second edn. W.B. Saunders, 1985.)

495

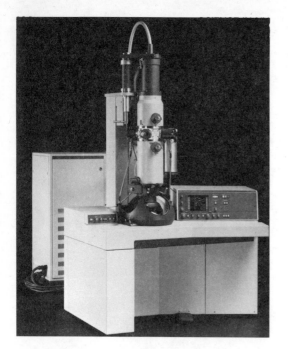

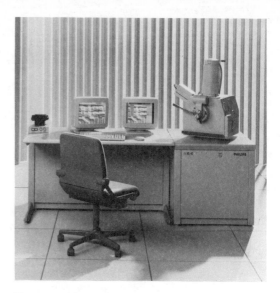

Photograph A.II.3. A scanning electron microscope. (Courtesy Philips Pty. Ltd.)

Photograph A.II.2. A transmission electron microscope. (Courtesy Philips Pty. Ltd.)

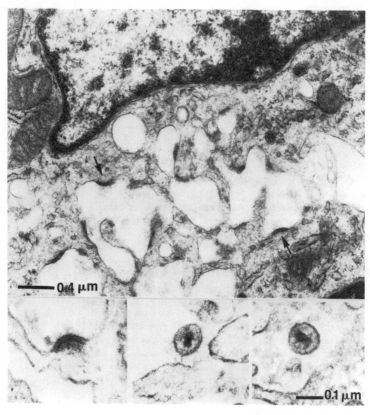

0.4 μm

0.1 μm

Photograph A.II.4. Transmission electron micrograph of a lymph node biopsy from an AIDS patient. (Courtesy Philips Pty. Ltd.)

2. *The substage,* which focuses and concentrates light on to the object. It contains a condenser (which concentrates light rays), a diaphragm, which controls the size of the aperture or opening through which the light passes, and a focusing control.

3. *The body,* which supports the stage and body tube. Focusing occurs by means of coarse and fine adjustment knobs (incorporated in the one knob on many modern microscopes). These move either the stage or the body tube up and down to enable the operator to focus the object so as to provide a clear image.

Compound light microscopes may be either monocular or binocular. The binocular microscope utilises two objectives at once so as to provide a three-dimensional image.

One refinement of the compound light microscope is the dual eyepiece (binocular), which generates much less eyestrain than the single eyepiece.

The Electron Microscope

For reasons which we will not go into here, the resolution of light microscopes is limited. The resolution of an electron microscope is very much greater, enabling objects as small as bacteria and viruses to be seen easily.

Two kinds of electron microscope exist — transmission and scanning types.

The **transmission electron microscope** passes a beam of electrons through a very thin specimen. It can achieve very high magnification, but only a very thin layer is in focus at any one time. One effect of this is to make the image of the specimen appear flat.

The **scanning electron microscope** focuses an electron beam on a portion of the specimen. This beam then scans over the specimen in a regular pattern, giving a highly detailed image of the specimen with the whole surface in clear focus.

The magnification achieved is better than that of the light microscope, but not as good as that achieved by a transmission electron microscope.

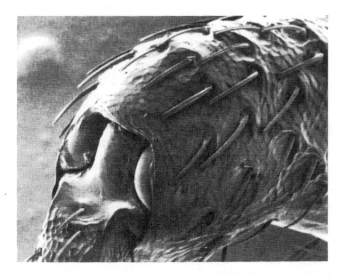

Photograph A.II.5. Scanning electron micrograph of the knee joint of an insect. (Courtesy Philips Pty. Ltd.)

Reference values for blood, plasma, serum of commonly used tests

Note: For some procedures the reference values may vary depending upon the method used, therefore differences occur between tests or laboratories.

	SI Units	Conventional (Older) Units
Bilirubin, serum		
Direct	1.7–6.8 µmol/L	0.1–0.4 mg/100 mL
Indirect	3.4–12 µmol/L (total minus direct)	0.2–0.7 mg/100 mL (total minus direct)
Total	5.1–19µmol/L	0.3–1.1 mg/100 mL
Carbon dioxide content, serum (adult)	24–30 mmol/L	24–30 mEq/L
Cell Counts		
Erythrocytes		
Males	$4.6–6.2 \times 10^{12}$/L	4.6–6.2 million/mm³
Females	$4.2–5.4 \times 10^{12}$/L	4.2–5.4 million/mm³
Leukocytes		
Total	$4.5–11.0 \times 10^{9}$/L	4500–11 000/mm³
Platelets	$150–350 \times 10^{9}$/L	150 000–350 000/mm³
Cholesterol, serum		
Total	3.9–6.5 mmol/L	150–250 mg/100 mL
Esters	0.68–0.76 of total cholesterol	68–76% of total cholesterol
Creatine, serum	15–61 µmol/L	0.2–0.8 mg/100 mL
Creatinine, serum	62–133 µmol/L	0.7–1.5 mg/100 mL

	SI Units	Conventional (Older) Units
Electrolytes: Bicarbonate		
serum (hydrogen carbonate)	23–29 mmol/L	23–29 mEq/L
Calcium, ionised, serum	1.05–1.30 mmol/L	2.1–2.6 mEq/L
Chloride, serum	96–106 mmol/L	96–106 mEq/L
Magnesium, serum	0.75–1.25 mmol/L	1.5–2.5 mEq/L
		1.8–3.0 mg/100 mL
Potassium, serum	3.5–5.0 mmol/L	3.5–5.0 mEq/L
Sodium, serum	136–145 mmol/L	136–145 mEq/L
Blood Gas Tensions (on basis of 1mmHg = 0.133 kPa)		
Carbon dioxide (CO_2)	4.655–5.985 kPa	35–45 mmHg
Oxygen (pO_2) arterial	9.975–13.3 kPa	75–100 mmHg
Glucose (fasting)		
Blood	3.33–5.55 mmol/L	60–100 mg/100 mL
Plasma or serum	3.89–6.38 mmol/L	70–115 mg/100 mL
Haematocrit		
Males, adult	0.40–0.54 mmol/L	40–54 mL/100 mL
Females, adult	0.37–0.47 mmol/L	37–47 mL/100 mL
Haemoglobin		
Males, adult	2.17–2.79 mmol/L	14.0–18.0 grams/100 mL
Females, adult	1.86–2.48 mmol/L	12.0–16.0 grams/100 mL
pH, arterial blood	7.35–7.45	7.35–7.45
	(general conversion as yet not made)	
Proteins, serum		
Total	60–80 g/L	6.0–8.0 grams/100 mL
Albumin	35–55 g/L	3.5–5.5 grams/100 mL
	0.54–0.85 mmol/L	
Globulin	25–35 g/L	2.5–3.5 grams/100 mL
Triglycerides, serum	0.4–1.5 g/L	40–150 mg/100 mL
	0.45–1.71 mmol/L	
Urea nitrogen		
Blood	7.1–14.3 mmol/L	10–20 mg/100 mL

Source: *Encylopedia and Dictionary of Medicine, Nursing and Allied Health,* edited by the late Benjamin F. Miller and Claire B. Keane, 3rd Ed. Philadelphia. W.B. Saunders 1983.

Reference values for common urine tests

Note: For some procedures the reference values may vary depending upon the method used.

	SI Units	Conventional (Older) Units
Albumin		
Qualitative	Negative	Negative
Quantitative	10–100 mg/24 h	10–100 mg/24 hrs
	0.15–1.5 µmol/24 h	
Creatine		
Males	0–0.30 mmol/24 h	0–40 mg/24 hrs
Females	0–0.76 mmol/24 h	0–100 mg/24 hrs
	(Higher during pregnancy and in children)	
Creatinine	0.13–0.22 mmol/kg body weight/24 h	15–25 mg/kg body weight/24 hrs
Creatinine Clearance		
Males	110-150 mL/min	110–150 mL/min
Females	105–132 mL/min	105–132 mL/min
17-Ketosteroids		
Males	21–62 µmol/24 h	6–18 mg/24 hrs
Females	14–45 µmol/24 h	4–13 mg/24 hrs
	(varies with age)	
Protein		
Qualitative	Negative	Negative
Quantitative	10–150 mg/24 h	10–150 mg/24 hrs
Specific Gravity	1.003–1.030	1.003–1.030

Source: *Encyclopedia and Dictionary of Medicine, Nursing and Allied Health*, edited by the late Benjamin F. Miller and Claire B. Keane, 3rd Ed. Philadelphia. W.B. Saunders 1983.

Some Australian examples of blocking agents

This information is based on a paper by Struan K. Sutherland which was published in *Chemistry in Australia*, September 1980, vol. 47, no. 9. We wish to express our gratitude to Dr Sutherland, not only for his ready agreement to allow us to use this material, but also for his updating of the original draft.

Although this book is not a physiology text, appendix V is included because of the difficulty in obtaining information about Australian venomous species. Most physiology texts available here are published overseas and give data on local species only. However, readers will need to have studied synapses, neuromuscular junctions and transmitter substances in their courses in physiology to fully appreciate and understand this appendix.

The nurse, and the community nurse in particular. is sometimes called upon as a resource in many areas of knowledge, including the following. We trust that the reader finds this information useful.

It is interesting to observe that Australian venomous species are among the most poisonous in the world. Examples include:

1. Potentially the most venomous snake, the small-scaled snake, which produces a venom similar to that produced by the taipan.
2. The most dangerous jellyfish — the box jellyfish or sea wasp.
3. The most poisonous octopus — the blue-ringed octopus.
4. The only spider in the world known to kill humans in less than 90 minutes — the Sydney funnel-web spider.
5. The high output of venom from many Australian snakes is an additional and important factor in their danger to humans.

Let us look at some of these in more detail.

Tiger snake venom

This is a complex venom, the main neurotoxin (a substance that is poisonous or destructive to nerve tissue) being notexin, which has two effects:

1. It is a strong pre-synaptic nerve blocker that prevents the recycling of synaptic vesicles.
2. It causes disintegration of muscle tissue.

Tiger snake venom also contains a very potent coagulant factor (a substance that causes the blood to coagulate or become clotted).

Taipan venom

This venom contains taipoxin, which is the second most potent venom yet isolated. It is similar in action to notexin, as in 1. and 2. above. Taipan venom can also convert prothrombin to thrombin in the absence of all other clotting factors, including calcium. Thrombin is the enzyme that converts fibrinogen to fibrin, the substance that forms the threads in a blood clot. This conversion to thrombin results in the formation of microclots in snake-bite victims, but it should be noted that such victims do not suffer from clinical blood clotting (thrombosis).

Brown snake

As with the taipan, brown snake's prothrombin is converted to thrombin by the venom, which also acts as a pre-synaptic blocking agent.

Note: The myolitic properties of tiger-snake venom (i.e. the degeneration of muscle tissue) has also been found to be a property of previously unsuspected venoms — those of:

- the copperhead snake
- the red-bellied black snake
- the Clarence River or rough-scaled snake

Red-back spider

The action of the venom of this spider appears to be identical to that of the black widow spider, i.e. the venom causes depletion of the acetylcholine reserves at motor nerve endings and hence acts as a blocking agent. It also acts at many other types of nerve endings, causing pain, sweating, high blood pressure, raised pulse rate, etc.

Sydney funnel-web spider

The most significant component of the venom of this spider is atraxotoxin, which causes widespread release of acetylcholine at nerve endings. This is effected by the venom, leading to direct stimulation of nerve fibres, thus producing action potentials in the motor nerve that tend to 'lock up' or paralyse the muscles. An anti-venom is now available for the treatment of funnel-web bites.

Box jellyfish or sea wasp

It is considered that the lethal factor in the venom of this creature probably interferes with membrane permeability at the target organs. It may also cause failure of the respiratory centre and electrical conduction disturbances in the heart. In addition, the venom causes severe skin damage at the site of the stings.

Blue-ringed octopus

This creature injects a toxic saliva, which causes paralysis. It contains tetrodotoxin, which blocks the movement of sodium ions and thus prevents action potentials from being generated.

Cone shellfish (Family conidae)
These creatures introduce a potent toxin into their victims by means of a small dart. The toxin in *Conus magnus* is a myotoxin (i.e. it affects muscles), which paralyses skeletal muscle by direct muscle membrane depolarisation.

In the case of *Conus geographicus*, one of the toxins present blocks the depolarisation of muscle fibres and another causes nerve block by inhibiting the movement of sodium ions.

Conversion factors

The SI system of units has been used throughout this book. However, the USA still uses the British system of units and American nursing and physiology texts reflect this.

This table is provided to assist the student to convert US units to SI units.

To convert		Multiply by
cmH_2O	to pascals	98
mmHg	to pascals	133.3
lb/in^2	to pascals	6895
lb/ft^2	to pascals	47.88
pounds	to newtons	4.45
ft^3	to m^3	2.832×10^{-2}
litres	to m^3	0.001
gallons	to m^3	3.785×10^{-3}
calories	to joules	4.186
kilocalories	to joules	4186
angstroms	to nanometres	10^{-1}
inches	to cm	2.54
feet	to cm	30.48

The periodic table

As was mentioned on p75, the periodic table is a type of filing system. It was first proposed by Mendeleev in 1869, long before anything was known of electrons or the structure of the atom. He noticed that the elements could be arranged in this way, since the properties of elements are *periodic* in nature — hence the title of this table. A couple of gaps existed, but this did not worry Mendeleev at all. He claimed that the gaps must be caused by elements which has not yet been discovered!

This may seem a little far fetched, but Mendeleev then proceeded to predict what the properties of those elements would be. These elements were later discovered (e.g. gallium and germanium) and found to have properties remarkably similar to those which Mendeleev had predicted.

The horizontal rows are called **periods**. The first of these can be seen (inside back cover) to consist only of the elements hydrogen (H) and helium (He). The second period starts with lithium (Li) and ends with neon and so forth.

The vertical columns are called **groups**. The two groups on the far left and the six groups on the right are numbered (we need not concern ourselves with the others, which are called the transition elements). The number in each case refers to the number of electrons in the outermost orbit of each atom of that element. Thus the members of Group 1, hydrogen (H), lithium (Li), sodium (Na), etc. all have atoms with *one* electron in the outermost orbit. Similarly, the members of Group 2, beryllium (Be), magnesium (Mg), calcium (Ca) etc. all have atoms with *two* electrons in the outermost orbit and so on.

Some of the groups are given names. Group 1 elements are called the alkali metals, Group 2 elements the alkali earth metals, Group 7 elements the halogens and Group 8 elements the noble metals.

Elements in the same group have similar chemical properties. For example, sodium (Na) and potassium (K) both react violently with water to produce hydrogen gas.

Periodic Table of the Elements

In each A group, the number of electrons ($\#e^-$) in the outer shell of each element is the same.

In each period, the identifying number (n) for the outer shell of each element is the same.

Key:

symbol
element
atomic number
atomic mass

Ru
Ruthenium
44
101.07

Group	1A	2A												3A	4A	5A	6A	7A	8A
Period 1	H Hydrogen 1 1.01																		He Helium 2 4.00
2	Li Lithium 3 6.94	Be Beryllium 4 9.01												B Boron 5 10.81	C Carbon 6 12.01	N Nitrogen 7 14.01	O Oxygen 8 16.00	F Fluorine 9 19.00	Ne Neon 10 20.18
3	Na Sodium 11 23.00	Mg Magnesium 12 24.31												Al Aluminium 13 26.98	Si Silicon 14 28.09	P Phosphorus 15 30.97	S Sulfur 16 32.06	Cl Chlorine 17 35.45	Ar Argon 18 39.95
4	K Potassium 19 39.10	Ca Calcium 20 40.08	Sc Scandium 21 44.96	Ti Titanium 22 47.90	V Vanadium 23 50.94	Cr Chromium 24 52.00	Mn Manganese 25 54.95	Fe Iron 26 55.85	Co Cobalt 27 58.93	Ni Nickel 28 58.71	Cu Copper 29 63.55	Zn Zinc 30 65.37		Ga Gallium 31 69.72	Ge Germanium 32 72.59	As Arsenic 33 74.92	Se Selenium 34 78.96	Br Bromine 35 79.90	Kr Krypton 36 83.8
5	Rb Rubidium 37 85.47	Sr Strontium 38 87.62	Y Yttrium 39 88.91	Zr Zirconium 40 91.22	Nb Niobium 41 92.91	Mo Molybdenum 42 95.94	Tc* Technetium 43 98.91	Ru Ruthenium 44 101.07	Rh Rhodium 45 102.91	Pd Palladium 46 106.4	Ag Silver 47 107.87	Cd Cadmium 48 112.40		In Indium 49 114.82	Sn Tin 50 181	Sb Antimony 51 121.75	Te Tellurium 52 127.60	I Iodine 53 126.90	Xe Xenon 54 131.30
6	Cs Cesium 55 132.91	Ba Barium 56 137.34	La* Lanthanum 57 138.91	Hf Hafnium 72 178.49	Ta Tantalum 73 180.95	W Tungsten 74 183.85	Re Rhenium 75 186.2	Os Osmium 76 190.2	Ir Iridium 77 192.22	Pt Platinum 78 195.09	Au Gold 79 196.97	Hg Mercury 80 200.59		Tl Thallium 81 204.37	Pb Lead 82 207.2	Bi Bismuth 83 208.98	Po* Polonium 84 (210)	At* Astatine 85 (210)	Rn* Radon 86 (222)
7	Fr* Francium 87 (223)	Ra* Radium 88 226.02	Ac* Actinium 89 (227)	Rf* Rutherfordium 104 (260)	Ha* Hahnium 105 (262)														

Lanthanide series

Ce Cerium 58 140.12	Pr Praseodymium 59 140.91	Nd Neodymium 60 144.24	Pm* Promethium 61 (145)	Sm Samarium 62 150.4	Eu Europium 63 151.96	Gd Gadolinium 64 157.25	Tb Terbium 65 158.93	Dy Dysprosium 66 162.50	Ho Holmium 67 164.93	Er Erbium 68 167.26	Tm Thulium 69 168.93	Yb Ytterbium 70 173.04	Lu Lutetium 71 174.97

Actinide series

Th* Thorium 90 232.04	Pa* Protactinium 91 231.04	U* Uranium 92 238.03	Np* Neptunium 93 237.05	Pu* Plutonium 94 (244)	Am* Americium 95 (243)	Cm* Curium 96 (247)	Bk* Berkelium 97 (247)	Cf* Californium 98 (251)	Es* Einsteinium 99 (254)	Fm* Fermium 100 (257)	Md* Mendelevium 101 (257)	No* Nobelium 102 (255)	Lr* Lawrencium 103 (256)

* All isotopes are radioactive.
( ) Indicates mass number of longest known half-life.
† All atomic masses have been rounded to .01.

(From Berlow et al. *Introduction to the Chemistry of Life.* Saunders College Publishing, Philadelphia. 1982.)

TABLE A. VII. 1. Electron configurations (arrangement of electrons) of the first 20 elements of the periodic table

H	1	1
He	2	2 (Complete outer shell)
Li	3	2,1
Be	4	2,2
B	5	2,3
C	6	2,4
N	7	2,5
O	8	2,6
F	9	2,7
Ne	10	2,8 (Complete outer shell)
Na	11	2,8,1
Mg	12	2,8,2
Al	13	2,8,3
Si	14	2,8,4
P	15	2,8,5
S	16	2,8,6
Cl	17	2,8,7
Ar	18	2,8,8 (Complete outer shell)
K	19	2,8,8,1
Ca	20	2,8,8,2

Bibliography

Arms, K. and Camp, P.S., *Biology,* W.B. Saunders, Philadelphia, 1987.

Australian Standards Association, Standard AS2500, *Guide to the Safe Use of Electricity in Patient Care,* 1986.

Black, J.M., Luckman, J. and Sorensen, K.C., *Medical-Surgical Nursing: A Psychophysiologic Approach,* fourth edition, W.B. Saunders, Philadelphia, 1993.

Brescia, F., *et al., Chemistry: A Modern Introduction,* fifth edition, W.B. Saunders, Philadelphia, 1988.

Brinkmeyer, S. *et al.,* 'Superiority of Colloid over Electrolyte Solution for Fluid Resuscitation (Severe Normovolemic Hemodilution)', *Critical Care Medicine,* May, 1981, vol. 9, no. 5.

Brunner, L.S. *et al., Textbook of Medical-Surgical Nursing,* Lippincott, Philadelphia, 1984.

Cree, L.A. and Webb, J.B., *Biology Outlines,* Pergamon Press, Sydney, 1984.

Emery, A.E.H., *Elements of Medical Genetics,* Churchill Livingstone, Edinburgh, 1979.

Giese, A.C., *Cell Physiology,* Saunders College Publishing, Philadelphia, 1979.

Greenberg, L.H., *Physics for Biology and Pre-Med Students,* W.B. Saunders Philadelphia, 1975.

Goldsby, R.H., *Cells and Energy,* Macmillan, New York, 1977.

Guyton, A.C., *Physiology of the Human Body,* sixth edition, W.B. Saunders, Philadelphia, 1984.

Guyton, A.C., *Textbook of Medical Physiology,* eighth edition, W.B. Saunders, Philadelphia, 1991.

Hal, E.J., *Radiobiology for the Radiologist,* Harper and Row, Maryland, 1978.

Hall, G.M., Body Temperature and Anaesthesia, *British Journal of Anaesthesia,* 1978, vol. 50, 39–44.

Hauser, C.J. *et al.,* 'Oxygen Transport Responses to Colloids and Crystalloids in Critically Ill Surgery Patients', *Surgery: Gynecology and Obstetrics,* June, 1980, vol. 150, no. 6.

Hearst, J.E. and Ifft, J.B., *Contemporary Chemistry,* W.H. Freeman, San Francisco, 1976.

Hillman, K., 'Fluid Resuscitation in Diabetic Emergencies – a Reappraisal', *Intensive Care Medicine,* (1987) 134–8.

Holbey, D.N. (ed.), *The Merck Manual of Diagnosis and Therapy,* fourteenth edition, Merck and Co., Railway, N.N., 1987.

Leahy, I.M. *et al., The Nurse and Radiotherapy: A Manual For Daily Care,* Mosby, St. Louis, 1979.

Le Veau, B., *Williams' and Lissner's Biomechanics of Human Motion,* third edition, W.B. Saunders, Philadelphia, 1992.

Luciano, D.S., Vander, A.J. and Sherman, J.H., *Human Function and Structure,* McGraw-Hill, New York, 1990.

McGilvery, R.W., *Biochemistry – A Functional Approach,* W.B. Saunders, Philadelphia, 1983.

Masterton, W.L. and Hurley, *Chemistry: Principles & Reactions,* second edition, Saunders College Publishing, Philadelphia, 1993.

Miller, B.F. and Keane, C.B., *Encyclopedia and Dictionary of Medicine, Nursing and Allied Health,* fifth edition, Saunders College Publishing, Philadelphia, 1992.

NSW Hospitals Planning and Advisory Authority, Seminar Report No. 40, *Safe Use of Electricity in Patient Care,* 16 August, 1983.

National Health and Medical Research Council Reports: *Code of Nursing Practice for Staff Exposed to Ionising Radiation, 1984. Recommended Radiation Protection Standards for Individuals Exposed to Ionising Radiation, 1981.* (Other, miscellaneous publications relating to the safe use of various diagnostic and therapeutic techniques.)

Nave, C.R. and Nave, B.C., *Physics for the Health Sciences,* third edition, W.B. Saunders, Philadelphia, 1985.

Novitski, E., *Human Genetics,* Macmillan, New York, 1982.

Oh, T.E. (ed.), *Intensive Care Manual,* Butterworths, Sydney, 1981.

Otto, J.H. *et al., Modern Biology,* Holt, Rinehart and Winston of Canada, Toronto, 1982.

Rackow, E.C. *et al.,* 'Fluid Resuscitation in Circulatory Shock: A Comparison of the Cardiorespiratory Effects of Albumin, Hetastarch, and Saline Solutions in Patients with Hypovolemic and Septic Shock', *Critical Care Medicine,* Nov., 1983, vol. 11, no. 11.

Selkurt, E.W. (ed.), *Basic Physiology for the Health Sciences,* Little, Brown, Boston, 1982.

Solomon, E.P. and Davis, P.W., *Human Anatomy and Physiology,* second edition, Saunders College Publishing, Philadelphia, 1990.

Spence, A.P. and Mason, E.B., *Human Anatomy and Physiology,* Benjamin/Cummings Publishing, Menlo Park, 1983.

Stern, C., *Principles of Human Genetics,* W.H. Freeman, San Francisco, 1973.

Sutherland, S.K., 'The Biochemistry and Actions of Some Australian Venoms with Some Notes on First Aid', *Chemistry in Australia,* Sept., 1980, vol. 47, no. 9.

Tiffany, R. (ed.), *Oncology for Nurses and Health Care Professionals,* Volume 1 Pathology, Diagnosis and Treatment, George Allen and Unwin, London, 1978.

Thomas, C.L. (ed.), *Taber's Cyclopedic Medical Dictionary,* twelfth edition, F.A. Davis Co., Philadelphia, 1980.

Tortora, G. and Anagnostakos, N., *Principles of Anatomy and Physiology,* Harper and Row, New York, 1990.

Walter, J., Cancer and Radiotherapy, Churchill Livingstone, Edinburgh, 1977.

Index

Where applicable, the letter 't' denotes 'table' and page numbers in bold signify key references.

(Tape shut)

REPLY PAID 5
Managing Editor, College Division
Harcourt Brace & Company, Australia
Locked Bag 16
MARRICKVILLE NSW 2204

TO THE OWNER OF THIS BOOK

We are interested in your reaction to *Science in Nursing*
by Laurie Cree and Sandra Rischmiller

1. What was your reason for using this book?

    _____ university course _____ continuing education course
    _____ college course   _____ personal interest
                                _____ other (specify)

2. In which school are you enrolled?_____

3. Approximately how much of the book did you use?
    _____ 1/4 _____ 1/2 _____ 3/4 _____ all

4. What is the best aspect of the book?

5. Have you any suggestions for improvement?

6. Would more diagrams help?

7. Is there any topic that should be added?

Fold here